P9-CFC-861

From Humors to Medical Science

A History of American Medicine

SECOND EDITION

John Duffy

University of Illinois Press · *Urbana and Chicago*

© 1993 by the Board of Trustees of the University of Illinois
Manufactured in the United States of America
1 2 3 4 5 C P 5 4 3 2 1

This book is printed on acid-free paper.

Library of Congress Cataloging-in-Publication Data
Duffy, John, 1915–
    From humors to medical science : a history of American Medicine /
John Duffy. — 2nd ed.
      p. cm.
    Rev. and expanded ed. of: The healers (McGraw-Hill, 1976).
    Includes bibliographical references and index.
    ISBN 0-252-01736-6 (cl : alk. paper). — ISBN 0-252-06300-7 (pb :
alk. paper)
    1. Medicine — United States — History.   I. Duffy, John, 1915–
Healers.   II. Title.
    [DNLM: 1. Education, Medical — history — United States.   2. History
of Medicine, Modern — United States.   WZ 70 AA1 D85f]
R151.D83 1993
610′.973 — dc20
DNLM/DLC
for Library of Congress   92-48760
                                                          CIP

To Corinne,

a loving wife,

excellent researcher,

and fine editor

Contents

Preface   ix

1. The Beginnings of American Medicine   1
2. The Eighteenth Century   13
3. The Medical Profession   31
4. Medicine in the Revolutionary Years   48
5. Early Nineteenth-Century Medicine   69
6. The Irregulars and Domestic Medicine   80
7. The Foundations of American Surgery   95
8. Early Leaders in Medicine and Surgery   120
9. The Education, Licensing, and Status of Physicians   130
10. Medicine in the Civil War   151
11. The Emergence of Modern Medicine   167
12. The Flowering of Surgery   188
13. Medical Education   203
14. The Medical Profession Organizes   214
15. The Advancing Front of Medicine   229
16. Surgery and Medical Technology since World War I   257
17. Medical Education since the Flexner Report   275

18. Women in Medicine   284

19. Minorities in Medicine   304

20. The Medical Profession in the Twentieth Century   313

21. The Community's Health   328

22. Whither Medicine?   345

   Notes   357

   Bibliography   391

   Index   405

Preface

THE HISTORY OF AMERICAN MEDICINE may not seem to lend itself to a grand theme, but medicine did assume certain distinctive characteristics in the United States. When the early colonists sought to recreate a British or European society in the New World, they endeavored to maintain class distinctions. Physicians with degrees from European universities were considered a class apart from surgeons, apothecaries, and other practitioners of medicine. Frontier conditions and the fluidity of American society soon tended to minimize, although not eliminate, distinctions among the various categories of medical practitioners. Without universities to teach physicians and in the absence of guilds to train surgeons and apothecaries, an apprenticeship system emerged in which the distinctions among physicians, surgeons, and apothecaries almost disappeared.

The American Revolution was at hand before the first two small medical schools appeared, and the number of medical schools did not grow appreciably until the early decades of the nineteenth century. Medical societies, which might have taken the role of the British guilds of surgeons and apothecaries in training and establishing standards for the profession, appeared by the mid-eighteenth century, but they won little support among medical practitioners. In the early years of the Republic these societies began to make gains and managed to push through a number of state laws regulating the practice of medicine. The Jacksonian era's emphasis upon egalitarianism, and its corollary, a suspicion of learning, ran counter to the movement for professionalization. Moreover, the several medical sects that sprang up in this period recognized that these laws were intended to restrict medical practice to orthodox physicians. The public, already suspicious of what they considered monopolies, agreed with them, and in consequence, the licensure laws were virtually eliminated by mid-century.

Without universities or guilds to train physicians and with only a handful of liberal arts colleges, the void in education was filled by the emergence of proprietary medical schools, most of which had either no connection or only a nominal one with an academic institution. Their quality varied, but since the schools depended solely upon fees for support, competition for students kept academic standards low. The last decades of the nineteenth century saw an increasing number of universities, a general rise in public education, and the application of the new scientific developments to medicine. The result was the reappearance of medical licensure laws, the merger of medical schools into universities, and the gradual rise of educational standards for physicians. Under the influence of people such as Dr. William H. Welch of Johns Hopkins and Abraham Flexner, who played a major role in bringing foundation money into the field of medical education, the early twentieth century marked the beginning of an emphasis upon research in medical training.

This emphasis, combined with America's growing wealth and population and the influx of outstanding medical scientists fleeing Europe's troubles, gradually enabled the United States to assume leadership in the medical world. Meanwhile, aided by a growing prestige and a reorganized American Medical Association, the American medical profession in the early twentieth century became a powerful political force. In consequence, far more than in any other country, physicians have shaped America's national health policy. The theme that emerges in the history of American medicine is the gradual evolution of a diverse group of unorganized medical practitioners into a remarkably powerful professional organization.

The present work represents almost fifty years of research and writing on the history of American medicine and public health. Lord Acton (1834–1902), the first editor of the *Cambridge Modern History*, was said to have been the last individual whose knowledge encompassed all fields of learning. Today no one can be an authority on all of the rapidly growing fields of medicine and the biological sciences, and I have relied to a considerable extent upon a wide range of historical sources and publications. In selecting from a vast mass of material I have had to make many difficult decisions, and a number of my readers may feel rightly that I have slighted their special field of interest or favorite historical individual.

When I wrote my original history of American medicine, *The Healers*, circumstances forced me to touch only lightly on the twentieth century. In the present version I have condensed and added the results of recent studies to the earlier material and placed much more emphasis upon the tremendous changes that have occurred during the past one hundred years. Any attempt to identify and trace major developments in the biomedical sciences during the twentieth century, a period when knowledge has been accumulating at an ever-accelerating rate, can only be tentative. The task has been made more difficult by the paucity of histories of biomedicine dealing with this period. In recent years the social aspects of medicine have attracted a great many historians. While this development is a welcome one, regrettably, there has not been a comparable interest in biomedicine.

Science, however, is only part of medicine. Despite all we have learned about pathogenic organisms, vectors, genetics, and human physiology, both normal and abnormal, the practice of medicine still remains an art conditioned by the society in which it is practiced. The fact that human beings are much more than the sum total of their parts places limitations on medical science, and medicine cannot be studied apart from its social context.

For the past fifty years I have read widely in medical journals and society transactions, public health records, newspapers, lay journals, historical-society collections, and all other sources for American medical history. My research extended to virtually every state in the Union. If I have given too little attention to the West, the explanation lies in the recency of its history. By the time the western states were coming of age, American medicine had begun to merge with that of Western Europe and lose its distinctive characteristics.

I am heavily indebted to a great many librarians throughout the United States who have cheerfully helped me in my search for materials. William D. Postell and staff members Cynthia H. Goldstein and Patricia S. Copeland of the Rudolph Matas Medical Library of Tulane University Medical School were particularly helpful during the latter stages of my writing. A number of my good friends and colleagues made invaluable suggestions: Dr. J. Harvey Young read the entire manuscript and made a major contribution to the book; Dr. Mason G. Robertson read several chapters on the twentieth century and was particularly helpful with medical developments; Dr. John E. Salvaggio read the chapters on medicine and surgery and provided invaluable information; Dr. Saul Jarcho helped with the chapter on twentieth-century medical education; and Dr. Gerald N. Grob gave me the benefit of his extensive knowledge of the history of mental health. My wife, Corinne, in this book as in my other publications, continued to straighten out my prose. My son, John, Jr., read the entire manuscript and proved quite helpful.

I have made a great many generalizations based upon my years of work in the field. Whatever the reaction of my readers, I take full credit or blame for these and for any errors that may have crept into the text.

CHAPTER I

The Beginnings
of American Medicine

A STARTLING CONTRAST exists between the economic and health conditions experienced by the early settlers and what they had been led to expect. By the time of settlement the seemingly incredible wealth of the New World had been trumpeted throughout Europe, and these glowing accounts of the newly discovered lands were underscored by the shiploads of gold and silver brought back by the Spaniards. Further convincing evidence was supplied by the early explorers and the Western European fishermen who were already exploiting the rich fishing grounds off the northeastern coast of North America. They recorded seeing vast forests, rich in furs and naval stores, and reported that land, the hallmark of the aristocrat, was there for the taking. Added to this felicitous picture were the equally enthusiastic accounts of the healthful air and wonder drugs to be found in the New World. These latter claims seemed to be confirmed by descriptions of the native Americans, who were invariably pictured as tall, strong, and healthy.

In truth the Indians first encountered by the whites did fit this category. Their mixed economy of hunting, fishing, and agriculture and their relatively sparse population saved them from the great epidemic diseases that plagued Europe.[1] In addition, a high infant mortality rate and recurrent periods of feasting and famine eliminated the weaker members of the tribes. The robust appearance of the native Americans and their ability to recover from major injuries helped to create a myth that their medicine had special virtues. While Europeans alternated between considering Indians "Noble Savages" and barbarians, native remedies continued to hold a strong appeal to all whites. Well into the twentieth century, pitchmen were peddling "Indian medicines" at American county and state fairs.

In terms of their way of life, the native Americans had an adequate medicine. They dealt rationally with fractures, dislocations, contusions, abrasions, and cuts, and they knew a good many useful herbals. Their medicine men, who employed rituals for calling on the help of the spirits, provided emotional support for the sick. Yet their medicine was based on the belief that sickness resulted from the work of spirits. Even when pragmatic remedies were used, these nostrums were an adjunct to ritual healing. It must be borne in mind, too, that the medicine man was a priest, and that healing was only a part of his function. Even more important, there was no native American medicine as such, since medical practices varied widely among the hundreds of Indian tribes. Effective botanical therapeutics used by one tribe were often unknown to neighboring groups, or even when known, their value might be negated by a tribe's utilizing the leaves rather than the roots or by incorrectly processing the plant. The limited knowledge available about native American medicine before the coming of the whites leaves ample room for conjecture.[2] A favorable view of Indian medicine may be found in *American Indian Medicine* by Virgil J. Vogel.[3]

In terms of the medical problems of the native Americans, their medicine was quite satisfactory, and it did not compare too unfavorably with the medical practices of sixteenth- and seventeenth-century Europe. The major difference was that Western medicine had already begun the shift from a spiritual to a rational basis. In the clash of cultures, the most significant impact of Europeans upon native American medicine was to transform it from a religious procedure with empirical overtones to an empirical procedure with religious overtones.

The white occupation not only changed Indian medicine, but it led to even greater changes in Indian health. The native Americans had little immunological defenses against white contagions, and smallpox, measles, tuberculosis, and venereal diseases wrought havoc among the tribes. One of the greatest killers, smallpox, may have paved the way for the Spanish conquest of Central and South America by killing an estimated three million natives in the sixteenth century;[4] it also may have been responsible for the epidemic that depopulated New England in 1616 and facilitated the settlement of that area; and it was the chief factor in the virtual elimination of the native Americans in the East during the colonial period. In 1679 Count de Frontenac referred to smallpox as the "Indian Plague," and from South Carolina in 1699 it was reported "to have swept away a whole neighboring [Indian] nation, all to 5 or 6 which ran away and left their dead unburied. . . ."[5]

The native Americans' susceptibility to smallpox led to its use as one of the early forms of germ warfare. In 1763 Pontiac, chief of the Ottawa, mobilized a group of Indian tribes and launched a well-coordinated attack on the British frontier posts west of the Alleghenies. Apprehensive over such successes, General Jeffrey Amherst suggested to Colonel Henry Bouquet that smallpox be sent among the disaffected tribes. Bouquet replied: "I will try to inoculate the —— with Some Blankets that may fall in their Hands, and take care not to get the disease myself." Subsequently, the British Army was billed by a private company for "Sundries got to Replace in kind those which were taken from people in the Hospital to Convey the Small-pox to the Indians."[6]

Whatever the merits of native American medicine, it was of little help to the early settlers. The London Company, which founded Virginia, assumed it was establishing a trading post comparable to those of the East India Company. Consequently the men recruited for the colony were soldiers and adventurers rather than sturdy yeomen farmers. The company took for granted that its men would obtain food and shelter by trading with or subjugating the natives. Consequently the first Virginia settlers had neither the skills nor the tools and agricultural implements needed to subdue the wilderness. When the original assumptions proved unfounded, starvation soon set in and remained a major problem for the first twenty-five years of settlement.

Initially, Virginia did provide a clean and healthful environment, but the settlers, jammed together for protection in a small fort, quickly befouled their living quarters with garbage and human wastes. With the arrival of the whites, the native population lost its freedom from the great epidemic and endemic disorders, for the settlers brought with them malaria, smallpox, typhoid fever, and a host of other contagions. The impact of these diseases upon the Indians was disastrous, and in the long run it was the major factor in reducing the Indian population.

The story of the first years in Virginia is one of constant starvation, sickness, and death. In the first place, the long voyage to the New World in small, crowded, and filthy vessels, usually taking from six to twelve weeks, exacted a heavy toll. The ships' food was dietetically unsound and often in short supply. Even if typhus and other fevers were not aboard, the lack of sanitation and poor food insured the presence of enteric complaints. Hence those passengers who escaped the many infections enroute could hardly avoid the omnipresent scurvy, and most settlers landed in a debilitated condition.[7]

Contemporary accounts of the early settlement of Virginia speak constantly of fluxes, fevers, bellyaches, and other ailments. The term "flux" was applied to any sort of intestinal complaint resulting in diarrhea. Bloody flux, as its name implies, was a more serious condition and encompassed such disorders as typhoid fever and various forms of dysentery. "Fevers" was a generic term covering a wide range of sicknesses, although certain fevers were often categorized as putrid fever, continued fever, or burning fever. The distinctive symptoms of the more common forms of malaria had already given that disease the name "fever and ague." Malaria was extensive in England and Holland in the seventeenth century, and its vector, the anopheles mosquito, could easily breed in the open water-caskets and buckets and the bilges of sailing vessels. The references to "burning fevers" in early Virginia have led to considerable debate among medical historians, who differ as to the exact nature of these fevers. The chief suspects are malaria, typhoid, and yellow fever, but Wyndham Blanton, a Virginia medical historian, has made an excellent case for typhoid as the most likely one.[8]

Regardless of which particular disorder was the most deadly, the mortality rate among the early Virginia colonists was horrendous. About nine thousand settlers had come to Virginia in the years from 1607 to 1625, but the total population in the latter year was somewhere between eleven hundred and twelve hundred. A few hundred had returned to England, but the rest had fallen prey to sickness and starvation. The first New England settlers, arriving in 1620, profited by the experience of the Virginians. Nonetheless, almost half of the Plymouth colonists died during the first winter.[9]

As a sound agricultural base was established and the food supply increased, health conditions improved. By the end of the colonial period, Americans probably enjoyed better health and a longer life expectancy than did Europeans. Yet life in general during the seventeenth and eighteenth centuries was both short and grim. In the colonies, as in Europe, parents accepted the loss of half of their infants and children as part of God's design, and people saw the hand of a wrathful God in the many epidemic diseases that winnowed all ages. The familiar summer fevers and fluxes were particularly hard on infants, while young and old fell prey to the "coffs," "Great Colds," "Pleurisies," and "Peripneumonias" of the winter months.

Strange and unfamiliar diseases have always aroused far more consternation than the more deadly and debilitating familiar ones. In the colonial period the omnipresent respiratory and enteric disorders were the major sources of sickness and death, but they received only scant mention in newspapers and other records. Among the fevers, malaria, which was endemic from New England to Georgia, undoubtedly was the leading cause of suffering and death, but it too, as with pulmonary tuberculosis, was accepted as a normal hazard. The disorder that most frequently terrified the colonies was smallpox. The incidence of this highly fatal contagion, which often horribly scarred the faces of those who survived its attack, rose steadily in Europe during the seventeenth century and peaked toward the end of the eighteenth. It may have been spread to one or more of the native American tribes before the settlement of North America, but in any case it arrived with the first settlers.[10]

While smallpox often proved disastrous to the colonists, it devastated the native Americans, literally destroying certain tribes. In the same way that it had swept through Central and South America in the sixteenth century, paving the way for the Spanish Conquistadores, so it proved an advance guard for the European occupation of North America. Why it should have been so deadly to the native Americans is still a matter of debate. Traditionally it has been accepted that whites had a measure of immunity to smallpox, whereas the Indians had none. Albert W. Crosby, however, argues that genetic susceptibility to the disease was not the issue. He maintains that the real problem was the inability of native American society, or any other virgin society, to cope with an unfamiliar pestilence. He suggests that Indian babies died when their mother's milk was no longer available; that with the high loss of young adults there was not enough help to keep the fires going and supply food and water; and that the medicine men, lacking any traditional means for dealing with smallpox, could no longer provide religious or moral support. The result was a complete breakdown of family and tribal society, with some individuals fleeing in panic and others fatalistically resigning themselves to death.[11]

The relative isolation of the American colonies from England and from each other prevented smallpox from becoming endemic, as it

did in England and on the Continent. But the intervals between outbreaks often permitted the rise of an entire generation of nonimmunes.
Smallpox was a highly contagious virus disease, and one attack usually
conferred a lifetime immunity. When smallpox was introduced into
one of the colonial ports, it was likely to strike everyone who had not
previously experienced an attack. Records of colonial towns and cities
show that during epidemics 60 percent or more of the inhabitants fell
sick and that the death toll ranged from 5 or 6 percent to as high as
20 percent of the community's population. Justifiably, a report of the
presence of smallpox in town was enough to cause a mass flight. In 1752
the Reverend Roger Price recorded in his diary that "the small pox is
broke out in Boston in a violent manner after two and twenty years
absence, it has occasioned almost a total Stagnation of trade So that
half the houses and shops in town are shut up and the people retir'd to
the country."[12]

Yellow fever was another disease that with good reason spread panic
in the coastal towns and cities. This malignant pestilence, which could
bring a horrible death through jaundice, high fever, and generalized
internal hemorrhages, struck at the colonies from New England to
Georgia from the 1690s to 1761. For some reason, probably related to
its incidence in the Caribbean, the fever did not appear again until 1793,
the beginning of a series of major attacks. In terms of overall morbidity
and mortality, yellow fever was a minor factor in the colonies, but its
dramatic nature gave it a prominent place in colonial records.

Two other epidemic diseases, diphtheria and scarlet fever, probably
caused more deaths than yellow fever, but they struck largely at children. By leaving the adult population relatively intact, these disorders
did not create widespread social and economic disruption. However,
this must have been small consolation to those parents who watched
their children, often gasping for breath, die one by one from what Noah
Webster called the "plague among children."[13] Fortunately, the two
diseases did not reach major epidemic proportions until 1735, and then
did not reappear on a large scale until a major pandemic in the 1850s.

The State of Medicine

In seventeenth-century England medical care was provided
by three major categories of practitioners, although the distinction was
never sharply maintained. In addition to these formal groups, a variety

of other individuals, including midwives, nurses, ministers, and folk practitioners, offered medical services. The highest-ranking of all practitioners were the physicians, a relatively small group of men, graduates of Oxford or Cambridge, who were members or licentiates of the Royal College of Physicians. Their training was largely theoretical and required only a minimal knowledge of anatomy and a limited amount of clinical work. At this time virtually nothing was known about physiology, and disease was generally assumed to be the result of some constitutional imbalance. For centuries the Galenic concept of morbid humors, one based on the humoral theory of the Greeks, had been the basis of medical thinking. In essence the theory attributed sickness to an imbalance or corruption of the four basic humors, blood, phlegm, black bile, and yellow bile. New theories, the iatrochemical and the iatrophysical, were coming into vogue, but medical practice still rested firmly on the humoral theory. Bleeding, blistering, purging, vomiting, and sweating, the so-called depletory regimen, long the mainstay of medicine, remained the standard practice. It was designed to restore the humoral balance or to eliminate morbid or corrupt humors.[14]

As university graduates, physicians were gentlemen, and their practice was restricted largely to the upper class. Below the physicians, and theoretically subject to them, were the surgeons. Surgeons, who worked with their hands, were considered tradesmen and received their training through an apprenticeship system. As early as 1462 barbers had been authorized to practice surgery, and in 1540 surgeons and barbers in England were joined by royal decree into the United Barber-Surgeons Company. It was not until 1745 that surgeons separated from the barbers to form their own guild.[15] The work of the surgeons and barber-surgeons was restricted largely to dealing with injuries, fractures, luxations, and with catheterizing, letting blood, excising cancers, dressing ulcers, opening abscesses, pulling teeth, and similar tasks. Occasionally surgeons were called upon to amputate, and the better ones might perform a lithotomy, the surgical removal of bladder stones. This latter procedure, however, along with couching for cataracts — wherein a sharp object was used to displace the clouded lens — was more generally handled by traveling lithotomists and couchers. Theoretically, surgeons could not practice medicine, but in fact they served as general practitioners to the lower classes.

On a par with surgeons, and subject also to the physicians, were the apothecaries, known in early days as "ye physicians cooke," since they compounded drugs. As was true in America, at least until World War II, apothecaries, or druggists, were often the first to be called upon for medical advice. In the seventeenth and eighteenth centuries physicians were virtually nonexistent insofar as the lower economic groups were concerned, and surgeons were in limited supply. Under these circumstances, apothecaries gradually began assuming the role of medical practitioners.

Physicians resented the infringement of apothecaries into medical practice, and their resentment culminated in a celebrated court case in 1703–4. An apothecary in London by the name of Rose was brought to court by the Royal College of Physicians on the charge of illegally practicing medicine. Suffice to say, he was acquitted, and the case, in effect, legalized the right of apothecaries to practice medicine. Relations between the two groups subsequently improved, and physicians began serving as consultants to the apothecaries.[16] Along with the practitioners already mentioned were a great many folk healers, including bloodletters, bonesetters, itinerant lithotomists and couchers, midwives, and herb doctors.

The American colonies saw the emergence of still another group, the minister-physicians. Although the Elizabethan Compromise had essentially settled the religious issue in England, the Stuart kings' attempt to move the Anglican church toward Catholicism led to a limited persecution of those ministers seeking to purify the church of Catholic influences. In part because they feared the possibility of being dismissed from the state church, many dissenting ministers in the seventeenth century began adding medicine to their university studies as an alternative way of livelihood.[17] While the first settlements usually included a physician or surgeon, a shortage of physicians soon developed in the rapidly growing colonies. The majority of colonists were motivated to come to the New World by economic, religious, or political considerations, but physicians, who tended to be conservative members of the upper class, had little incentive to chance life in the colonies. In both Puritan New England and the Anglican colonies to the south, ministers — usually the best-educated individuals in the community — were called upon to deal with the physical as well as the spiritual ills of their flocks. The study of medicine was still largely theoretical at this time, and most ministers, Anglican or Puritan, had access to at least one or two medical books.

The minister-physicians played a particularly strong role in New

England. The leading physician in early New England was Deacon Dr. Samuel Fuller, a passenger on the Mayflower in 1620. Fuller was equally well versed in theology and medicine, having studied in Leyden, one of the leading medical centers in Europe. His reputation as a physician was such that his help was requested by the governors of the Salem and Charleston colonies during times of serious illness.[18] Another outstanding minister-physician was the Reverend Thomas Thacher, who learned his theology and medicine from Charles Chauncy, the second president of Harvard. Despite his staunch Puritanism, Thacher earned his place in history by writing the first medical publication in America, a broadside entitled *A Brief Rule to Guide the Common People of New England how to order themselves and theirs in the Small Pocks, or Measles.*[19] Throughout the seventeenth century and continuing into the eighteenth, medicine in New England remained the domain of ministers and government leaders, apprentice-trained physicians, midwives, and folk practitioners.

The role of the New England ministers in medicine is clearly shown by the experience of Giles Fermin, the first New England physician, who arrived in 1632. Fermin had studied medicine at Cambridge although he does not appear to have taken a degree. He apparently found ministerial competition too great for he wrote in 1639 that he was "strongly sett upon to studye divinitiae . . . for physick is but a meene helpe."[20]

The Virginia colony was well supplied with physicians in its early years. To their credit, the directors of the London Company responsible for the first settlement of Virginia recognized the need to keep the colonists healthy. Specific instructions were given as to the location of the settlement and the number of physicians and apothecaries. Two "chirurgeons" (surgeons) were included in the first group of settlers. One, Chirurgeon General Henry Wotton, was described as a gentleman-chirurgeon, and the second, Will Wilkinson, who was probably a barber-surgeon, was simply listed along with the bricklayer and the barber. The first two physicians in the colony were Dr. Walter Russell, arriving in 1608, and Dr. Lawrence Bohun, in 1610. Bohun remained only one year and was replaced by Dr. John Pott, described as "a Master of Arts and . . . well practised in Chirurgerie and Phisique." Indicative of the status of physicians, Dr. Pott served as a member of the Governor's Council.[21]

The enormous death rate during the early years in Virginia arose from unanticipated conditions and clearly was not due to want of medical care. Ironically, as economic conditions improved, the caliber of physicians in terms of education and training declined. Once the London Company's charter was revoked in 1624 and the Crown assumed control, medical care became an individual responsibility. While surgeons or physicians occasionally chose to settle in Virginia, henceforth the majority of Virginians received their medical care from barber-surgeons, apothecaries, midwives, ministers, and colonial physicians trained through an apprenticeship system.

Whereas Britain paid only minimal attention to its early colonies, the Dutch government was quite paternalistic. The New Amsterdam (New York) colony, benefiting from the experiences of both Virginia and Plymouth, avoided the heavy losses from sickness and disease. In 1630 a midwife arrived in the colony and was soon succeeded by several barber-surgeons. The first physician came to the colony in 1637. This was Dr. Johannes La Montagne, a Huguenot refugee and a graduate of the University of Leyden, the leading medical center in Western Europe.[22]

New York, under both Dutch and British administrations, had a relatively liberal policy and tended to attract better-qualified physicians than did the other colonies. Among them was Dr. Samuel Megapolensis, who, following graduation from Harvard, sailed for Holland and took degrees in medicine and theology at the University of Utrecht. On his return to New York he assumed a pastorate and tended to both the spiritual and medical needs of his flock. Another leading physician was Dr. Adriaen Van der Donck, best known for his observations on New World medicinal plants and the medical practices of the native Americans.[23] The ability of New York to draw medical personnel from diverse areas can be seen in a committee of physicians and surgeons appointed by Governor Henry Sloughter in 1691 to assist in an autopsy. The group was headed by a Dutchman, Dr. Johannes Kerfbyle, and included a Scotsman, a German, two Englishmen, and a Frenchman.[24]

Despite a relatively high number of physicians with first-rate degrees, by 1700 medical care in New York, as in the other colonies, was provided by a variety of empirics and a few apprentice-trained physicians. Although the colony continued to draw a number of university-trained physicians, by the eighteenth century the majority of colonial physicians were products of the apprenticeship system.

With some variations, the patterns of medical care in New England

and New York held true for all of the colonies in the seventeenth century. It is well to bear in mind, too, that colonial medical care was not far removed from that in Britain and on the Continent. The major difference lay in the regulation of physicians and surgeons. Colleges and guilds operating under royal charters in the homelands set standards for physicians and surgeons, whereas in the colonies only tentative efforts were made to regulate medical practice. A Virginia law first passed in 1639 provided for the arrest of any physician charging an unreasonable fee and permitted the courts to censure a physician for refusing aid to the sick or for neglecting a patient. In 1649 Massachusetts General Court resolved that all medical practitioners, midwives included, should follow "the known approved Rules of Art." A similar measure was enacted when the British took over the Dutch colony of New Amsterdam in 1664.[25]

The only references to a license to practice medicine occur in some of the county records in Massachusetts, but no mention is made of any specific requirements. Since the laws and resolutions were rather vague and no provision was made for their enforcement, it is safe to assume that the practice of medicine was open to all. Despite the lack of regulation, the colonies were not overrun by quacks and empirics as was the case elsewhere. It is true that a shortage of trained physicians existed. Formal medical education, however, was acquired largely through lectures and books, and a high percentage of ministers and government leaders were well versed in the prevailing medical theories and practices, thus insuring that the colonists received medical care that was as good as that in Europe. Moreover, Americans, as Daniel J. Boorstin has pointed out, are a practical people, and colonial physicians who acquired their knowledge through an apprenticeship were less inclined to apply a medical theory dogmatically and more likely to rely upon experience and observation.[26]

In their detailed study of the town of Portsmouth, New Hampshire, J. Worth Estes and David M. Goodman show how the apprenticeship system provided the town with trained physicians until well into the nineteenth century. Dr. Clement Jackson (1705–88) and his students dominated medical practice in the town for almost sixty years. His apprentices, however, were far from the illiterates encountered in the West during the nineteenth century. Several of them attended Harvard College, and almost all of Jackson's students were active in colonial affairs. The emphasis upon education in New England probably helped the area to avoid the worst abuses of the apprentice training system that characterized the later period.[27]

The colonial experience also made it virtually impossible to maintain any distinctions among physicians, surgeons, and apothecaries. University-trained physicians usually ranked high in colonial society and frequently served on the governors' councils and held other responsible positions. Nonetheless, they were forced to become general practitioners, since they could not rely on apothecaries to compound their drugs or on surgeons to dress injuries and ulcers, let blood, and perform other manual procedures. Surgeons, and the few apothecaries who arrived in the seventeenth century, soon assumed the title "doctor" and took over the general care of the patients, including prescribing and dispensing drugs. Obstetrics remained in the hands of midwives throughout the colonial period, although physicians were called in difficult cases. By the end of the seventeenth century in the American colonies the stratification that characterized European medicine was weakening, and the apprenticeship system was beginning to emerge as the basic form of medical training.

CHAPTER 2

The Eighteenth Century

B<small>Y THE EIGHTEENTH CENTURY</small> the colonies were established on firm economic foundations, and colonial society was beginning to resemble that of Great Britain. Accumulating
wealth and the emergence of a leisure class helped to sharpen class
distinctions and to promote higher education, a prerequisite to the development of a professional class. Beginning with Harvard in 1636, nine
colleges were established by the time of the Revolution, but professional schools lagged behind. Only two small medical schools had been
founded by the end of the colonial period and law schools awaited the
post-Revolution era. Young colonials seeking the best medical education were compelled to complete their studies in Edinburgh, London,
or Paris. Nonetheless, physicians were beginning to organize medical
societies and to promote licensing laws.

The seventeenth century has been described as the century of genius,
one in which individuals made fundamental discoveries in mathematics,
physics, and other areas. It culminated in Isaac Newton's discovery of
the law of gravity, the basic principle that helped to explain the work-
ings of the universe. Newton's brilliant work convinced philosophers
in other areas that they too could find the one fundamental principle.
Reflecting this intellectual milieu, the eighteenth century was preemi-
nently an age of medical theorizing, one in which philosophers set off
on a fruitless quest to find the one universal law of health. The previous
century had set the stage by introducing two new theories: the iatrophysical, which saw locomotion, digestion, and respiration as purely
mechanical processes and envisioned the body as a machine motivated
by a "life force" circulating through the nerves; and the iatrochemical,

which assumed that chemistry was the basis of physiology and saw acids and alkalis as the basic bodily substances. To the iatrochemical school, sickness was the result of abnormal chemical reactions, as evidenced by the formation of gallstones and urinary calculi.

The eighteenth century witnessed the appearance of several new theories, including vitalism, tonism, solidism, tension, and homeopathy. Fortunately, it also saw significant developments in clinical medicine, and the rise to prominence of intelligent practitioners, such as Thomas Sydenham in England and Hermann Boerhaave in Holland, both of whom emphasized observation and experience. Sydenham accepted a modified version of the Galenical or humoral theory but relied to a large extent upon observation and common sense. In the midcentury, Boerhaave, an outstanding Dutch clinician, also preached moderation. He was an eclectic, willing to borrow from any medical system, but he emphasized the need for closely observing the patient and taught that the function of the physician was not to combat nature but to assist it in curing the patient. Unfortunately the moderating influence of Sydenham and Boerhaave was eclipsed late in the century by the extreme views of John Brown and Benjamin Rush. Both Brown and Rush advocated rigorous therapies—a development that did little to help the public image of the medical profession in the nineteenth century, and, as will be seen in subsequent chapters, proved even worse for the patients.

Medical Practice

Colonial physicians, the majority of whom had little academic training, paid limited attention to the new medical theories and continued to base their practice on a modified humoral system. In terms of twentieth-century medicine, scarcely any eighteenth-century therapy could be called moderate. The basic treatment consisted of bleeding, blistering, purging, vomiting, and sweating—all designed to restore the proper balance of body humors or to rid the body of putrid or peccant humors. William Douglass, probably the best-trained physician in early eighteenth-century Boston, wrote that the New England medical practice "was very uniform, bleeding, vomiting, blistering, purging, anodyne, etc. if the illness continued there was repetendi, and finally murderandi." The practitioners, he added, "follow Sydenham too much in giving paragoricks after catharticks, which is playing fast and loose."[1]

Douglass was guilty of hyperbole, since recent studies of ledger books of several late eighteenth-century practitioners reveal a much more moderate practice. Moreover, many sensible physicians in all centuries have used discretion in applying the prevailing medical theory. J. Worth Estes, a medical historian, examined the books of four colonial New England physicians and found that two country physicians bled only about 5 percent of their patients and that the Boston physicians rarely resorted to bloodletting.[2]

Estes's same study shows that the four colonial physicians used about 225 medications compounded from about 100 different raw materials. Cathartics (rigorous laxatives), such as rhubarb, aloes, castor oil, and mercury compounds, were the most commonly prescribed drugs; ipecac and antimony compounds were used for sweating and vomiting, and camphor and opium as pain relievers. The most general use for opium, however, was to relieve the omnipresent diarrheas of earlier days. Cantharides (dried Spanish fly), which caused blisters when applied to the skin, was another frequently used therapeutic. The blistering process was thought to draw out the poisons or bad humors from the body. In the southern colonies, cinchona bark, the substance from which quinine is derived, was the common antidote for "fevers."[3] Since malaria was the most common fever, and quinine is a specific for all forms of malaria, the "bark," as it was often called, was assumed to be a specific for all fevers.

Notwithstanding Estes's limited study, colonial records abound with complaints of patients dying from excessive purging and vomiting. The prescription for a patient suffering from rheumatism in 1720 illustrates this point all too well. On the first day the patient was to be purged twice. On the second day he or she was to be bled twelve to fourteen ounces of blood, preferably from the foot. A day or so later the patient was to be purged twice more. On the days when purging or bleeding was not carried out, the patient was to be given various powders and herbal concoctions. If nothing else, this treatment must at least have had the merit of distracting the patient's attention from the pains of rheumatism.[4]

Even a casual survey of medical prescriptions as reported in correspondence, diaries, and journals makes one shudder at the implications in phrases such as "brisk purging" or "copious bleeding." In addition to depletory forms of therapy and a wide range of botanicals and other therapeutics, eighteenth-century medicine included an extensive use of nauseating substances (the well-known *dreckapotheke*). Syrups made from sheep's "Purles" or cow's dung were not uncommon, and they were widely used in poultices. The Reverend Cotton Mather, who kept abreast of the latest medical developments, wrote that human excreta was "a Remedy for Humane Bodies that is hardly to be paralleled," and that urine had virtues far beyond all the waters of medicinal springs.[5]

With physicians in short supply and subject to little regulation, folk practitioners and quacks supplied much of medical care, and the quacks undoubtedly contributed to the public suspicion of the medical profession. An Anglican missionary in 1709 reported that one of his colleagues had died after "a pretended Phisitian" had prescribed a medicine that "work't so violently that it gave him 100 vomits and as many stools . . . which soon carried him off, and caused him to purge till he was Interr'd."[6] Dr. Alexander Hamilton encountered a former cobbler who, having chanced to "cure an old woman of a pestilent disease," decided that medicine was more profitable than shoe repairing and "fell to cobling of human bodies." William Smith in his history of New York wrote, "Quacks abound like locusts in Egypt, and too many have recommended themselves to a full and profitable practice and subsistence."[7] Since the line between folk medicine and orthodox practice was not sharply drawn, miracle drugs could readily find support in legislatures. The Virginia House of Burgesses, for example, gave £100 to one Mary Johnson for discovering a cure for cancer and another £250 to Richard Bryan for his remedy for the "dry gripes," the common name for lead poisoning.[8]

Much of the home care was provided by women, and undoubtedly they also formed a large percentage of the folk practitioners. Midwifery, and to a large extent the care of children, was left almost exclusively to women. Physicians were called only in difficult obstetrical cases, although upper-class women in the later eighteenth century increasingly resorted to doctors. Since few educated women practiced as midwives or folk practitioners, there is scant evidence of their work. Among those for whom we have a record was Elizabeth Hubbard Stiles of Newport, Rhode Island, who was described by Benjamin Rush as having "considerable medical & chirurgical Skill by which she was enabled to do much good." Most women with an interest in medicine cared only for their families and friends and called in physicians for serious illnesses. The diary of Elizabeth Sandwith Drinker of Philadelphia provides an excellent account of one of these home practitioners, since it describes both her own medical activities and those of the family's physicians.[9]

While medicine was only an incidental interest to Mrs. Drinker, Elizabeth Coates Paschall (1702–67), the wife of a Philadelphia merchant, was well acquainted with medical literature, discussed medicine with the local physicians, and freely treated members of the community as well as her own family. Between 1740 and 1765 she compiled a book containing 212 recipes, nearly all of which were medicinal. These remedies present an excellent picture of eighteenth-century domestic medical practice. Typical of folk medicine, her recipe book makes no reference to the use of bloodletting, laudanum, or mercury, and nine of the remedies included the use of animal and human wastes.[10]

Although gross anatomy was well delineated by the eighteenth century, major surgery was still limited to emergency situations. No sharp division existed between physicians and surgeons in the colonies; hence physicians were expected to deal with fractures, luxations, wounds, and abrasions, and to dress ulcers, lance boils, let blood, and give enemas. Amputations of limbs were the most common of major procedures, although on rare occasions a breast would be excised because of cancer. Individuals with the inclination and manual dexterity would occasionally perform a lithotomy (the removal of urinary calculi) or paracentesis (surgical puncture of a body cavity for the aspiration of fluid), but these were considered major operations. In 1732 the *South Carolina Gazette* reported that a naval surgeon had drawn ten quarts of water from the abdomen of a seaman, and that the operation had been observed by the surgeons of all His Majesty's ships in the harbor. And when Dr. John Jones of Newark, New Jersey, performed a lithotomy in 1767, the operation was done "before several very eminent Gentlemen in the Practice of Physick and Surgery." [11]

Toward the end of the colonial period, surgeons were becoming more venturesome, as a fee bill issued by the New Jersey Medical Society shows. Among the procedures listed on the bill were trepanning, removing cataracts, "extirpation of tonsils," correction of "Harelip" and "Wryneck," and amputations of limbs and breasts, excision of tumors, paracentesis, and lithotomy.[12] It is difficult to know how many physicians had the skill or courage to attempt some of these more serious procedures. The chances are that they would not have had too many opportunities, since in the days before anesthesia only the most desperate of patients would have been willing to submit to major surgery. Most physicians performed surgery only out of necessity, usually contenting themselves with routine services. A few of them, those with special skills, gradually gained reputations for their surgical or obstetrical work and began to concentrate in these areas. By the Revolution, doctors such as William Shippen, Jr., in Philadelpia, William Moultrie in Charleston, and James Lloyd of Boston were well known for their work in obstetrics. Nonetheless, they still considered themselves primarily as physicians; the formal specialities of surgery and obstetrics were still in the future.

The Practitioners of Medicine

As of the midcentury, medical practice was in the hands of a diverse group of practitioners, but a small, articulate professional body was beginning to emerge. These physicians constituted the best of the four main categories of medical practitioners. They were a rather amorphous group representing the better-trained and more intelligent physicians. They achieved their status by a combination of formal preparation, ethical conduct, and demonstrated success in medical practice. Included among their ranks were those men with medical degrees from British or European universities; those who had served an apprenticeship under a well-trained physician and then studied medicine abroad; and graduates of American colleges who had subsequently read medicine under an established practitioner. Occasionally, entrance to their ranks was gained by individuals whose sole training was an apprenticeship but who had demonstrated enough skill and interest in medicine to win the approbation of their medical colleagues.[13]

As the eighteenth century wore on, there was a growing professional consciousness among the better physicians, and they began drawing together to exchange medical information and provide mutual support. Aside from professional reasons, they faced intensive economic competition from the large number of less-qualified practitioners. This competition came largely from the second category, the run-of-the-mill apprentice-trained practitioners who constituted the majority of colonial doctors. The best of these, as already noted, sought additional training and tended to move upward. Many of these empirically trained physicians provided satisfactory medical care and were highly regarded in their communities. A newspaper obituary of Dr. Roelof Kierstede of New York City in 1751 described him as a "Gentlemen eminent in his Profession, altho' not skill'd in the technical Terms thereof, which often drew on him the Contempt of his Brethren, yet his great Knowledge in Simples, his extensive Charity and successful Cures to poor People has made his Memory precious to them, and his death a real public loss."[14] To offset the Kierstedes were an even larger number of poorly trained doctors who were only vaguely acquainted with anatomy and the prevailing medical knowledge, and who eked out a miserable living through medicine or practiced on a part-time basis to supplement their incomes as farmers, planters, or merchants.

The third group encompassed the practitioners of folk medicine and the outright quacks. With a limited knowledge of folk medicine and some acquaintance with simples or herbal remedies, anyone could set up as a medical practitioner. Success was best achieved if the would-be doctor first treated a number of patients with self-limiting disorders. Yet many of the folk doctors, a group that included bonesetters, herbalists, and midwives, were both skilled and knowledgeable. In the seventeenth and early eighteenth centuries quacks were relatively few, but their numbers steadily increased with the growing affluence of the colonies. Since orthodox medicine could neither prevent nor cure most of the disorders troubling patients, it is not surprising that the public turned to anyone who could promise relief.

In the last category of practitioners, but certainly not the least, were the omnipresent minister-physicians. Despite the growing number of professional and lay doctors, ministers continued to provide medical services—in some cases out of necessity and in others by choice—to members of their congregations and to the public at large. Anglican missionaries sent to the American colonies in the eighteenth century by the Society for the Propagation of the Gospel often found their knowledge of medicine to be an effective way of reaching potential church members. In 1716 the Reverend Mr. Henry Lucas reported from New England that his "little knowledge in Physick" had given him "a great Opportunity for conversing with Men by whc. I have done that, whc. by preaching I could not have done." Other ministers discovered that medicine was an effective means of supplementing their income.[15]

Ministers to German congregations in Pennsylvania and other colonies also found their congregations wanting more than spiritual consolation. The Reverend Mr. Henry Melchior Muhlenberg in a bitter moment likened himself to a "privy to which all those with loose bowels come running from all directions to relieve themselves." Fortunately he was well prepared to handle complaints of both spirit and bowels, since he had been trained in medicine in Halle.[16] The role of minister-physician brought a mixed reaction from congregations. In some cases the members were glad to be relieved of providing full support for their ministers and were happy to secure medical assistance. A few congregations, however, objected to receiving medical bills from their pastors, feeling that healing the sick was a normal responsibility for one whose life was presumably dedicated to the great Healer.

As a well-educated class, the ministerial profession contributed notably to colonial medicine. Thacher's broadside on smallpox was the first of a series of articles and pamphlets by ministers on medical subjects. One of the best of these was a pamphlet published by Cotton Mather following a measles epidemic in 1713 that killed five members of his household. It included an excellent clinical description of the disease, warned against excessive treatment, and noted that the sequelae could often be more dangerous than the disease itself. He stressed the need for the patient to have complete rest, even in mild cases, adding: "Let him not be *well too soon*, and throw himself into a *Fever*, and throw away his *Life*, as many have inconsiderately and presumptuously done." [17]

Mather's chief claim to fame in the medical area lies in his sponsorship of inoculation or variolation in the colonies. Somewhere in antiquity it had been discovered that taking pus from the pustules of an active smallpox case and inserting it under the skin of a healthy person resulted in a relatively mild case. The individual so inoculated would henceforth be immune to the disease. This procedure is known as variolation, from the technical name for smallpox, *variola*, to differentiate it from the present-day technique of vaccination. Variolation was an old folk practice in isolated rural areas of England and the Continent and in other parts of the globe. It did not arouse much interest in the medical world until a series of letters from Constantinople describing the procedure was published by the Royal Society between 1714 and 1716. [18]

Mather, who kept up with the *Proceedings* of the Royal Society, was intrigued since he had already heard of the procedure from his slave Anesimus. He decided to try it at the first opportunity. In 1721, when several ships from the West Indies introduced smallpox into Boston, Mather circulated a letter to the local physicians urging them to try inoculation. The only physician to respond was Dr. Zabdiel Boyleston, who promptly inoculated his own son and a number of other children. The townspeople and the local doctors were outraged at the idea of spreading a deadly disease, and Mather complained in his diary of "the vile Abuse which I do myself particularly suffer . . . for nothing but my instructing our base Physicians, how to save many precious lives." [19]

Led by Dr. William Douglass, who accused Boyleston of mischievously "propagating the Infection," the medical faculty generally condemned inoculation, while the clergy tended to support it. Not all of the latter were in agreement, however, for one minister called inoculation "a distrust of God's overruling care" and another suggested that freeing people from the fear of smallpox would tend to promote "Vice and Immorality." [20] Douglass, as a conservative physician, felt that smallpox was too dangerous a disease for experimentation and that inoculation had not been properly tested. Beyond the specific issue of inoculation, the clash between Douglass and Mather represented a larger conflict between the physicians, whose growing professionalism caused them to resent interference in medical matters, and the ministers, led by Mather, who firmly believed in their right to control life in the community.

In any event, the statistics gathered by the Selectmen of Boston at the end of the epidemic demonstrated that the case fatality among the 300 individuals inoculated was only 2 percent, compared to 14 percent for those who caught the disease naturally.[21] The success of the Boston experiment led to a steady increase in the use of inoculation. Smallpox inoculators traveled from town to town, often taking an inoculated child with them to provide the necessary virus. Unfortunately, while those inoculated usually suffered only a mild case, they were capable of passing a virulent disorder on to anyone with whom they came in contact. The result was that inoculators frequently started a full-scale epidemic, leading colony after colony to pass laws prohibiting inoculation. When smallpox was present or threatening, the laws were usually held in abeyance. As the value of inoculation became more apparent, by 1760 the laws were rewritten to regulate the procedure and provide for a minimum quarantine period for those inoculated. The repeated introduction of smallpox during the Revolutionary War led to inoculation becoming a general practice. George Washington, faced with repeated smallpox outbreaks among his troops, in February 1777 ordered the entire army inoculated.[22]

An interesting aspect of Mather's role in introducing smallpox inoculation was his rationale for so doing. The introduction of the early microscopes in the seventeenth century made it possible to see microscopic "worms," leading Athanasius Kircher (1602–80), a leading microscopist, to postulate that these tiny "animals" were the cause of disease. His idea, known as the animalculae theory, received only limited attention until Pasteur and Koch in the late nineteenth century demonstrated its validity. Mather was familiar with the theory, and he was convinced that these pathogenic animalculae were the cause of smallpox.

In *The Angel of Bethesda*, a major medical work that Mather began writing in the 1720s, he provided a clear and lucid description of the germ theory, suggesting the specificity of these animalculae and their means of transmission, and even pointing out that healthy bodies could often resist their invasion. His originality is further shown in a pamphlet published in 1722 in which he noted that the animalculae ordinarily entered the body through the respiratory system and thus quickly reached the vital organs. In the case of inoculation, he wrote, the contagion was introduced only at the periphery, giving the body time to mobilize its defenses against the invader.[23] Although in one heated debate, Dr. Douglass dismissed Mather as a credulous layman, in point of fact Mather was probably the most original medical thinker in the colonial period.

Among the other minister-physicians to contribute to medicine were the Reverend Mr. Jabez Fitch, who collected and published an excellent statistical account of the great "throat distemper" epidemic of the 1730s, and the Reverend Mr. Jonathan Dickinson, who also wrote a first-rate account of the disease.[24] From their detailed clinical descriptions it becomes clear that diphtheria was not the new disease it was thought to be in the 1730s. One can scarcely leave the minister-physicians without mentioning John Wesley's *Primitive Physick*. This classic do-it-yourself medical book went through thirty-two English and seven American editions between 1747 and 1829. In it Wesley counseled against excessive bloodletting and strong drugs, a factor that undoubtedly helped its sale. The book's sale was further enhanced by the fact that it enabled patients to save fees. From earliest days Americans had an aversion to paying medical fees, an attitude that helps to explain the proliferation of domestic medical books in the nineteenth century.

Despite occasional clashes between doctors and ministers on the score of medical practice, in a number of communities they worked together. The Reverend Mr. Robert McKean of Perth Amboy was elected the first president of the New Jersey Medical Society when it was founded in 1766, and during the first ten years of its existence six of its thirty-six members were pastor-physicians.[25] By the opening of the nineteenth century, medicine had become more professionalized and the status of the minister in the community was on the decline. In consequence, the minister-physician began to disappear and was supplanted by the overseas medical missionary.

As might be expected, colonial physicians contributed little to advance the general field of medicine. They did, however, help lay the basis for an effective American medical profession and made significant contributions in other areas. Generalities about medicine scarcely give us a picture of the physician's life in colonial times, but we can gain some insight from the lives of outstanding personalities. In terms of original medical thought, it is likely that two laymen, Cotton Mather and Benjamin Franklin, rank at the top among colonials. Mather's *The Angel of Bethesda*, however, was not published until the twentieth century, and, while he promoted inoculation in the colonies and commented wisely on other medical matters, his ideas did not affect the development of medicine. Franklin's work, too, was essentially applying common sense—in his case "uncommon" sense—to the medicine of his day, but he did make specific contributions to the field of medicine. As with Mather, he strongly supported inoculation and was wary of all forms of quackery. Exercise and fresh air, he wrote, were invaluable in preventing diseases, a very important objective, he wrote, "since the cure of them by physic is so very precarious."[26]

Franklin's good sense is best shown in connection with electricity. While his experiments with it are common knowledge, what is not so well known is that he tried to use electricity to stimulate paralyzed muscles. In 1757 he used it on several patients and discovered that although they showed an immediate improvement for two or three days, by the fifth day they become discouraged and discontinued the treatment. Franklin concluded that while electrical treatments might have value in the hands of a skillful physician, he had serious doubts as to their effectiveness. Franklin's work with electricity led to his appointment to a special commission in Paris to study the claims of Franz Anton Mesmer, who had purportedly discovered a substance called animal magnetism. Through Franklin's own experiments with patients, he had come to some understanding of what we call psychosomatic medicine today. The commission dismissed Mesmer's claims after Franklin shrewdly pointed out that the successes attributed to Mesmer were largely due to the imagination of the patients.[27]

Franklin's best-known contribution was his invention of bifocal lenses in 1784 to avoid carrying two pair of glasses. In his later years he suffered acute pain from recurring bouts with urinary calculi (bladder stones), and he devised a flexible silver catheter in place of the customary rigid one. He was also one of the first to recognize the need to continue taking cinchona bark for at least two or three weeks after the malarial fever had abated. Among the other medical topics on which Franklin made acute observations were the heat of blood, deafness, infant mortality, and medical education. Franklin was a shrewd promoter, and he deserves major credit for founding the Pennsylvania Hospital, probably the oldest hospital in the original American colonies still in operation. Dr. Thomas Bond of Philadelphia, who had been trying unsuccessfully to raise funds by popular subscription, was advised to see Franklin. Franklin inveigled the colonial legislature into enacting a bill to match funds raised by private subscription and then used the promise of government money to persuade private donors to contribute.[28] The hospital would have been established eventually, but Franklin greatly speeded the process.

The emphasis given to two laymen in the foregoing paragraphs should not minimize the contributions of a number of first-rate minds in the medical community. Dr. William Douglass, whose opposition to Mather on the inoculation issue has been mentioned, was a dogmatic and assertive Scotsman with a medical degree from Leyden. He was an able individual who wrote an excellent clinical account of a scarlet fever outbreak in Boston in 1735–36. This clear description of the disease is important since it was published twelve years before the famous English physician, Dr. John Fothergill, wrote his classic account of scarlet fever. Douglass also had an active interest in natural history and collected several hundred botanical and mineral specimens in and around Boston.

Douglass was one of four colonial physicians whose work was recognized by the international natural history circle. The second of this group was Cadwallader Colden, who took an M.A. at Edinburgh before the university offered medical training and then headed to London for his medical education. He emigrated to the colonies and settled in New York. Since botanical remedies constituted the major part of materia medica, physicians with intellectual curiosity often tended toward the study of botany. Colden's interest in botany led him to read Linnaeus's *Genera Plantarum*, and he quickly mastered the Linnaean system of plant classification. Subsequently Colden's work in describing and classifying plants in the New World brought him to the attention of the two leading European naturalists, Linnaeus and Gronovius.[29]

Colden practiced medicine only briefly, but he was acutely conscious of the need to raise the status of the profession and constantly urged government support for medical education and research. At this time virtually nothing was known about the great epidemic disorders. Hippocrates in his *Airs, Waters, Places* had stressed the role of environment in disease causation. Since scientific minds in the seventeenth and eighteenth centuries were turning to observation and the collection of statistics, this method was applied to meteorological phenomena. In consequence, physicians and lay observers began keeping exact records of daily changes in temperature, humidity, and so forth in order to correlate them with the rise and fall of particular epidemics. In 1720 Colden published *Account of the Climate and Diseases of New York*, the first of a series of similar works that continued well into the second half of the nineteenth century.

His most important medical work was an essay, written after New York City had suffered a mild yellow fever epidemic, entitled *The Fever Which Prevailed in the City of New York in 1741–42*. He first reviewed the history of yellow fever and then turned to the unsanitary conditions in the city, which he believed were responsible for the disease. He noted that the disorder invariably appeared in the vicinity of docks—where dirt and filth tended to accumulate—and in low-lying areas where the city had built upon swampy ground. He questioned the traditional belief that the high morbidity and mortality among infants and children was due to eating fresh fruit, pointing out that deaths were far fewer among country children who had greater access to fruit. The real cause, he wrote, was the deleterious atmosphere and the unsanitary condition of the city.

Having stated what he believed were the conditions predisposing people to epidemic fevers, Colden then made a series of specific recommendations to the city officials. The city must make arrangements to drain all low-lying damp grounds and see to it that "all the filth and nastiness of the town be emptied into the stream of the river." The deplorable sanitary and drainage conditions, he said, resulted from leaving the responsibility for drainage in the hands of private individuals. The solution was to make the city responsible, "then every one, since it would cost him no more, would be desirous and careful to have his cellar clean and dry, and his nostrils freed from an offensive stench." He stressed the need for conscientious officials, "men of Known industry, and zeal for the welfare of the town." [30] The force of Colden's logic and his prestige as Surveyor-General of the Province and a member of the Governor's Council gave his recommendations real meaning. In May 1744 the Provincial Assembly enacted "A Law to Remove and Prevent Nusances [*sic*] within the City of New York." On the basis of this law, the Common Council of New York City promulgated a sweeping sanitary ordinance and followed up by appropriating funds for cleaning the city. The preamble to the city ordinance stated the principle that was to dominate public health for the next 150 years: "the health of the Inhabitants of any City Does in a Great Measure Depend upon the Purity of the Air of that City and that when the Air of a City is by Noisome Smells Corrupted, Distempers of many kinds are thereby Occasioned." The law established a table of fines for each offense against the sanitary code and divided the revenues between the individual responsible for prosecution and the church wardens.[31] The system worked well up to the time of the Revolution, although its success was more likely due to the tradition of cleanliness among the town's inhabitants.

Colden's thesis was scarcely an original one. A good part of it was borrowed from *De nosiis paludum effluviis*, a classic work published in 1717 by the Italian clinician and epidemiologist, Giovanni Maria Lancisi. Yet Colden obviously kept abreast of the current medical literature, he was receptive to new concepts, and his ideas on sanitation were applied on a relatively large scale. His essay on fever is not only the first significant writing on sanitation in the American colonies but, more important, it bore fruit.

The third of this group of Scottish physicians to make a name for himself in botany was Dr. Alexander Garden of Charleston. Garden, however, was a naturalist first and a physician second, and his major contributions relate to botany and zoology. The fourth of these botanist-physicians was Dr. John Mitchell of Urbana, Virginia. Educated at Edinburgh and Leyden, he settled in Virginia until ill-health forced his return to England in 1746. While in America he wrote several papers on botanical subjects and was well known in the European natural history circle. In England he published his *Map of the British and French Dominions in North America*. This map, which remained the standard work for many years, was used in settling British and French claims in the peace treaty ending the American Revolutionary War.

Mitchell's medical contribution, although indirect, was to have a strong impact upon nineteenth-century medical practice. Following outbreaks of yellow fever in Virginia in 1737 and 1741, he wrote an essay on the disease, which he sent to Benjamin Franklin for presentation to the Society for the Promotion of Useful Knowledge. Many years later this manuscript came to the attention of Dr. Benjamin Rush, who used it in preparing his lectures on medicine. Rush reread the manuscript during the 1793 yellow fever epidemic in Philadelphia and became convinced on the basis of Mitchell's experience that his own therapy had been too mild. The result, as will be seen later, was to be of major consequence to thousands of American practitioners and their patients.

Another Scot interested in botany but who was primarily a physician was Dr. John Lining of Charleston. Lining's best-known work is a description of the yellow fever outbreak in Charleston in 1748, a careful and precise clinical account in which he sought to correlate weather conditions with disease. Lining also deserves credit for his efforts, even if not successful, to investigate physiology. During the summer of 1740, he wrote, "as opportunity served, I weighed myself every hour, second or third hour, through the day, to investigate the differences of the urine and perspiration in the different hours of the day, under different circumstances." [32] Admirable as was his intent, the answers to his research would have to await a vastly improved technology and fundamental breakthroughs in science.

There were other physicians, too, who dabbled in botany — and other botanists who dabbled in medicine. John Bartram, for example, made his name in natural history, but to support himself he had to farm and occasionally practice medicine. Among physicians who concentrated their attention upon medicine was Dr. John Bard, recognized as New York City's leading practitioner before the Revolution. After a private education, he had been apprenticed to Dr. John Kearsley, an irascible English surgeon in Philadelphia. Subsequently Bard moved to New York where he quickly established a fine reputation. He published several excellent papers on medical topics, and along with Dr. Peter Middleton he performed the first dissection of a human for teaching purposes in America. In recognition of his long and active career, he was elected the first president of the Medical Society of the State of New York at its organization in 1788. [33]

John Bard's son, Samuel, continued his father's tradition. After graduation from King's College (Columbia), in 1760 he was sent abroad to study medicine, and he immediately encountered one of the hazards facing colonists who ventured across the Atlantic. His ship was captured by a French privateer, and young Bard spent five months in a French prison until he was released through the efforts of Benjamin Franklin. Undeterred by this experience, Bard studied medicine in London and Edinburgh, acquired an M.D. in the latter city, and returned to join his father in medical practice. He wrote a first-rate paper on diphtheria, a disorder that had become quite common following the pandemic of 1735–40.

Philadelphia produced several excellent physicians, at least two of whom rank with the best in the colonies. Dr. John Redman (1722–1808) was educated in Philadelphia, served an apprenticeship under Dr. John Kearsley, studied at the University of Edinburgh, and took a medical degree from the University of Leyden. He was an able physician but is best known as the preceptor of such outstanding physicians as John Morgan, Benjamin Rush, and Casper Wistar. John Morgan (1735–89), one of the first of these apprentices, far outshone his teacher. After attending a private academy, he spent six years apprenticed to Dr. Redman. During his apprenticeship he enrolled in the College of Philadelphia (University of Pennsylvania) and in 1756 completed both the apprenticeship and his college degree. He promptly joined the Pennsylvania Provincial forces and served as a surgeon until the end of the French and Indian War.

Recognizing the need for additional medical study, Morgan decided to complete his medical education in Europe. As was true of many young colonists going abroad, he headed for Britain and the Continent armed with letters of introduction from Benjamin Franklin. He spent a year studying under the two Hunters, John, the outstanding British surgeon, and his brother William, the leader of British obstetrics. He also came under the influence of the prominent Quaker physician, Dr. John Fothergill. From London, Morgan moved on to spend two years taking an M.D. at the University of Edinburgh. He then embarked on a grand tour of Europe, stopping off in Paris for three months to study medicine before going on to Italy where he made a courtesy visit to the great anatomist Giovanni Morgagni. Before returning to America in 1765, Morgan was elected to membership in several leading medical and intellectual societies in London, Edinburgh, Paris, and Rome. From the standpoint of his American contemporaries, the most signal honor was his membership in the British Royal Philosophical Society. While in London, Morgan, encouraged by Dr. Fothergill, initiated plans to establish a medical school and a medical society on his return to Philadelphia. In both of these projects he succeeded.[34]

Along with Morgan, the other outstanding Philadelphia physician of the late colonial period was William Shippen (1736–1808). Shippen graduated from the College of New Jersey (Princeton) in 1754 and studied medicine under his father, William Shippen, a prominent doctor in his own right. In 1757 the young Shippen sailed for Britain. He spent three years working with Dr. William Hunter and at the same time was fortunate enough to enter the breakfast circle of the Quaker reformer, Dr. John Fothergill. Following the pattern of the better colonial physicians, he completed his medical education by taking an M.D. from Edinburgh and studying briefly in Paris and Montpellier.

Urged on by Fothergill, who gave him a number of anatomical drawings and casts, Shippen returned to Philadelphia where he began offering the first formal anatomy course in the American colonies, in November 1762. Although he used Fothergill's teaching materials, he relied largely upon the dissection of human subjects, a practice that caused considerable popular resentment and on several occasions led to his dissecting rooms' being mobbed. Despite this problem, the course proved successful, and Shippen soon added a course in midwifery for medical students and prospective midwives. With the return of Morgan a medical school was established. Regrettably, Morgan and Shippen became embroiled in a personal controversy that peaked during the Revolutionary War and, as will be seen later, plagued them for the rest of their lives.

One can scarcely leave Philadelphia without some mention of Dr. Thomas Bond (1712–84). A native of Maryland, Bond served an apprenticeship with Dr. Alexander Hamilton of Annapolis and then crossed the Atlantic to study medicine on the Continent. He began practicing in Philadelphia around 1734 and gained a fine reputation as a surgeon and physician. During his lifetime he published two excellent clinical papers, but his chief claim to fame lies in his role as the prime mover in promoting the Pennsylvania Hospital and his long association with it. In 1766 he began giving lectures on clinical medicine in the hospital. Although he was not on the faculty of the newly organized medical school, the students were advised to attend Bond's lectures. Aside from his contributions to medicine, Bond is equally well known for his leadership in founding the American Philosophical Society in 1768.

In addition to those physicians mentioned, many others kept abreast of European developments and promoted professional societies, hospitals, and medical education. An interesting question is precisely why so many physicians dabbled in botany and other areas. Was the demand for their services limited, or did they feel a sense of frustration with their inability to deal with the omnipresent ailments and infections that brought death to so many of their patients? Whatever the case, the eighteenth century saw the better American physicians beginning to make contributions in medicine and the sciences, and becoming aware of their need to join together for professional purposes.

CHAPTER 3

The Medical Profession

T HE HALLMARK of a profession is formal specialized academic training, and, except for theology, professional
training came late in the colonies. In the seventeenth and early eighteenth centuries Leyden was the great center for medical education
in northern Europe, but by the second half of the eighteenth century
Edinburgh and Glasgow were supplanting Leyden, and the London
hospitals were offering excellent clinical and surgical training. Since the
London hospitals did not offer medical degrees, colonists seeking to
further their medical education usually went first to London for one to
three years and then headed to Scotland for a medical degree. The University of Edinburgh alone granted 117 medical degrees to Americans
between 1747 and 1800.[1] Interestingly, the university's medical school
was in a seemingly contradictory position of offering easy mail-order
degrees and at the same time providing the best education for those
students anxious to learn medicine.

Medical Training in the Colonies

In the colonies a medical degree carried prestige, but it was
no guarantee of professional competence. Aside from men who acquired degrees rather than a medical education, individuals with only
a brief tenure at one of the Scottish universities not infrequently assumed the title of doctor on arriving in the colonies. Although there
was no formal teaching of medicine in the colonies until shortly before
the Revolution, two medical degrees were awarded. In 1663 the General Court of Rhode Island conferred a medical degree upon one John

Cranston in the process of licensing him to "administer physicke and practice chirurgery." One section of the act read that Cranston "is by this Court styled doctor of physick and chirurgery." Sixty years later, Yale bestowed a medical degree upon a man named Daniel Turner in return for a gift of books.[2]

The start of formal medical education in America came in 1750 when John Bard and Peter Middleton of New York offered a private course in anatomy. Other physicians who gave lectures in anatomy were Thomas Wood in New Brunswick, New Jersey, in 1752 and William Hunter in Newport, Rhode Island, in 1754 and 1756. The first formal academic work in anatomy was provided by Dr. Samuel Clossy at King's College in 1763, although the school at that time had no medical curriculum. By this date William Shippen and John Morgan in Philadelphia were moving ahead with plans to establish a medical school. Shippen envisaged an independent medical college and thought he was laying the basis for it by offering private courses in anatomy and obstetrics on his return to Philadelphia in 1762. He anticipated that when Morgan returned from Britain with his degree, the two men would jointly establish the college. Morgan, however, disregarded his friend Shippen and pushed ahead with his own plan for organizing a medical school in conjunction with the College of Philadelphia, a course of action that led to bitter enmity between the two men.

Immediately on his return to Philadelphia in 1765, Morgan contacted several of the trustees of the college and proposed that they establish a school of medicine. Impressed by his recommendation, the trustees appointed him professor of medicine and gave him permission to present the May commencement address. This address, "Discourse upon the Institution of Medical Schools in America," marks the high point of Morgan's career. He first criticized the apprenticeship system and excoriated the majority of American physicians, whom he accused of slaughtering their patients through ignorance "and laying whole families desolate." He next pointed to the advantages offered by Philadelphia — skilled physicians, a hospital, a college, and a central location. Turning to medical education, he emphasized that physicians needed to study both liberal arts and science. Reflecting the new European ideas, he declared that medicine was a science and required both clinical observation and physical experiments. Flying in the face of accepted colonial practice, he declared that physicians should not be required to combine medicine, surgery, and compounding drugs, for each of these was a separate profession.[3]

Morgan's appeal was successful, and in 1766 the first colonial medical school was founded. Unfortunately Morgan scarcely mentioned Shippen in connection with the proposed school and sought to take full credit for initiating the project. In addition to embittering relations between the two men, the result was to antagonize Shippen's many friends and in the long run to hurt Morgan's reputation. The first faculty consisted of Morgan, professor of botany and the practice of medicine; Shippen, professor of anatomy; and William Smith, the provost of the college, who gave a course in natural and experimental philosophy. Dr. Thomas Bond, although not officially a member, taught clinical medicine. In 1768 Adam Kuhn was appointed professor of botany and materia medica, and the following year Benjamin Rush joined the faculty as professor of chemistry. Two years after the school opened, the first students graduated. By this time the total enrollment numbered about forty students. Typical of teaching methods down to the end of the nineteenth century, the first chemistry professor simply read back the notes he had taken in William Cullen's classes at the University of Edinburgh.[4]

The example of Philadelphia stirred physicians in New York City into action. The two Bards, John and Samuel, had reservations about their city as a site of medical education. The senior Bard regretted the lack of a hospital, and his son, Samuel, noted that the city had no medical library. Nonetheless, Samuel Bard, along with several other physicians, in 1767 petitioned King's College to follow the path of the College of Philadelphia. In response the King's College trustees established a full medical training program and appointed six professors: Samuel Clossy, professor of anatomy; John Jones, surgery; Peter Middleton, physiology and pathology; James Smith, chemistry and materia medica; John V. B. Tennant, midwifery; and Samuel Bard, medical theory and practice. All of these men had studied abroad, and each achieved some measure of distinction. For example, Bard wrote the first American textbook on obstetrics; Jones served in the Revolution and wrote the first American work on surgery; and Tennant was a member of the Royal Society.[5]

In his inaugural address in 1767, Dr. Middleton briefly surveyed the history of medicine and rejoiced that by opening the school "we may in a great measure prevent the future necessity of long and perilous voyages to Europe, as well as large Remittances of money, which never more returns." At the initial commencement in May 1769 Dr. Bard spoke on the duties of a physician, and his discourse, which was published, is considered the first American tract on medical ethics. His urgent plea for an infirmary or hospital led the provincial governor, Sir Henry Moore, to subscribe £200 toward the project. The graduates of the Columbia and Philadelphia schools received bachelor's degrees in medicine. In 1770 Columbia granted the first doctorate in medicine to Robert Tucker.[6]

Despite troublesome times foreshadowing the approaching revolution, both institutions prospered. Graduates of the two colleges ordinarily received an M.B. degree, which was awarded following two courses of lectures. The two courses, however, were identical, although the students were expected to have served a preceptorship with a practicing physician for at least two years. The doctorate in medicine required a minimum of seven years of medical practice and the completion of a satisfactory thesis. Between 1768 and 1774 the College of Philadelphia awarded twenty-nine M.B. degrees and five M.D.'s. King's College in this same period conferred twelve M.B.'s and two M.D.'s.[7] The outbreak of the Revolutionary War interrupted formal medical education, but both institutions eventually reopened.

Colonial Hospitals

The first hospital built in the British American colonies was constructed in 1612 in Virginia near the falls of the James River. It was described as an eighty-bed structure with lodging "for the sicke and lame, with keepers to attend them for their comfort and recoverie." It is thought to have burned during the Indian uprising of 1622, and, when the Royal government assumed control of Virginia in 1624, no effort was made to replace it. Probably the next colonial hospital was a small military hospital erected in New Amsterdam in 1658.[8] The history of hospitals in the English colonies during the next one hundred years is rather vague, and the claims for priority in the founding of hospitals depend largely upon how one defines a hospital.

Until well into the nineteenth century the line between hospitals and almshouses was not sharply defined. Even institutions originally designed to provide care and treatment for the sick often became filled with the aged poor and chronically ill. Local authorities were always compelled to make some provision for the sick poor, and the standard practice was to employ a physician, either on a yearly basis or as the occasion arose. Since sick strangers and impoverished individuals frequently had no residences, communities were forced to either buy or rent houses for this purpose. By the eighteenth century the larger towns had established almshouses and appointed physicians to serve them. In describing these institutions, the terms "almshouse" and "hospital" were used interchangeably, leading to much of the present confusion.

It is precisely this confusion that lies at the crux of the dispute as to priority between Charity Hospital of New Orleans and the Pennsylvania Hospital. While Charity was founded in 1736, some sixteen years before the Pennsylvania Hospital, the supporters of the latter institution claim that Charity was an almshouse in the early years. Before taking up this question, it will help to glance at the history of hospitals in Louisiana. The French settled in Louisiana around 1699 and established several military hospitals. The Company of the Indies, the French equivalent of the Virginia Company, was quite paternalistic, sending surgeons, apothecaries, midwives, and ample medical supplies to its colony. When a hurricane destroyed the hospital in New Orleans in 1722, a new, larger one was immediately built, one that during the sickly season of 1723 held over eight hundred patients. The company invited the Ursuline Sisters of Rouen to assume control of the hospital, and in 1727 a mother superior and five nuns arrived. They continued to administer the hospital until 1770. This institution, known as the Royal Hospital, received support from the French and Spanish governments until it was closed with the American occupation in 1804.[9]

The Royal Hospital accepted civilian patients in the early days, but, as the colony grew, governing officials objected to the expense. In response, a sailor and boat-builder named Jean Louis willed his entire estate to found a hospital. In 1736 a small temporary building was acquired for patients while a new brick hospital was under construction. During the ensuing years the hospital was rebuilt several times, eventually becoming the first state-operated hospital in the United States. This hospital was given various names, but at all times it was a "charity" hospital. Eventually the name Charity Hospital became official.[10]

Those who argue that the Pennsylvania Hospital is the oldest existing hospital in the United States maintain that Charity was more of an almshouse than a hospital. The truth is that all hospitals in the eighteenth century were designed to care for sick strangers and the poor. It is true that Charity held many chronically sick poor, but it always provided medical care for those who could not be treated in their homes. It is well to bear in mind that as late as 1900 respectable people expected to be treated in their own homes and to die in their own beds. While almshouses were designed to shelter the poor, they also provided care for the sick. For example, the Philadelphia Almshouse, founded in 1729, ultimately became the Philadelphia Hospital, the forerunner of the Philadelphia General Hospital (Blockley Division). Dr. Robert J. Hunter, historian of the hospital, argues that the almshouse was "a hospital in every sense . . . an institution where people with many kinds of illness were receiving medical care."[11] New York City and Charleston established similar almshouses in 1736.[12] These almshouses were primarily welfare institutions and provided medical care only incidentally to their main purpose.

In addition to almshouses, another precursor of modern hospitals was the pesthouse, lazar, or lazaretto. These institutions, which date far back, were designed to protect the public by isolating infectious disease cases rather than to help the patient. At least as early as 1702 Boston was removing smallpox patients to the pesthouse. In 1717 Massachusetts established a pesthouse on Spectacle Island to isolate "infectious persons" arriving by sea. In 1738 a pesthouse was established on Bedloe's Island in New York harbor. Subsequently the city council appointed John Brown, a "Laborer," as "Overseer and Manager."[13]

As mentioned earlier, it is likely that the oldest institution in the thirteen original colonies still in existence today is the Pennsylvania Hospital. This was the one founded through the joint efforts of Dr. Thomas Bond and Benjamin Franklin. Unlike the almshouses, which admitted all deserving poor, the hospital stipulated first that no patients should be admitted "whose Cases are judg'd incurable, Lunaticks excepted; nor any whose Cases do not require the particular Conveniences of an Hospital." A second regulation forbade the admission of persons with infectious diseases unless special rooms were provided for them, and another stated that sick women could not bring their children into the hospital with them. After stating the procedures by which the poor would be admitted, the regulations added that if there was room to spare, the managers of the hospital could admit private patients "at such reasonable Rates as they can agree to." While caring for private patients was secondary to the main purpose of the hospital, this is the first instance where provision was made for their admission.[14]

The regulations also throw light on early hospital conditions. Patients were forbidden to "swear, curse, get drunk, behave rudely or indecently, on Pain of Expulsion after the first Admonition." They were also enjoined from playing cards, dice, or other games, or from begging. Ambulatory patients were expected to assist in nursing, washing, cleaning, "and such other Services as the Matron shall require." [15]

In order to gain legislative support for the hospital, Franklin had persuaded three physicians, Lloyd Zachary, Thomas Bond, and Phineas Bond, to offer gratuitous service for three years. Once the precedent of free service was established, the practice continued. Aside from gaining a measure of prestige, the hospital physicians were allowed to bring apprentices or students into the hospital for clinical training at a charge of one English guinea per year. [16]

During the first fourteen months the hospital admitted 64 patients, of whom 32 were listed as cured, 4 were discharged after being helped, 2 left voluntarily, 6 were removed by their friends, 5 died, 5 were discharged as incurable, and 1 was dismissed for "irregular Behavior." The largest category of patients were the 37 admitted with "Ulcers, with Caries &c.," and the second largest number of admissions were "Lunatics." Of the 18 mentally ill patients admitted, 2 were discharged as cured and 3 as improved. Only 2 patients were admitted with "fevers," but the refusal to accept individuals with infectious disorders probably accounts for this small number. Among the other categories of patients were those with "Dropsies," "Scorbutick" (scurvy) and "scrophulous Diseases," "Ague," "Falling Sickness," "Consumption" (pulmonary tuberculosis), "Flux" (dysentery), and cancer. [17]

The success of the Pennsylvania Hospital encouraged the medical society in New York to found a similar institution. The society's physicians recognized that an institution designed exclusively for treating the sick would provide clinical training for apprentices and students, while responsible citizens saw it as a means for providing good medical care. The founding of King's College Medical School and Dr. Bard's stirring appeal in 1769 provided the needed impetus. Led by Bard and other physicians, the Society of the Hospital in the City of New-York was organized and granted a charter. The sum of £800 was raised by private subscription, and the provincial legislature was persuaded to grant an annual allowance of £800 annually for twenty years. Construction of the hospital began in 1773, but it was destroyed by fire shortly before it was completed. The legislature quickly appropriated another £4,000 and construction began anew. The time was scarcely propitious, however, for the Revolutionary War began before the building was finished. Wartime and postwar problems created a succession of problems, and it was 1791 before the New York Hospital officially opened.[18]

Before leaving the subject, brief mention should be made of inoculation hospitals. These, in effect, were much-improved versions of the pesthouses and arose from a recognition that persons undergoing variolation needed medical attention and, more important, were a potential threat to the community. A number of these hospitals were opened by private physicians or "inoculators" who used their own homes or other buildings. In times of smallpox epidemics provincial governments or cities occasionally opened inoculation hospitals. For example, during a smallpox outbreak in 1764 the province of Massachusetts opened two of them. By the time of the Revolution inoculation hospitals were scattered throughout the colonies. Aside from inoculation hospitals, pesthouses, and almshouses, only two hospitals, the Pennsylvania Hospital and Charity Hospital in New Orleans, were operating at the end of the colonial period.

Medical Licensure

The principle of regulating the practice of medicine is an old one, dating at least as far back as the Code of Hammurabi, nearly two millennia before Christ. In late medieval England, since education was in the hands of the church, the licensing of physicians came under ecclesiastical jurisdiction. During the Renaissance, the regulation of doctors gradually shifted to the universities and to the early professional guilds, such as the Royal College of Physicians and the various "Companies" of surgeons and apothecaries. The colonists were familiar with the principle of licensure, but it was not until the eighteenth century when colonial America began to mirror the urban culture of England that the first call for the licensing of medical practitioners was sounded. A few tentative steps had been taken in the seventeenth century, but there is no evidence that the early measures were enforced.

The American apprenticeship system, which emphasized common sense and sound practical experience, may well have provided a better basis for learning medicine in the eighteenth century than years of formal academic study and reading. American medical practice benefited from the elimination of the distinction between physicians and surgeons and the greater reliance on clinical training. In contrast, university-trained physicians were far better versed in the subtle philosophical distinctions between various medical theories than in clinical medicine. Certainly many colonials, laypeople and practitioners alike, believed this. An intelligent and conscientious individual trained under an able physician was more likely to make a good doctor than a mediocre person with the best of medical degrees, or even a university graduate whose mind tended to revel in philosophical abstractions. All one can say is that an intelligent person will usually do well, but the better the training the greater will be his or her professional skill.

The assumption that empirically trained colonial physicians were at least as good as their university-trained colleagues was strengthened by the fact that too many physicians were guilty of adhering to a particular medical theory regardless of its consequences to their patients. Fortunately only a few doctors were like the eighteenth-century Scottish physician reputed to have said that he was not going to practice unphilosophical medicine merely because his patients died. The question arises as to the quality of those medical graduates who migrated to the colonies. Some of them, as we have seen, were able individuals, but it is likely that the best graduates had little incentive to migrate, and in any case they probably preferred to stay close to the centers of medical learning.

One of the wisest of American medical historians, Richard H. Shryock, raised an important question about the colonial apprenticeship system. Why, he asked, if practical training was so effective, were so many of the better practitioners calling for the regulation of medical practice and the establishment of medical schools?[19] Without exception colonial physicians who had studied abroad and were in a position to make a comparative judgment of colonial medical practice were usually the harshest in their criticism of colonial doctors. Men such as William Douglass, John Morgan, William Shippen, Peter Middleton, and Samuel Bard all favored formal education and licensing requirements for physicians.

The first eighteenth-century law relating to physicians was more concerned with protecting patients than raising the caliber of medical care. The Virginia legislature in 1736 enacted a law specifying charges for medical services. A standard fee was set for visits in town, and fees based on mileage were established for out-of-town calls. Significantly, in light of the earlier discussion, university-trained physicians were allowed to charge twice the fees established for apprentice-trained doctors. This Virginia measure may be called the first "truth-in-advertising law," since it required physicians to specify the drugs prescribed on their bills. The law was allowed to lapse at the end of two years, and, although in the succeeding years three more bills to regulate medical fees were introduced, none of them passed.[20]

In New York the first law regulating medicine applied only to midwives. A 1739 municipal ordinance required all midwives to "take the Oath of a Midwife," one that specified how they should conduct themselves. Since the law said nothing about examinations, the concern of the legislators evidently was with moral and ethical conduct rather than medical qualifications. One section of the law showed that obstetrics was still clearly in the woman's domain, since the oath included a vow not to "open any mystery appertaining to your Office, in the presence of any Man, unless Necessity . . . constrain you to do so."[21]

Agitation to license physicians began in New York in the 1750s. A newspaper correspondent in 1753 pointed out that some type of regulation was necessary to prevent "the dismal havock made by quacks and pretenders." Urged on by prominent physicians and with the help of Cadwallader Colden, at that time a member of the Governor's Council, in 1760 the Provincial Assembly passed the first colonial medical licensure law.[22] The measure was well written, since it required that applicants for a medical license be examined by government officials assisted by reputable physicians. Despite the soundness of the law, little effort was made to enforce it. No record appears of anyone convicted of practicing medicine without a license, and, judging by the newspapers in the ensuing years, quacks and charlatans continued to abound in New York City.

Twelve years later, in 1772, the New Jersey Medical Society secured the enactment of a medical licensure law on a provincewide basis. The provisions of the law closely followed those of the 1760 New York City measure, and it is quite likely that the end results were the same. In New Jersey as in New York, there is no evidence to show that the law was enforced. Aside from one or two other abortive attempts to secure medical regulation (for example, a licensing bill was defeated in South Carolina in 1765), nothing further was accomplished in the colonial period, and the advent of the Revolution meant that medical licensing would have to await more orderly times.

Medical Societies

One of the first signs of an emerging professional consciousness is the development of professional organizations. As already indicated, among colonial physicians this awareness developed around the mid-eighteenth century, although several medical societies existed briefly before this time. At least three were established in Boston, all of them through the initiative of Dr. William Douglass. The first two met in a desultory fashion, but the Medical Society of Boston, organized in response to the great "Throat Distemper" (diphtheria and scarlet fever) epidemic that swept through New England beginning in 1735, survived for almost twenty years. Occasional references in the Boston *Weekly News-Letter* furnish the little information known about the society. Between 1755 and 1781 no less than ten other societies were established in Massachusetts, culminating in the founding of the Massachusetts Medical Society in 1781.[23]

New Yorkers may have formed a medical society, for a notebook of John Bard mentions in 1749 delivering a medical essay before the Weekly Society of Gentlemen of New York. James J. Walsh, medical historian of New York, states that about this same time a group known as the Physical Society was comprised largely of physicians.[24] Since physicians always constituted a substantial part of membership in scientific societies, it is likely that neither of these organizations was exclusively medical.

It was not intellectual companionship that motivated South Carolina's physicians to organize. In June 1755 the physicians in Charleston, South Carolina, met under the leadership of Dr. John Moultrie in order to promote "the better Support of the Dignity, the Privileges, and Emoluments of their Humane Art." The announcement in the *South Carolina Gazette* asserted that physicians were summoned to the homes of patients "under the greatest Inclemencies of the Weather," but that they were "often slowly and seldom sufficiently paid." In a commentary upon the practice of medicine, the statement read that the physicians did not "think the Payment of an Apothecary's Bill a sufficient Reward to him who acts in the three distinct Offices of Physic, Surgery, and Pharmacy." In view of the foregoing, the members of the society had resolved to make no further visits unless they received a reasonable fee, payable on each visit.[25]

This bold proclamation stimulated a series of letters to the newspapers, some satirical and others highly derogatory of the profession. The storm of outrage that greeted the physicians' statement apparently had its effect, for nothing further was heard of either the medical organization or its proposals. The complaints of the practitioners were undoubtedly justified, but part of the problem lay in the excessive number of practitioners in the city. When Benjamin Rush sounded out Dr. Lionel Chalmers in 1772 about coming to Charleston to practice medicine, Chalmers discouraged him. "In this town," he wrote, "there may be 11,000 to 12,000 persons . . . and we have between 30 and 40 persons who practice Physick, most of whom, tis true, have not much to do. . . ."[26]

Surprisingly, Philadelphia, which was the scientific center in the later colonial period and the home of the first medical school, never had a medical association of any consequence before the Revolution. The only one was a short-lived group, the Medical Society of Philadelphia, organized largely by Dr. John Morgan in 1767. By this date Morgan had already antagonized many of the older physicians by his brashness, and he compounded his error by not including them among the founding members. To make matters worse, he did not invite the two Shippens to join. In consequence the society survived until 1768 when its twelve members merged with the American Society, one of Philadelphia's two scientific organizations, and became the American Society's medical committee.[27] The best physicians in Philadelphia, who would normally have been organizing a medical society, were too active in general scientific pursuits to concentrate upon medicine. For example, physicians constituted a high percentage of the membership of the American Philosophical Society, the second scientific association. Thus the very activity and interest in scientific inquiry in Philadelphia mitigated against the development of a strong medical organization in these years.

The most effective medical organization in the colonial period was the New Jersey Medical Society, founded in New Brunswick in 1766. It holds the distinction of being the only colonial medical society to survive the Revolution. In 1790 it was incorporated as the Medical Society of New Jersey, a name it holds today. In their initial statement the fourteen founding members spoke of the "low State of Medicine in New Jersey" and dedicated themselves to discouraging "quacks, mountebanks, imposters or other ignorant pretenders of medicine." The fierce competition from quacks, irregulars, and poorly trained practitioners in these years kept medical fees very low, and, as was true of virtually all newly organized medical societies, the first action of the New Jersey group was to draw up "A Table of Fees and Rates."[28]

The fee bill, as was the case in Charleston, brought outraged protests, and four months later the society rescinded the requirement that members adhere to it. While the fee bill did not help the financial status of the physicians, it does give us an insight into medical practice. For one or two visits in town the physicians, like the English apothecaries, charged only for the medicines administered. For daily visits over a long period of time, the fee was ten shillings per week. The charge for out-of-town visits was based upon the distance traveled. As noted earlier, the first president of the society was a minister-physician and the membership included several other ministers. Their inclusion in the medical society speaks well for the status of the minister-physician as late as 1766. Although the society failed in its aim to raise medical fees, it did succeed in promoting a licensure law.[29]

In Connecticut two local societies were organized in the 1760s. A small group of physicians in Norwich in 1763 considered requesting authority to license physicians but decided the time was not ripe. Some thirty physicians in Litchfield County were more adventurous. They organized in the town of Sharon in 1767, and two years later petitioned the legislature for licensing authority. The effort was fruitless, for the newspapers and public arose in protest, accusing the doctors of seeking a monopoly. Sharon lies close to the borders of New York and Massachusetts, and its members included physicians from both provinces, giving the Sharon Medical Society the distinction of being the only interprovincial medical association.[30]

The Public Image of the Physician

A great deal of ambivalence has always existed in the public mind with respect to the medical profession. The same individuals who may denounce the profession collectively will not infrequently swear by their own physicians. One can find this same ambivalence in the colonial period, but the suspicion of physicians and medicine in general tended to increase as the years wore on. Historians generally agree that the caliber of physicians in the early years was reasonably high, but that as it became clear that medicine was no royal road to success, the number and quality of physicians declined. Throughout the seventeenth century physicians were often in short supply, and it was common for towns to ask colonial governors to recruit doctors to provide medical care and train apprentices. When the local physician died in Portsmouth, New Hampshire, the selectman sought to induce a physician to settle in the town by offering a servant, food, candles, and fees for medical services to the poor.[31]

Almost one-third of the physicians who practiced in seventeenth-century Massachusetts had migrated to the colony. In the eighteenth century the percentage of immigrant physicians fell to 3.9 percent. In consequence medical practice fell into the hands of colonial doctors, most of whom had no formal training.[32] Joining the apprentice-trained physicians were a multiplying number of folk doctors, bonesetters, herbalists, and a variety of quacks. The preface to the 1760 medical licensure law in New York begins: "Whereas many ignorant and unskilful persons in Physic and Surgery . . . do take upon themselves to administer physick, and practice surgery . . . to the endangering of the lives and limbs of their patients. . . ." A few years later Dr. Peter Middleton deplored the presence of so many quacks and empirics, and wondered why medicine "should be the receptacle and resource for the refuse of every other trade and employment."[33] Possibly more significant than the quantity of physicians was the widespread skepticism of medical theories and the drastic measures employed by some of even the best-trained practitioners. In a day when medical degrees were earned largely through attending lectures and reading, any educated individual could acquire some knowledge of medicine and be in a position to pass judgment upon his physician. While intelligent physicians used discretion in applying various forms of therapy, too many medical graduates never questioned the precepts they had learned. To compound the situation, public disagreements among physicians over the cause, nature, and cure of diseases only served to increase public skepticism.

Criticism of the medical profession fell into two categories. First were the denunciations of incompetent practitioners by their better-educated colleagues. Dr. William Douglass's comments on the profession in Boston, for example, or those of Dr. Middleton, mentioned above, were typical. The second were the often bitter comments of laymen. John Oldmixon wrote that the Virginians "have but few Doctors among them, and they reckon it among their Blessings, fancying the

Number of their Diseases would increase with that of their Physicians."
When John Watts was asked about the possibility of a medical lecture-
ship in New York in 1764, he wrote that there was little hope, explaining, "we have so many of the Faculty already destroying his Majestys
good Subjects that in the humor people are, they had rather one half
were hanged . . . than breed up a New Swarm."[34] Colonial newspapers
carried frequent stories of individuals dying as a result of medical treatment, or poems and stories satirizing the medical profession. Suspicion
of the medical profession, however, was in no sense unique. Even the
ministry was beginning to lose its status by the opening of the eighteenth century, and for the next two hundred years Americans had little
regard for any profession. William Byrd in 1706 expressed a widespread
view when he described New Jersey as "a Place free from those 3 great
Scourges of Mankind, Priests, Lawyers, and Physicians."[35]

Despite strong competition, once a physician was established in a
middle- or upper-class practice, his financial and social position was
usually satisfactory. This, however, ordinarily presupposed that he had
a well-to-do family or excellent medical connections. The economics of
medicine were undoubtedly one of the factors that drove many physicians into becoming planters, merchants, government officials, and,
occasionally, ministers. The average physician usually had to supplement his income by farming or operating a small business.

Since dissatisfied patients are most likely to make public their complaints, the physician-patient relationship was probably better than the
tirades against the medical profession would indicate. Despite public
criticisms of the profession, the services of physicians were always in
demand, and the majority of patients had faith in their doctor. In the
first place, although most medical disorders are self-limiting, patients
and physicians alike tended to assume that the cure was brought about
by the treatment. In the second, many of the drugs administered by
physicians, such as cinchona bark (quinine), digitalis, opium, and a host
of emetics and cathartics, were effective. The following description of a
late eighteenth-century physician may be somewhat romanticized, yet
it does help to counteract the many diatribes against the medical profession: "He also wears a full suit of a rich brown color, with cambric
ruffles, silk stockings, and gold buckles at this knees and shoes. His is
a small wig, or hair, curled and powdered at the sides, with a black silk
bag behind, a three cornered hat, and a gold-headed cane. As he picks

his way, with quick, but careful steps, through the muddy streets, his hat is completely off at the meeting of every townsman, and every child in his particular case. . . ." [36]

William Douglass, who was so scornful of his fellow practitioners in Boston, nonetheless wrote that he could "live handsomely here by the incomes from my practice." He classified his patients into four categories: families who paid him an annual fee; occasional patients needing immediate help; almshouse or free patients; and native New Englanders from whom he had difficulty collecting fees. [37] His criticism of the New England patients was not without some validity, since Americans, at least until the twentieth century, have generally been reluctant to pay medical fees.

Another indication of respect were the many physicians who held high positions in civic and provincial governments. In this connection, the historian Whitfield Bell raises an interesting point. Why was it that with a few exceptions, most notably Cadwallader Colden in New York, such physicians took so little interest in public health or made so few efforts to secure medical licensure laws? [38] The most likely answer is that the climate of opinion in the colonies was scarcely conducive to any form of government regulation except in emergency situations. Quarantine and isolation measures were accepted when epidemics threatened, but in normal times they received short shrift. And with the public doubtful about all professions, and medicine in particular, there was little chance for any professional group to determine public policy or to gain the right to regulate either its practice or its practitioners.

The relationship between male physicians and their female patients is always a delicate one, and the charges and countercharges in court records show that colonial physicians had at least their share of moral problems. A North Carolina practitioner and ordained minister was rumored to have "poysoned a man [in order] to lye with his wife." He brought suit for character defamation, and, since he continued to practice, the suit must have been successful. In 1736 a widow sued a neighbor for saying she "had often lain & coppulated with" her physician. Another Carolina physician sued a libeler who had accused him of impregnating a black slave. [39] The court records and the newspapers report many such cases, but one can only assume that medical practitioners, then as now, reflected the general level of morality.

One last point should be mentioned. For most colonial doctors, medicine was simply a means of livelihood, more of a trade than a profession. As a result, they felt no particular obligation to provide free care for the poor. No dispensaries or clinics existed, and, although individual physicians undoubtedly did some charity work, it was not the general rule. The deserving poor who received medical care did so at the expense of the township or community. The occasional newspaper obituaries stating that a deceased physician had rendered help to the poor implies that this conduct was not typical.

In summary, many physicians were respected and affluent members of their community, but this respect arose from their social position and personal qualities rather than their status as physicians. The majority of doctors had no formal training and were poorly paid. At least until the mid-eighteenth century they had little professional consciousness and held only a limited concept of professional ethics or responsibilities. By the Revolution the situation was beginning to change, but the road ahead was still a long one. The public in the eighteenth century accepted physicians on these terms; they liked and respected individual doctors, but they were suspicious of medical theories and practices and had serious reservations about the profession as a whole.

CHAPTER 4

Medicine in the Revolutionary Years

THE PANOPLY AND ACCOUTREMENTS of war — brilliant uniforms, colorful flags, bands, and marching men — and the courageous actions of individuals and armies have always made wars a subject of fascination to readers. The words glory, valor, and victory carry a far more heroic connotation than the words disease, casualties, and death, which explains why millions of words have been written about wars, but only a small fraction of this number has been devoted to describing the medical and health aspects of soldiering. Accounts of the American Revolution are no exception. Of all the journals kept by participants, not one of them deals more than cursorily with military medicine. Ironically, even the physicians and surgeons who recorded their experiences were more intrigued by marching and battles than with their aftermath. Possibly the most complete journal written by a physician was that of Dr. James Thacher of Massachusetts, but Thacher too wrote primarily of his military, rather than medical, experiences. Of the four men who served as medical directors of the Continental forces, only Dr. John Morgan, who sought to vindicate himself from the charges that led to his dismissal, wrote anything about his medical work. Fortunately, despite the paucity of medical writings and the lack of medical journals, we can glean enough from the wide variety of historical sources relating to the Revolution to draw a reasonably accurate picture.

Altogether approximately fourteen hundred physicians and surgeons enrolled in the American armies during the Revolution, but many served in a purely military capacity. In addition to their role in the war, physicians also were active in the events leading to the outbreak of hostilities. The first Provincial Congress of Massachusetts, for example, included no less than twenty-one doctors. One of them, Joseph Warren, helped spread the alarm to Lexington and Concord, and another, Benjamin Church, was appointed the first medical director of the Continental army. Five physicians, Josiah Bartlett and Matthew Thornton from New Hampshire, Oliver Wolcott from Connecticut, Benjamin Rush from Pennsylvania, and Lyman Hall from Georgia, signed the Declaration of Independence.[1] Several others achieved high military rank, including Arthur St. Clair and James Wilkerson, both of whom subsequently served as commander-in-chief of the army, and Dr. John Thomas, major general and commander of the Northern Army of 1777. As might be expected in a time of divided loyalties, many physicians remained loyal to Great Britain and others sought to maintain a measure of neutrality.

The overall picture of army medicine is one of general confusion, since the colonials had neither an effective central government nor a national army at the outset. The armies commanded by Washington and his officers consisted of the Continentals, or regulars, and the colonial militia, the latter usually drawn from the particular area of conflict. During the first years the war was fought largely in New England and the middle colonies and during the later years in the South. At first the provincial governments provided some elementary medical services for their militia. Subsequently the Continental Congress created its own army and medical department and began to superimpose a limited central authority over the provincial forces. This latter proved difficult, and it was not until 1781 that the Continental Medical Department was able to extend its medical jurisdiction over the southern colonies. To complicate matters, a sharp conflict immediately developed between the Medical Department of the Continental army and the regimental surgeons. The militia regiments had their own surgeons, few of whom had any experience with military injuries or diseases, and to make matters worse, many were political appointees.

The health, medical care, and welfare of the troops depended upon a number of factors: the ability of the commanding officers; the quality of the regimental surgeons and general hospitals; the availability of food, clothing, and medical supplies; and the willingness of Congress or the provincial legislatures to provide adequate appropriations. A weakness in any one of these areas could and did cause a great deal of unnecessary suffering. The ration prescribed for the soldiers was generous for its day. Each man in the Massachusetts forces was supposed to receive a daily allotment of a half-pound of salt beef, a half-pound of pork, a pound of bread, and one gill (a half-pint) of rice, peas, or other "equivalent." An additional weekly allowance of six ounces of butter, a half-pint of vinegar, and one-sixth pound of soap was also provided. This ration could be replaced with a weekly ration of seven pounds each of fresh beef and flour, when it was available. A similar ration was subsequently prescribed for the Continental army. Unfortunately, the lack of trained cooks and the unsanitary conditions under which the food was prepared negated much of the value of this diet. Furthermore, wartime inflation, inadequate appropriations, and other factors often drastically reduced the available food supply.[2] The rapid movement of troops as the balance of war shifted placed enormous strains on the local economy, and inadequate transportation compounded the problem. One hospital might be desperately short while ample supplies were available only fifty or a hundred miles away. Repeatedly hospitals had to be evacuated as the battle lines surged back and forth, adding to the confusion and further complicating supply problems.

As might be expected, the quality of medical care varied widely from region to region. The multiplicity of forces in the field, the short-term enlistments, and the amorphous medical organization makes it almost impossible to know the exact number of sick, wounded, and dead. Throughout the war years, thousands of soldiers furloughed because of sickness or injuries never returned. How many of these subsequently died will never be known. The vicissitudes of battles and campaigns also add to the difficulties of ascertaining exact figures. Disastrous defeats so scattered some forces that one can only estimate the number of dead, wounded, and deserted.

Notwithstanding these difficulties, it is possible to come up with a reasonable estimate of casualty rates. Louis C. Duncan, a military historian, has estimated that during 1776 the American forces consisted of 47,000 Continental troops, whose enlistment was for one year, and 27,000 militia, who had volunteered for terms ranging from a few days to several months or more. Of this total, about 1,000 were killed in battle or died from their injuries, 1,200 suffered wounds, 6,000 were taken prisoner, 10,000 died from disease, and several thousand either deserted or simply disappeared. Army records for August of the following year show that about 26 percent of Washington's forces maneuvering around Philadelphia were sick. Dr. James Thacher, who participated in the fighting from Breed's Hill to Yorktown, estimated the total American deaths during the entire war at 70,000, roughly 10,000 per year for the seven years of military activities, 1775–81. Duncan considers this figure reasonable, but he doubts that it includes the thousands of sick who simply went home and for whom we have no records.[3]

The most exhaustive study of casualties during the Revolutionary War was undertaken by Howard H. Peckham of the University of Michigan with the help of his graduate students and research assistants. He estimated the probable deaths from 1775 to 1783 at 25,324. Of these 6,824 were killed in battle, an estimated 10,000 died in camp, and approximately 8,500 died in prisons. His statistics show that the Revolutionary War was second only to the Civil War in terms of deaths in relation to the total population, and that the ratio of deaths to the number of men who bore arms was almost as high.[4]

Every observer agrees that the ratio of sick to battle casualties was very high. Dr. James Tilton, a Delaware physician who later became surgeon general of the army, declared that "we lost not less than from ten to twenty of camp diseases for one by weapons of the enemy."[5] Most other contemporary estimates place the figure closer to nine to one — approximately nine deaths from sickness for each one resulting from battle action. American casualties were higher than those for the British. The British troops, however, were veterans whose enlistment period was twenty years. Most of them had already encountered and survived the main camp diseases, and they were better disciplined and backed by a more effective medical service.

The major disorders affecting the American forces were smallpox, dysentery, respiratory complaints, malaria, and the so-called camp fevers, probably typhus and typhoid. Smallpox was always a serious threat in the colonies, but the long years of war at the midcentury and the more general use of smallpox inoculation tended to make it both more familiar and less dangerous. Even so, the mobilization of thousands of young men, many from relatively isolated areas, led to widespread outbreaks of smallpox and other diseases. In June 1776, John Adams wrote from Philadelphia almost in despair: "The small pox! the small pox! What shall we do with it? I could almost wish that an inoculating hospital was opened in every town in New-England."

The disease was a constant factor in the early military actions and well may have been decisive in the unsuccessful attempt to capture Quebec in the winter and spring of 1775–76. When the American forces were attempting to regroup in June 1776, General John Sullivan reported to General Washington: "There are some regiments all down with the small-pox—not a single man fit for duty," and a day later Benedict Arnold reported that half of his forces were sick, "mostly with the small-pox." [6] The two American armies converging on Quebec were forced to make long, hard marches through the wilderness in bitter weather and on limited rations. These difficulties might have been surmounted, but the widespread dysentery and smallpox virtually precluded any chance for victory. Fortunately, after the first two years most of the soldiers had either survived smallpox or been inoculated. Henceforth, although flaring up on occasions, smallpox was no longer a major problem.

In addition to smallpox, the chief diseases afflicting Washington's forces besieging Boston in the fall of 1775 and those of General Gates before Ticonderoga in the summer of 1776 were "bilious, remitting and intermitting fevers with some of the putrid kind; dysenteries, diarrhoeas, with rheumatick complaints." The remitting and intermitting fevers were undoubtedly malaria, and the bilious and putrid fevers were most likely typhoid and typhus. Typhus has never been a serious problem in the United States, but it was probably responsible for a good share of the "putrid" camp fevers. Typhoid, which arrived with the early settlers and exacted a steady toll from the American population until well into the twentieth century, is another likely suspect. Malaria troubled soldiers in all sectors, but it was present in its most acute form in the southern colonies. Northerners campaigning in the South were particularly susceptible, although the fever represented a hazard to all men. As early as 1776 Congress ordered its medical committee to send three hundred pounds of Peruvian bark (cinchona) to the Southern Department. During the siege of Yorktown, according to Thacher, the New England soldiers in particular suffered heavily from malaria.[7]

Dysentery has been a concomitant of every military campaign, and invariably its incidence has been highest at the outset of hostilities. The explanation is that the incidence of dysentery correlates closely with discipline and the effectiveness of sanitary regulations. The troops gathered around Boston in the first years of the war were notorious for urinating and defecating in the areas surrounding their camps, leading Washington to comment that the New Englanders were "an exceedingly dirty and nasty people."[8] In this respect the New Englanders were no worse than any other soldiers. Poorly disciplined troops neither build adequate latrines and sanitary facilities nor use the available ones, with the result that in short order they contaminate their water supply. The famous English army surgeon Sir John Pringle (1707–82) had stressed the necessity for providing proper sanitary facilities and strictly enforcing their use, but the lesson has had to be relearned in every war since. Discipline was a major problem in the colonial armies, and few officers recognized the value of camp hygiene. The more able ones learned from bitter experience, but progress was slow. Although the incidence of enteric diseases dropped off slightly as the fighting continued, the rapid turnover in the American forces brought about by short-term enlistments meant that diarrheas and dysenteries were a constant factor in reducing the effectiveness of colonial troops.

The extent to which disease rather than battle wounds was a major source of casualties is clearly shown by the hospital reports. For example, during March 1780 a military hospital in South Carolina reported 302 admissions. Of these, only 12 patients had gunshot wounds; the rest were admitted for a wide range of medical complaints, with enteric disorders, typhoid, malaria, and rheumatic complaints leading the list.[9] The constant shortage of supplies in the colonial armies meant that malnutrition and exposure were significant factors in the health of troops. An inadequate diet undoubtedly accounts for much of the diarrheas, and lack of adequate clothing and shelter help to explain the relatively large number of rheumatic complaints.

The history of the organization of American medical services from the opening of hostilities to the end of the war presents a confusing picture. The province of Massachusetts was the first governing body to take firm and definite action to raise troops and to provide for their medical care. In February 1775 the provincial legislature appointed Drs. Joseph Warren and Benjamin Church to study the medical needs of the Massachusetts militia, and the following month it voted funds for medical supplies and hospitals. When it became apparent that many regimental surgeons were not qualified, the Massachusetts Committee on Public Safety appointed an eight-man medical committee to examine them.[10] This action, by weeding out the worst of the surgeons, may help to account for the relatively good health of the New England troops compared to those from the middle and southern colonies.

In May 1775 the Second Continental Congress assumed charge of the colonial militia besieging the British force in Boston, but it was not until July 27 that Congress resolved to create "an Hospital" (hospital system or medical department). This Medical Department was headed by a Director General and Chief Physician at a salary of four dollars per day. The staff consisted of 4 surgeons, 1 apothecary, 20 surgeon's mates, 1 clerk, 2 storekeepers, and 1 nurse for every 10 sick men.[11] Since Massachusetts was the mainstay of the colonial forces, the position of director fell to Dr. Benjamin Church, a prominent Boston physician and active patriot. Church and his successors faced an almost impossible task. The medical staff had no familiarity with military medicine and only limited surgical experience, drugs and medical supplies were in chronically short supply, and the relationship between the regimental surgeons and the Medical Department was never clearly established. As the drug shortages became more evident, in September 1775 Congress established a Medical Committee to deal with the problem. This congressional committee and its successors gradually assumed more authority over the Medical Department, determining such matters as personnel, internal disputes, and inoculation policies.

A basic problem confronting the Medical Department was the failure of Congress and the provincial legislatures to appropriate sufficient funds for personnel, equipment, and supplies. Military commanders and legislators have traditionally underestimated the needs of sick and wounded soldiers, at least for the first year or so of wars. Even Washington did not immediately realize the value of medical services. As late as January 1777 he marched his army from Trenton to Princeton without taking a single surgeon or telling his medical officers of the move.[12]

On assuming charge, Director Church's first action was to take control over the thirty-odd hospitals located in private homes and miscellaneous buildings. He promptly began consolidating these hospitals into what was termed the General Hospital and ordered the closing of regimental hospitals. The regimental surgeons resented this infringement on their authority and took their complaints to Congress. In the meantime Church was desperately trying to build a competent staff, standardize procedures, systematize records, and find much-needed medical and hospital supplies. As criticism of Church's work mounted, Washington ordered an investigation, but before its work was completed Church was discovered to have been in treasonous correspondence with a British officer. A letter he entrusted to his mistress to pass on to the British was intercepted and his career came to an abrupt end. He was dismissed from his post and jailed, but neither the Articles of the Continental army nor the Continental Congress included provision for dealing with treason. John Adams wrote in disgust that no one knew what to do with Church, since there were neither laws nor courts to try him. The problem was solved when Church's health failed, and he was allowed to sail for the West Indies. In a tragic finale to his life, the ship was lost at sea with all hands.[13]

On October 16, 1775, Congress selected Dr. John Morgan as the new medical director. Morgan was able, energetic, and well qualified, but personality problems helped bring about his downfall. On assuming his duties he found virtually no records of the number of patients in hospitals and a deplorable shortage of supplies. The department had only a handful of medicines, two hundred bandages, almost no surgical instruments, and scarcely any blankets. Morgan immediately began scouring the countryside for supplies and appealing to private individuals and local and provincial governments for help. By this means he managed to acquire limited supplies for the Medical Department staff, but he was not able to help the regimental surgeons. It should be pointed out that regiments were usually recruited from a single community or area and the surgeons were appointed by the commanding officer. A few surgeons brought their own medicines and surgical instruments, but many of them assumed they would be supplied by the army. Unfortunately, Congress not only neglected to provide adequate funds for the Medical Department, but it had made no provision for the regimental surgeons. Unaware of this, the regimental surgeons accused Morgan of hoarding supplies.[14]

Except in Massachusetts and one or two of the other New England states, little effort was made to insure that regimental surgeons were qualified. Morgan described many of them as "unlettered, ignorant, and rude to a degree scarcely to be imagined." Some of them, he added, had no training in physic and had never seen an operation. In view of the heroic practices of even the best physicians, a lack of training might not have been quite so bad. Dr. Thacher, one of the leading army surgeons, and two of his colleagues handled a case of rattlesnake bite by forcing the patient to swallow repeated doses of olive oil and rubbing the affected leg with mercurial ointment. Within two hours, Dr. Thacher reported, the patient was saved. Dr. William Eustis of Massachusetts treated a patient shot through the lungs with repeated and liberal bloodletting. The patient's survival was attributed "to the free use of the lancet and such abstemious living as to reduce him to the greatest extremity." [15]

Despite such rigorous therapy, there was a large and useful body of medical knowledge available, and Morgan was justified in seeking to improve the caliber of regimental surgeons. His efforts to do so merely added to their bitterness and dissatisfaction. As if Morgan did not have problems enough, shortly before he assumed office Congress appointed Dr. Samuel Stringer as Director of the Hospital in the Northern Department but failed to define his relationship to Morgan. Stringer promptly began lobbying Congress to strengthen his position. Thus Morgan found himself involved in a fight with Stringer while at the same time struggling to gain jurisdiction over the regimental surgeons, who were also appealing to Congress.[16] Instead of resolving the problem, Congress created yet another hospital system, one headquartered in Williamsburg, Virginia. Meanwhile, Morgan's old rival, William Shippen, Jr., who had useful contacts in Congress, had been appointed Director of the Hospital for the Flying Camp, the name assigned to some ten thousand militia called up from the surrounding provinces to protect New Jersey. Shippen's exact status was not made clear, and he soon began encroaching upon Morgan's authority. Morgan, who was fully engaged in fighting against potential rivals within his department and battling with the regimental surgeons, on January 9, 1777, suddenly found himself dismissed.

Morgan, who had worked indefatigably at his job, was taken by surprise, and immediately demanded a hearing. His sense of outrage reached new bounds when he learned that he was to be replaced by his old enemy Shippen. The ensuing personal vendettas between the two men brought at least one benefit. In trying to clear his name and at the same time tear down his old enemy, Morgan published *A Vindication of His Public Character in the Station of Director-General*, one of the few medical sources providing an insight into medical conditions during the war.

The military events of 1776 made clear the need for an army based upon more than one-year enlistments. Congress responded by reorganizing the military forces and creating a new Continental army for 1777, one in which soldiers enlisted for three years. By this date both Congress and Washington had become aware of the needless suffering of the sick and wounded and its impact upon the effectiveness of the fighting forces. Consequently William Shippen took over as medical director under far more auspicious circumstances than his two predecessors. In the first place, Morgan had started to bring some order to the Hospital Department and demonstrated the role that a good medical system could play. In the second, Shippen had a more polished and affable personality and was far more skillful in dealing with people, a particularly useful asset for a medical director dependent upon Congress for funding.

Dr. Benjamin Rush, a member of Congress's Medical Committee who had been impressed by the operation of the British army medical service during the fighting around Philadelphia, urged that the Hospital Department be reorganized. Shippen, working with Dr. John Cochran, drew up a proposal that, like the plan of his predecessor Morgan, was based largely upon the British system. It involved both a considerable increase in medical personnel and relatively large pay raises, provisions likely to meet opposition in Congress. Strongly supported by the Medical Committee and General Washington, the reorganization was pushed through Congress on April 1777. It provided for a director general and three deputy directors. The director general headed the Hospital Department and was personally responsible for the Middle Department. The three deputies were responsible for the Northern, Eastern, and Southern departments. The Northern Department was headed by Dr. Jonathon Potts, the Eastern by Dr. Isaac Foster, and the Southern by Dr. William Rickman. Working directly under Shippen, Dr. Benjamin Rush was appointed surgeon general of the Middle Department. The exact status of the Southern Department was not made clear, although Congress apparently intended it to remain more or less autonomous. The evidence indicates that its deputy director, Rickman, was inadequate, but he had enough political connections to hang on to his job until 1780.[17]

The reorganization also set up a regular chain of command reaching from the regimental surgeons to the director general. Regional hospitals were established in every district and a chief medical officer was appointed for each army in the field. In addition to coordinating hospital and medical care, this official theoretically was given supervisory powers over the regimental surgeons. Although the new program was a marked improvement, and Congress, if somewhat belatedly, was providing more generous support, the basic problems remained. The enmity between the regimental surgeons and the hospital surgeons continued unabated, with the regimental surgeons reluctant to surrender control of their patients to the general hospitals. Washington repeatedly had to order them to submit regular weekly reports to the Hospital Department. The actions of the regimental surgeons were not based solely on infighting between the two groups of surgeons, for eighteenth-century hospitals had a horrible reputation, and the sick and wounded were always reluctant to leave their comrades. The British had learned that soldiers recovered much faster and were less likely to catch "hospital fever," the scourge of early hospitals, when they were cared for within their own regiments.[18]

While Congress had increased the budget for drugs, it did not provide the Hospital Department with a commissary general to handle food, clothing, bedding, and other items needed for the sick. In the fall of 1777 many patients could not rejoin their units for lack of clothing, but it was not until November 19 that the Hospital Department was authorized to draw on army commissaries. Serious shortages of all supplies, intensified by the steady inflation of Continental currency, continued to be a problem throughout the war. The morale of the Hospital Department, which continued to be torn by professional dissension, was further damaged by the failure of Congress to give military status to physicians and surgeons. In the early years of the war they had neither military rank nor the privileges of military officers, and it was 1780 before Congress allowed physicians to draw allowances for clothing and rations comparable to those of line officers.[19]

As if the administrative and other problems were not bad enough, everyone in the Hospital Department with any political influence carried his problems to Congress, and the latter, through its various medical committees, had no hesitancy about intervening in departmental affairs. For example, when justifiable criticisms were made of conditions in the Alexandria hospital under direct control of Dr. Rickman of the Southern Department, Director General Morgan was prevented by Congress from taking any action. A more serious instance of political interference involved Drs. Rush and Shippen. Lack of discipline was a major problem in the American forces, and Rush, as surgeon general for the Middle Department, was particularly incensed by his inability to control his patients and by what he considered the general slackness in the army. He was a man of passionate convictions and was quick to form opinions. He blamed Washington for the lack of discipline and, as a result, became involved with the Conway Cabal. Because Shippen did not or could not remedy certain hospital conditions that Rush brought to his attention, the latter soon engaged in a vendetta against him.

Shippen did not want for enemies; Dr. Morgan was already dedicating himself to this cause and complaints of all types were pouring into General Washington's headquarters and to Congress. Rush was serving in Congress when he was appointed to his army medical post and was in a position to cause serious trouble. Shippen was not without his own political support, but what probably enabled him to hold onto his job until January 1781 was the sheer vindictiveness of the attacks by Morgan and Rush. Had the two men been less personal in their criticisms, they might have driven Shippen from office sooner. As it was, Shippen won the first round, and Rush was compelled to resign from the Hospital Department on January 30, 1778.[20] Thus with sickness and disease rampant and drastic shortages of all supplies, the Medical Department was crippled by infighting at the top level and by the continuing clashes between the Hospital Department staff and the regimental surgeons at the lower level.

Meanwhile, Director Shippen carefully avoided field campaigns and battles, seldom visited hospitals, and appears to have had limited concern for the army patients. At a time when the sick and wounded were suffering from want of food and other essentials, he was accused of profiteering on hospital supplies. After Rush made this charge public, Congress in 1778 reacted by separating the procurement of hospital supplies from Shippen's office. The following year Morgan brought additional charges of misconduct. A long legal battle ensued in which a military court finally acquitted Shippen. Congress, after reviewing the findings of the court-martial in the summer of 1780, was not convinced of his innocence and merely resolved to discharge Shippen from arrest rather than to confirm the court's decision to acquit him. Morgan and Rush, still not satisfied, continued their attack, and on January 3, 1781, Shippen, having saved a measure of face, quietly resigned.

The last of the wartime medical directors was Dr. John Cochran, who, after moving to New Jersey, helped establish the New Jersey Medical Society in 1766 and became its president in 1769. On Washington's suggestion, he had been appointed Physician and Surgeon General of the Middle Department under Shippen. He had collaborated with Shippen in the reorganization plan in 1777 and was largely responsible for the final overhaul of the Hospital Department, which

Congress enacted in October 1780. Although Shippen was reconfirmed as director that same fall, he was already contemplating resigning, and it was Cochran who placed the department on a relatively effective basis. Under the new organization, the semiautonomous geographical divisions were eliminated and full authority was concentrated in the hands of the director. The duties of the regional deputy directors were assumed by three chief hospital physicians who could be assigned wherever needed. In March 1781 Congress took the final step and placed the Southern Department under the supervision of the director general.

Dr. Cochran, an exceedingly capable individual, managed to avoid the personality clashes that had troubled the department since its inception, and his tenure of office was relatively peaceful. This is not to say that all was well: shortages of all sorts continued to plague the department; inflation was rampant; and the Continental Congress was scraping the bottom of the barrel for additional sources of funds. From the beginning of his administration Cochran was forced to plead desperately for additional medical and hospital supplies. In March 1781 he reported that one of the hospitals had been compelled to allow ambulatory patients to beg for food, and that conditions were not much better in the other hospitals. On April 2 he wrote that he had received no pay for twenty-three months. Fortunately in 1781 military action ceased and in the succeeding years the army steadily dwindled away. Despite many difficulties, Cochran remained on the job until the peace treaty was signed. By this time the majority of sick and wounded had been discharged.[21]

The end of the Revolution brought a wave of optimism and patriotism, but the immediate effect of the war was to reduce intellectual contacts with Britain and Europe. The medical profession in particular suffered a severe setback. Before the Revolution the better colonial physicians completed their education in the London hospital schools and the universities of Edinburgh and Glasgow. The war severed this connection, and the intense patriotic spirit that followed independence discouraged its renewal. The wartime closing of the two small American medical schools left medical education almost exclusively to the apprentice system. Even worse, the bitter division between Tories and Patriots led many of the best-trained physicians to leave the country. Some elected to go with the withdrawing British forces and others were expelled. In the immediate postwar years, a patriotic committee in Charleston, South Carolina, banished thirteen physicians classified as "obnoxious persons" and levied heavy fines on two others. Among those expelled was Dr. Alexander Garden, America's leading naturalist.[22]

One might assume that the lessons learned in dealing with wartime injuries and sicknesses and the close contact with experienced British and French military surgeons would have provided some compensation for these disadvantages, but there is little evidence to this effect. From the standpoint of medicine and surgery no significant advances were made during these years. Drs. Morgan and Shippen, two of the best minds, were preoccupied with their army medical roles, and Benjamin Rush was more concerned with politics than medicine. The latter, a true representative of the eighteenth-century age of enlightenment, at least made a few shrewd observations based on his limited military experience. As an avowed exponent of cleanliness and moderation, he argued that the sickness and death that characterized army camps could be avoided by correct hygienic procedures and better food. He warned officers to avoid crowding too many men in a tent and suggested that "unnecessary fatigue" would invite disease. In an age when bathing was commonly assumed to place one's health at risk, he recommended that the soldiers bathe twice a week.[23] He also noticed the psychological effect of victory upon the troops, citing the excellent health enjoyed by officers and men in the British fleet following their decisive defeat of the French in April 1782. The same held true, he wrote, of the men of the Philadelphia militia who joined Washington's army shortly before the American victory at Trenton. Although they had little experience with an outdoor life, these troops slept in tents and barns—and occasionally out in the open—during the winter months with scarcely any sickness.[24]

The Immediate Postwar Years

Despite the setback caused by the Revolution, the immediate postwar years did see a quickening of scientific and educational activity. The rapid expansion in population and wealth that helped the colonies win their independence convinced Americans that theirs was a glorious destiny as the growing spirit of nationalism emerged in full flower in the early national period. Physicians, along with other American scientists, equated political democracy with the free spirit of scientific inquiry and were convinced that American science, untrammeled by political restrictions, would soon lead the world. In part these hopeful beliefs, as Brooke Hindle pointed out, reflected the weakness of the American intellectual position. The new nation had only one scientist with an international reputation and no educational or scientific societies of consequence. All scientific activities had been disrupted by the war, the efforts of the best minds diverted, and the essential contact with Great Britain cut off.[25]

Either unaware of or undaunted by these problems, the medical profession quickly recovered. Pre-Revolutionary medical societies such as those of New Jersey, Connecticut, New York, and Philadelphia were revived and new ones sprang into existence. Although beset by difficulties, the medical colleges in Philadelphia and New York resumed operation, and Harvard added medicine to its curriculum in 1782. Four years later the Philadelphia Dispensary opened its doors, to be followed in 1791 by the New York Dispensary. Based on the European pattern, these dispensaries were philanthropic agencies designed to give free outpatient care to the poor and at the same time provide a measure of clinical training for physicians and their students. In 1791 the New York Hospital accepted its first patients, inaugurating an era of hospital building.

Despite the general suspicion of Great Britain, intellectual ties were reestablished, for a common language and culture inevitably led Americans to renew their intellectual allegiance to the mother country. Even that arch-patriot Dr. Rush observed: "What has physic to do with taxation or independence?" The new ties that had been formed with France and the Continent during the Revolution proved too tenuous to threaten the cultural relationship with Great Britain. Moreover, the Continent was soon to be torn by twenty-five years of revolution and war, and England had temporarily taken leadership in medicine and surgery under the guidance of men such as John and William Hunter.

Dr. Benjamin Rush, the American Hippocrates

America had many able physicians at the end of the eighteenth century, but without doubt the one who epitomized American medicine in his day was Dr. Benjamin Rush.[26] His importance lies not only in his dominant role in medicine but in his profound influence upon American medical practice, an impact that continued to be felt far into the nineteenth century. While scarcely typical of early American physicians, he represented much of the best—and some of the worst—

of his day. His family background, which had embraced a wide variety of Protestant religious concepts ranging from Quakerism to Anglicanism, gave him a strong social conscience that was reflected in his humanitarian interests. Although christened in the Anglican faith, his moral ideas were profoundly shaped by the Reverend Samuel Finley, a Presbyterian minister who ran Nottingham Academy, a boarding school where the young Rush spent five years. Subsequently Rush entered the College of New Jersey, or Princeton, and graduated a year and a half later at the age of fifteen. Shortly thereafter he was apprenticed to Dr. John Redman, an outstanding Philadelphia physician and another staunch Presbyterian who would help form Rush's character. In the course of spending five and a half years with Dr. Redman, Rush attended the lectures on anatomy given by Dr. William Shippen, Jr., in 1762 and subsequently enrolled under Shippen and Morgan at the College of Philadelphia.

Medical competition in Philadelphia was keen, and Rush soon realized that he needed a European medical degree if he were to succeed. Encouraged by his preceptors, in August 1766 he set forth to enroll in the University of Edinburgh. Shortly after taking his medical degree in June 1768, he headed south to London to continue his studies. Here he spent some five months attending William Hunter's anatomy lectures and making the acquaintance of a wide circle of leading British physicians, a group that included Sir John Pringle, the famous army surgeon, and Drs. John Fothergill and John Coakley Lettsom. The latter two are best known for their humanitarian interests and philanthropic endeavors, qualities that appealed to Rush. When Rush learned that Benjamin Franklin was in London, he promptly called on him. Franklin, always happy to help young Americans, took him under his wing, and in short order Rush was attending receptions and dinners with the outstanding artists and literary figures of the day, men such as Sir Joshua Reynolds, Oliver Goldsmith, and Samuel Johnson.

Armed with letters of introduction from Franklin, early in 1769 Rush spent several weeks in Paris, where he considered the medicine to be fifty years behind that of England and Scotland, and then set sail for home. With assistance from some of the local physicians, he soon established a successful practice — a practice that was greatly helped by Rush's appointment immediately on his return from Europe to the position of professor of chemistry in the College of Philadelphia. As the break with Great Britain steadily widened during the tumultuous years of the 1770s, Rush flung himself into politics. His activity in Pennsylvania affairs led to his election to the Second Continental Congress where he signed the Declaration of Independence and developed a taste for political intrigue. During 1777–78 he served briefly in the army, but his fulminations against Dr. Shippen and General Washington soon led to a demand for his resignation. Rush was not solely to blame, but he displayed an unusual rashness and lack of discretion.

In the years following the Revolution, Rush turned his efforts toward moral and humanitarian reforms. He was a strong advocate of both private and public education, and he fought for prison reform, temperance, the abolition of slavery, and the elimination of all forms of tobacco. In the meantime he maintained a substantial practice and continued to play an active role in medical teaching. The combination of his political, philanthropic, and medical activities soon gained Rush a reputation as America's outstanding physician.

It was in this period that Rush began to formulate his personal philosophical approach to medicine. In the seventeenth century, as medicine sought to break away from traditional thinking, physicians such as Thomas Sydenham (1624–89) had substituted a nosological approach to medicine, i.e., they began by assuming that disease entities existed and then sought to classify disorders on the basis of symptoms. Since symptoms and syndromes come in an infinite variety, nosographic texts were soon publishing longer and longer lists of supposed diseases. Instead of clarifying the medical picture, the result was to compound the confusion in medical circles. As Rush reflected on medicine over the years, he rejected the nosological approach, or concept of disease entities, and consciously or not, returned to the traditional monistic pathology, which explained all diseases in terms of one fundamental cause. In lecturing to his students Rush constantly warned against espousing any particular medical doctrine. In 1801, for example, he declared that "undue attachment to great names" had led to the establishment of "a despotism in medicine," and he urged that progress in medicine could be achieved only by free inquiry. At the University of Edinburgh Rush had been greatly impressed by William Cullen, one of the most influential medical professors of his day and a philosopher who believed in systematization. Ironically, two of his students, John Brown and Benjamin Rush, developed medical systems that profoundly, if not disastrously, affected medical practice for two or three generations.

The impetus that led Rush to formulate his medical doctrine was the great yellow fever epidemic in Philadelphia during 1793. Beginning in this year, a series of devastating yellow fever epidemics struck every major American port from Boston southward. The disease had been absent from America for over thirty years, and the medical profession was at an utter loss to explain or treat the fever. Along with his colleagues in 1793, Rush was overwhelmed with patients and was desperately seeking some form of effective therapy. At first he tried a cooling regimen supplemented by moderate purging and bleeding, but it seemed of no avail. After fruitlessly consulting the leading medical authors and trying various other forms of therapy, he recalled an old manuscript that Franklin had given him describing a yellow fever outbreak in Virginia in 1741. In it Dr. John Mitchell reported how the stomach and intestinal tract in yellow fever was filled with blood and putrefying matter. Until this matter was purged away, he had written, it was impossible to procure a "laudable" sweat. Mitchell further declared that the physician should not be deterred from decisive action by an "ill-timed scrupulousness about the weakness of the body."[27]

Rush was familiar with Dr. Thomas Young's "Ten-and-Ten," a horrendous purge of ten grains of calomel and ten grains of jalap, a violent herbal cathartic. Although it had been used by the army during the Revolution, Rush had qualms about administering it to anyone weakened by yellow fever. Late in August he encountered a patient with yellow fever who was apparently on the point of death and who had been deserted by his family and friends. Rush in desperation administered a large dose of mercury and jalap, and to his surprise the man showed signs of recovery. Delighted with the result, he began experimenting with even larger quantities until he was prescribing three doses, each consisting of ten grains of calomel and fifteen of jalap, to be given at six-hour intervals. Along with this, he combined bloodletting and a cooling regimen of cold baths, cold drinks, and cool air. It is likely that the first few individuals on whom Rush tried this therapy either did not have yellow fever or had only a mild form of the disease. Whatever the case, Rush became convinced that he had solved the problem. He immediately proclaimed the new doctrine and, over considerable opposition, his views carried the day. Rush's success in promulgating his thesis meant that for years to come, particularly in the West and South, massive purging and bloodletting were to characterize American medical practice.

Rush's purported success in 1793 led him gradually to formulate his concept of the unity of disease. By 1796 he was informing his students that fevers resulted from three factors: a predisposing debility; an external or internal stimulus acting upon the body; and a "convulsive excitement" in the walls of the blood vessels. This "convulsive excitement," he had become convinced, was the essence of fevers and the common feature of all diseases. "Where I formerly said there was only one fever," he declared in a lecture, "I will [now] say there is but one disease in the world." Having concluded that the underlying cause of all illness was vascular tension, Rush assumed that the way to relieve the tension was by bleeding. The centuries-old practice of bleeding had shown clearly that a restless, feverish patient when bled sufficiently would within a few minutes lose the flushed skin, delirium, high temperature, and other characteristics of fever. He would, moreover, break out into a sweat, long accepted as an indication that the fever was broken.

Since Rush believed that one of the hindrances to the development of medicine had been an "undue reliance upon the powers of nature in curing diseases," a thesis that he blamed upon Hippocrates, he resolved after 1793 to take whatever measures were necessary to save the patient's life.[28] A phrase that one finds repeatedly in early nineteenth-century medical journals epitomizes Rush's approach: "Desperate diseases require desperate remedies." He believed that the body held about twenty-five pounds of blood, well over double the actual quantity, and he urged his disciples to continue bleeding until four-fifths of the patient's blood was removed. When massive purging caused the bowels to bleed, Rush felt the purge was doing double duty. The patient's welfare was the prime objective, and if it was necessary to give the individual violent cathartics and to relieve the person of six to eight pints of blood over a two- or three-day period, Rush did not intend to be fainthearted.

One of the more surprising aspects of the 1793 epidemic is that Rush's medical views should have gained so many adherents. The evidence is clear that the yellow fever epidemic in Philadelphia exacted an enormous death toll. In light of the prevailing medical knowledge, Rush and his colleagues could have done little to reduce the number of deaths, and Rush's heroic therapy undoubtedly compounded the suffering and mortality. Yet Rush emerged a popular hero from the outbreak. While a number of his colleagues died and several fled, Rush remained resolutely at his post seeing a hundred or more patients a day. When a slight fever attacked him, he had himself purged and bled, and before he was fully recovered he was again seeing patients. The best explanation for his popularity lies in his personality. He was a warm, humane individual, positive and enthusiastic in his beliefs, and these qualities, plus his reputation as America's leading physician, gave credence to his medical doctrine. Against his better qualities, Rush was a complex personality, rigid and self-righteous, and he pursued his medical thesis with a fanatical zeal.[29]

The tragedy is that his personality obscured the views of other, more observant and perceptive physicians. Several of his colleagues in Philadelphia—Drs. Adam Kuhn, Edward Stevens, Joseph Goss, and James Hutchinson—were all opposed to purging and bleeding and generally followed a mild supportive policy, the only course that could have been of any help at that time. Dr. James Currie, who was as busy as Rush during the outbreak, wrote a pamphlet describing yellow fever and the best means that he had found to combat it. In contrast to Rush, Currie declared that the disease was a specific contagion spread by contact with the sick or their personal belongings. He decried the burning of gunpowder and tar as a preventive and advised his readers to practice personal hygiene, moderate their diet, exercise mildly, and to get plenty of fresh air. He too rejected bloodletting and purgation and advocated a moderate treatment emphasizing the relief of symptoms and the principle of making the patient as comfortable as possible. Since little could be done for yellow fever patients once the disorder was established, it is unfortunate that the voices of moderation went virtually unheeded.[30]

Rush represents a transition between the eighteenth-century age of reason and the nineteenth-century age of science. He had a philosophic bent that made him seek fundamental causes, and his medical training encouraged this tendency. Although he was a keen clinical observer, Rush had little interest in pathology and laboratory research. He related to people, and he was happiest when dealing with patients. As indicated, he had broad intellectual interests and dabbled in many fields. His social consciousness may well have been responsible for his political activities. While he had a barely perceptible influence upon political events, his election to various political offices, his status as a signer of the Declaration of Independence, and his brief services as an army medical officer all added to his public exposure and helped enhance his medical reputation.

By 1800 Rush was considered the greatest American physician. His students were spreading his fame throughout the United States, and his reputation was adding to the luster of Philadelphia as the leading medical center in the country. When he died in 1813 he was eulogized as the American Hippocrates. As a transitional figure, however, his fame was short-lived. Within ten years of his death his ideas were questioned, and within thirty they were almost universally condemned. In the twentieth century a more balanced picture of him has emerged. By viewing him in light of his era, we can understand the factors that led him into error in his medical reasoning, and we can appreciate his many contributions. While his assumptions may not have been correct, Rush, by emphasizing personal and public hygiene, gave impetus to the public health movement of the nineteenth century. His shrewd clinical observations and ideas with respect to psychiatry were well in advance of his day. For the next century and a half scientists were to withdraw into their laboratories, unlike Rush who felt that all educated men should participate actively in government.

CHAPTER 5

Early Nineteenth-Century Medicine

IN THE HISTORY OF MEDICINE two separate streams flow side by side. One represents the evolution of medical theories, the gradual accumulation of knowledge, and the major figures involved in the application of that knowledge. Parallel to this, and frequently having little relation to it, was the practice of the average physician. To a cynical observer, it would appear that in each age medical theorists simply sought to justify existing medical practices in terms of the prevailing philosophic or scientific concepts. All aspects of society were undergoing revolutionary changes in the early nineteenth century, but medical knowledge and practice lagged far behind. Medicine could not advance until progress had been made on a broad front of the biological and chemical sciences. In consequence, public suspicion of orthodox medicine tended to increase during the first decades of the century.

Medical practice was little changed from what it had been in the eighteenth century, consisting largely of bleeding, blistering, purging, vomiting, and sweating. The agents to procure these results varied and the emphasis frequently shifted from one to another, but the basic therapy remained relatively unchanged. While the theorists argued, the average practitioner, with only a minimum of theoretical knowledge, clung to a vague combination of humoralism and solidism; the former was concerned with the body juices and the latter sought to relax or stimulate the nerves and blood vessels. Thus cures could be achieved through eliminating the bad or vitiated humors and/or stimulating or relaxing the nerves and muscles. The only question that troubled physicians was not whether to resort to these depletory tactics, but to what degree. Physicians and their patients shared a general assumption that body and mind were intimately related, and that the normal body balance could be disrupted by individual physiological factors and by the physical and cultural environment. The administration of therapeutics was designed in part to correct specific symptoms and in part to reassure the patient that the physician was doing something. The results of traditional remedies such as bleeding and purgation left no doubt in the patient's mind that they were working.[1]

Bleeding was usually the initial therapeutic, whether the patient was a child or adult, and few doctors questioned its value. The major debates were over the method, quantity, and location from which to take blood. Venesection, leeching, scarification, and cupping were the standard procedures for drawing blood. Venesection, as the name implied, was simply the opening of a vein. Scarification was performed by a small instrument with a spring mechanism that made a series of small cuts. Scarifying was frequently combined with cupping. Wet cupping consisted of heating a small glass vessel and placing it over the scarified area. As it cooled, the resulting vacuum drew blood from the cuts. Dry cupping was the same procedure, but it was intended to draw blood to the surface.[2]

Among the drugs, calomel, or mercurous chloride, was known as the "Sampson of Materia Medica." Depending on the dosage, it was either a laxative or purgative, although the dosages were usually large enough to act as a purge. Prescriptions often called for enough calomel to cause salivation or to "touch the gums," both symptoms of acute mercurial poisoning. A southern physician, Dr. Edward H. Barton, stated that he had seen many individuals from the same family die of mercurial mortification and declared that in the face of this evidence, many practitioners were convinced that if calomel did not do the patient any good, it would at least do no harm. Nor was the use of calomel restricted to the South and West. A computer study of 549 prescriptions written by three New Jersey physicians in 1854 showed that calomel and mercury in other forms were prescribed ninety-five times. One physician prescribed for his own child twelve doses of two grains of calomel administered during a twenty-four-hour period. The three other drugs most often prescribed were opium, ipecac, and camphor, the latter two often prescribed in conjunction with opium. Ipecac was widely used as a diaphoretic and emetic, and camphor for its anodyne and narcotic effect.[3]

Blistering consisted of placing mustard plasters, Spanish fly (cantharides), or some other substance on the skin with the intention of causing a second-degree burn. The blisters frequently became infected, and the resulting suppuration was assumed to be the poisons or "bad humor" being drawn from the body. Blistering, along with the other depletory measures, was scarcely a mild form of treatment, but it was made more painful by the many physicians, particularly in the South and West, who heeded the advice that the sicker the patient the more drastic the therapy.

Yet in these same years it was becoming evident to many perceptive physicians that neither the prevailing medical theories nor traditional forms of therapy were of much value, and increasingly they turned to clinical experience. By this date hospitals were growing in number and size, and clinicians were able to observe hundreds of patients. In Paris a group of young physicians brought to the forefront by the French Revolution began using new techniques and instruments to turn diagnosis into a fine art. By applying statistics to diagnoses and following patients into the postmortem rooms, they soon discovered that the traditional forms of therapy were not only useless but in many cases positively harmful.

The impact of the French Clinical School was first felt in Louisiana where the Creoles still looked to France for intellectual leadership. Although Louisiana was acquired by the United States in 1803 and became a state in 1812, its population remained predominantly French for many years. As English-speaking Americans flooded into the state, the two groups inevitably clashed. American physicians were largely apprentice-trained or else had taken a relatively easy degree from one of the American medical colleges. The Creoles carried on the European tradition of university training, which required a physician to spend as much as fourteen years acquiring his medical degree. With some justification they considered the Americans both crude and virtually illiterate. To make matters worse, the Anglo-American doctors generally espoused the doctrines of Benjamin Rush, scorning the healing power of nature and firmly believing in direct and drastic action. When confronted with a sick patient, they unhesitatingly gathered their purges and emetics, couched their lancets, and charged the enemy, prepared to bleed, purge, and vomit until the disease was conquered.[4]

The Creole physicians did not completely escape the pernicious influence of the great French bloodletter of this period, François-Joseph-Victor Broussais (1772–1838), but they generally believed the role of the physician was to assist nature in making the cure. They were averse to wholesale bloodletting and were reluctant to use calomel and other powerful and dangerous drugs. The wide differences in the medical practices of the two groups can best be seen in their approach to yellow fever. The Société Médicale de la Nouvelle Orléans requested two of its members to report on a yellow fever epidemic that struck the city in 1817. The ensuing report stated that the only methods that had proved of benefit were tepid baths to reduce the fever, "gentle evacuants, acid drinks with cream of tartar, tamerind, orange juice and lemon juice; whey, emollient clysters and purgatives."[5] The regimen recommended in this report was for its day a sensible and moderate one, and it continued to form the basis for the treatment of fevers by the Creole physicians in the succeeding years.

The Americans, however, had little use for the policy of moderation, and their methods were in sharp contrast to this mild, supportive treatment. Dr. M. L. Haynie of St. Francisville, Louisiana, wrote with contempt that the Louisiana French were "extremely averse" to the use of mercury or the lancet because of their "want of correct physiological knowlege." Confident of his own understanding of physiology, Dr. Haynie stated that bleeding was essential "to ease the heart and arteries" and that mercury was the most effective stimulant in relieving prostration. His dosages of mercury, he continued, were proportioned to the violence of the disease, usually one hundred to two hundred grains an hour. He then epitomized what has been called the heroic school of medicine by declaring: "It is but trifling with the life of a man, to give him less of a remedy than his disease calls for."[6]

The existence of two cultures in Louisiana discouraged the mutual exchange of ideas for about two generations. The Creoles held themselves aloof from the uncultured Americans, maintaining their own societies and French-language publications. By the midcentury, however, the better medical men in both groups were recognizing each other's merits, and the Creole practice was exerting a moderating influence upon American practices. Meanwhile, by 1830 the Paris Clinical School was beginning to modify the practice of physicians in the East. France had supplanted Great Britain as the mecca for medical students, and American physicians returning from Paris were soon championing the cause of moderation. Some 105 American physicians studied in Paris during the 1820s and another 222 in the 1830s. The list of those studying medicine in France in the 1830s is a virtual catalogue of the outstanding names in American medicine, men such as Jacob Bigelow, James Jackson, Jr., Oliver Wendell Holmes, John Collins Warren, Valentine Mott, Alexander H. Stevens, Josiah Clark Nott, and Willard Parker. All told, almost 700 American physicians spent some time in France in the years from 1820 to 1860.[7]

While in Paris these young Americans learned the use of the stethoscope and the art of diagnosis, and they took advantage of the unrivaled opportunities for clinical observation and anatomical work. They brought back with them a skeptical approach to traditional therapy that gradually permeated the American medical profession. Jacob Bigelow was one of the first to express this new outlook. In an address before the Massachusetts Medical Society in 1835 he discussed what he called the "self-limited" diseases, disorders that once entrenched in the system could not be affected by the art of medicine but that ran their course and eventually disappeared. The existence of these diseases, he said, probably explained why able practitioners employing totally different methods could each claim success for their treatment or why infinitely small homeopathic doses often succeeded. While Bigelow suggested that only a few disorders fell into this category, he made the point that some diseases could be cured by nature alone, a view of medicine directly opposite to that which Rush had taught. Significantly, Oliver Wendell Holmes wrote subsequently that Bigelow's essay "had more influence on medical practice in America than any other similar brief treatise."[8] By the 1840s medical practice among the more able physicians had generally swung away from the policy of active interference to one of caution and moderation. Bloodletting was definitely on the wane, and calomel was beginning to lose its role as the mainstay of medication.

It is an oversimplification to ascribe this beneficial development solely to the influence of French and European physicians. Change was in the air, and one can cite any number of physicians who refused to be carried away by a particular system and who modified the teachings of their preceptors by using their own powers of observation. Mention has already been made of Drs. Kuhn and Stevens and others in the 1790s who opposed Benjamin Rush's debilitating treatment. The medical care given George Washington in 1799 has often been cited as an illustration of heroic therapy. Washington, who was suffering from an acute infection of the throat, probably streptococcal, was given the full treatment. He awoke early in the morning of December 14 feeling quite ill and sent for Dr. James Craik. In the meantime he asked his overseer to bleed him. On Dr. Craik's arrival, he blistered Washington's throat with cantharides, applied leeches to the throat and behind the ears, ordered an enema, and, when these measures proved unavailing, he twice let blood. It was clear that the patient was in a serious condition, and by three in the afternoon two other physicians had been summoned, Gustavus Richard Brown and Elisha Dick. Although Washington had already been blistered, bled three times, and given several doses of calomel and tartar emetic within the space of a few hours, the two senior physicians, Craik and Brown, over the objections of young Dr. Dick, decided more bleeding was necessary. On this occasion another thirty-two ounces was taken, the blood coming thick and slow. Although the physicians continued their efforts, Washington's condition rapidly worsened, and he died at ten o'clock that night.[9] Whether or not Washington at his age and condition could have survived the infection is doubtful, but the debilitating and dehydrating measures taken by his medical attendants could only have hastened his death.

Aside from the picture of orthodox medical treatment provided by the description of Washington's last hours, a letter from Dr. Brown gives a glimpse into the soul-searching that existed among conscientious physicians. He wrote to Craik subsequently expressing regret over the bleeding and suggesting that Dr. Dick was probably right in opposing it. He described Dick as a sensible man who used common sense rather than books in practicing medicine. Brown's most significant comment indicates that Dr. Dick was literally despairing of medical practice, for Brown concluded: "He is disposed to put up his lancet forever and turn nurse instead of Doctor, for he says one good nurse is more likely to assist nature in making a cure than ten Doctors will by his pills and lancet." [10]

Many other physicians, too, were growing increasingly skeptical of the prevailing medical practices. Dr. Jacob Heustis, a military surgeon who served in New Orleans, was horrified at the cavalier way in which mercury was administered to men suffering from yellow fever during an outbreak in 1812. It was not prescribed by weight or grains, he wrote caustically, for that would have been unworthy of "the characteristic liberality and boldness of its great advocate and supporter

[Rush]." Instead it was given by the spoonful, and "few survived to tell the mournful story."[11] Twenty years later Dr. Edward H. Barton of Louisiana bitterly criticized all aspects of drastic medicine: "It makes me shudder when I hear of 'heroic practice'; heroism in war is built upon the slaughter of our fellow creatures; it is little less in physic."[12]

The two great epidemic diseases in nineteenth-century America, yellow fever and Asiatic cholera, also played a role in moderating therapy. Yellow fever virtually disappeared from the northeastern states after 1806, but it struck with increasing intensity along the south Atlantic and gulf coasts, reaching its peak in the 1850s. Although a few physicians dissented, bleeding, calomel, and other drastic measures remained the standard treatment until the late 1830s. The introduction of the alkaloid quinine in 1820 proved a boon in the South where malaria was endemic. Unfortunately the concept of the unity of fevers was still widely accepted, and it led in the late 1830s to a vogue for prescribing massive doses of quinine for yellow fever. In 1844 the *New Orleans Medical Journal* announced that in the treatment of fevers the use of purgatives and emetics had moderated and been replaced "by the more prompt and bold administration of tonics, above all the sulphate of quinine." "Quinine, instead of calomel," the *Journal* declared, "is now considered in the South, the *Sampson* of the *Materia Medica*."[13]

A series of major yellow fever outbreaks from 1853 to 1855 finally convinced many southern physicians that active interference in the case of yellow fever was more harmful than beneficial. At the end of the great yellow fever epidemic of 1853, the *New Orleans Medical and Surgical Journal* conceded that the quinine treatment, like its predecessors, was of little value.[14] Quinine, bloodletting, and calomel still had their advocates, but there was a rising consensus that a mild, supportive treatment combined with good nursing was all that could be done.

The second American scourge was Asiatic cholera, a filth disease that gained a foothold three times in the nineteenth century. Improvements in transportation and the emergence of large, crowded, and dirty cities, which provided an ideal environment for enteric disorders, were responsible for the three major cholera epidemics. As with yellow fever, the physicians could neither prevent nor cure the disease. Since a rapid dehydration is the worst aspect of cholera, the traditional depletory forms of therapy only worsened the patient's condition. During the first two outbreaks, in 1832 and 1849–50, heated debates over medical treatment occurred among physicians, but essentially the question was how best to utilize the standard therapeutics. Opium was the traditional treatment for enteric or diarrheal complaints, and arguments raged over the best way to combine opium with calomel, bloodletting, and emetics.[15] In New York City during 1832 groups within the medical profession openly clashed. The Board of Health's Special Medical Council recommended calomel, opium, brandy, and cayenne pepper. Another group of physicians advised freely purging with calomel and aloes or scammony. Still a third group published *The Cholera Bulletin.* On July 23 its editor sarcastically classified his fellow physicians as "the Bleeders, the Calomel Brigade, the Opium Foragers, [and] the Guard of Leechers and Blisters." His major criticism, however, was against those who applied one form of therapy either indiscriminately or exclusively, for he concluded that the lancet, opium, calomel, tobacco, and the other therapeutics were valuable; the problem was how to use them.[16]

When cholera returned almost twenty years later, the same arguments ensued, with each doctor stressing his own variant. However, as was the case with yellow fever in the 1850s, the arguments suggest a general moderation of practice, a tendency to consider the weakened state of the patient and to follow a more supportive program. Within a few years this policy was becoming more general, and when Asiatic cholera returned a third time, in 1866, the treatment tended to be simpler and more effective. For example, Dr. Warren Stone, a well-known New Orleans physician and surgeon, announced in 1866 that he had found it beneficial to give cholera patients as much ice water as they wished, a great step forward in dealing with a disease that dehydrated its victims.[17]

The almost universal prescription of calomel for cholera (and almost every other ailment) was based upon long-established beliefs. One was the miasmatic thesis, which maintained that an invisible miasma or "noxious substance" arising from filth, putrefying matter, or the bowels of the earth corrupted the body's humors. Calomel, along with jalap and other purgatives, was counted on to drive out these so-called vitiated humors. It was also assumed that calomel would help to restore the normal balance of the basic bodily humors. In addition, the liver had long been blamed for many bodily ills, and postmortems showing the liver of cholera victims to be engorged seemed to confirm the liver's role in illness. The obvious solution was to stimulate the flow of bile by large doses of calomel. So widely held was this belief that calomel continued to be prescribed into the twentieth century.[18] Regardless of the therapeutic value of mercury, it is important to keep in mind that intelligent physicians sought a rational explanation for the use of their therapeutics. And it is precisely this fact that differentiated the medical profession from the empirics.

The work of the French Clinical School, the observations of intelligent physicians, and the impact of yellow fever and Asiatic cholera all played a role in helping to bring about the transition from excessive and drastic forms of therapy to a policy of moderation and support for the patient. One last factor needs to be considered: the role of the public. Medical practice in any society and at any time depends to a considerable degree upon the public's wants and demands. While the medical profession today deserves much of the blame for the excessive use of antibiotics, steroids, and tranquilizers, it is equally true that patients share it with them. Most patients expect their physicians to do something, and if they are not given an injection or prescription, they are likely to look elsewhere. In the nineteenth century patients were conditioned to calomel and bloodletting, and a physician who did not resort to either or both of these would have been considered remiss. Yet, just as perceptive physicians had their doubts about heroic therapy, so did many laypeople. This skepticism increased in direct ratio to the spread of drastic medical measures. In fact the most zealous advocates of bleeding and purging were the ones most instrumental in turning popular opinion against the practice. Public opinion in this regard was one step ahead of the profession. As much as anything else, it was the decision by many patients to turn from the advocates of rigorous therapy to herbalists, homeopaths, hydropaths, and other medical sects eschewing heroic practices that led orthodox physicians into reconsidering their position.

In the care of the insane, American medicine tended to reflect European developments. The Enlightenment and the new spirit of humanitarianism that led men such as Philippe Pinel of France and William Tuke in England to offer alternatives to the cruelty and neglect of the insane stimulated a number of sensitive and intelligent Americans to take similar action. The Pennsylvania Hospital admitted insane patients as early as 1751, and in 1773 the colony of Virginia opened the Eastern State Hospital in Williamsburg to provide for the mentally ill.[19] The first major breakthrough in treatment in America, however, did not come until 1789 when Dr. Rush petitioned the authorities of the Pennsylvania Hospital to provide better facilities for the insane. Rush represented a new school of medical thought, one that considered mental illness a somatic disorder and hence curable. Although we may look askance at the heroic regimen of bloodletting, purging, and other forms of therapy to which he subjected his patients, Rush, in considering mental disease treatable, was moving in the right direction.

The late eighteenth and early nineteenth centuries saw the emergence in Europe and America of the so-called moral treatment. An outgrowth of humanitarianism, it assumed that kindness, a cheerful environment, and proper respect for the patient's physical well-being would restore the mentally ill to health. Rush conceded some value to the moral treatment, but he believed the major emphasis should be placed upon physical medicine. The moral treatment was first applied in a few private institutions catering to middle- and upper-class patients, and the results exceeded the hopes of its advocates. Whereas mental patients formerly had been considered incurable and had been simply chained in dark basements or attics, it now appeared that half or more responded to treatment. At Bloomingdale Asylum in New York, the Pennsylvania Hospital in Philadelphia, the Hartford Retreat, and other institutions, the moral treatment swept the day.[20]

The apparent success of this new form of therapy, which for the first time offered hope for the insane, led to the establishment of a host of state asylums in the period from 1825 to 1860. The individual chiefly responsible for this development was Dorothea Lynde Dix (1802–87). In 1841, on becoming aware of the atrocious conditions under which most of the insane poor were kept, she launched a campaign in Massachusetts that led to the expansion and renovation of the Worcester State Hospital. Encouraged by this success, she expanded her activities by going from state to state, systematically exposing the deplorable condition of the insane poor, gaining support from newspapers, prominent citizens, and legislators, and then fighting for the creation of state hospitals. As she swept through the United States, she left a host of insane asylums in her wake.[21]

Ironically, the success achieved by Dix and her supporters almost proved self-defeating. The moral treatment, which seemed to work so well when physicians and asylum superintendents were treating patients of their own class, broke down in the case of immigrants and native-born poor. Mutually acceptable moral values were a fundamental aspect of the moral treatment and required that the healer and the patient belong to the same class; but when class distinctions were intensified by differences in culture, communication between doctors and patients broke down completely. If this were not enough, the number of the insane poor rose in direct ratio to the increasing degree of urbanization. The number of insane poor may have been even greater since the problems confronting the newcomers pouring into the cities placed enormous stresses upon them. Consequently, the newly created insane hospitals were overwhelmed with patients from the start, so that even the best-intentioned hospital authorities could do little more than provide custodial care. Fortunately there were a few exceptions such as the two New York institutions, the Lunatic Asylum at Utica and the Asylum for the Chronic Insane in Willard, the former concentrating upon curable cases and the latter providing good medical care for the permanently ill.[22]

Even in the private institutions, by the midcentury it was becoming clear that the moral treatment at best had only limited value. This factor, combined with the almost complete failure in treating the poor, gradually undermined the concept that the insane could be helped. With medicine unable to find a satisfactory explanation for mental illness, the assumption gained strength that it was a genetic or hereditary ailment and hence incurable. The general pessimistic attitude toward the insane in the second half of the nineteenth century meant that, while they were no longer treated with deliberate cruelty, neither did they receive active therapy.

CHAPTER 6

The Irregulars and Domestic Medicine

DOMESTIC MEDICINE, folk practitioners, and irregular
doctors have always played a significant role in providing medical care for Americans, and this was certainly true in the
nineteenth century. Precisely how much care was provided in this manner is difficult to say, but it may well have exceeded that given by
orthodox practitioners. The disastrous results of heroic medical practice and the decline in prestige of orthodox physicians helps to account
for the flourishing of medical sects in the early nineteenth century.
There are other factors, too, that account for the rise of the irregulars.
The colonial period had been one in which any person who could read
could be his own physician, lawyer, or theologian. As American society
became more complex and specialized, a conservative reaction developed. The egalitarianism of the age of Jacksonian democracy was in
part an effort to return to those simpler days when every American was
self-sufficient—his own lawyer, physician, carpenter, and cartwright.
The organization of medical societies with their fee bills symbolized
the decline of individual independence. Although most physicians were
unable to make a decent living, newspapers and journals in the early
nineteenth century constantly inveighed against the high cost of medical care. Medical fees in themselves were not excessive, but, when added
to indirect costs—those involved with transportation—they were costly
in relation to domestic medicine. America was a rural nation, and for
either the doctor or patient to travel several miles by horseback or
buggy was expensive of time and effort.[1]

The Thomsonians

The first individual to capitalize on the growing suspicion of the medical profession was Samuel Thomson (1769–1843). As a young man growing up in rural New Hampshire, Thomson had seen his mother die from what he believed were the mercurials and the harsh therapy of the orthodox physicians. When his wife became sick and was subjected to the customary bleeding and drugging, Thomson dismissed the physicians and called in two herb doctors whom he credited with saving her life. He decided to learn about herbals and eventually left the farm in 1805 to become an itinerant herb practitioner. In the succeeding years he gradually formulated his medical system. Based on a vague misunderstanding of Galenic medicine, he surmised that cold was the source of all disease, and that the only cure was heat. The restoration of heat was accomplished initially by steam baths and then the use of so-called "hot" botanicals such as cayenne pepper. He likened the digestive system to a stovepipe that occasionally becomes clogged with soot. To clean it out and restore its proper functioning, he resorted to botanic emetics, purgatives, diuretics, and sudorifics.

As Thomson's practice grew, he incurred the enmity of the regular physicians. Their reaction was predictable since Thomson constantly denounced them, claiming their medical training was designed to see "how much poison [could] be given without causing death." In addition, he opposed bloodletting, blistering, and the administration of mercurials, arsenicals, and other mineral drugs. Probably the gravest affront to the physicians was Thomson's success in building a practice at a time when few doctors could make a decent living. One of the regulars charged Thomson with murdering a patient, but the jury acquitted him.

In 1812 Thomson published a brief account of his method and gradually expanded it in a series of pamphlets. His culminating work was a book published in 1822 entitled *New Guide to Health; or Botanic Family Physician* . . . .[2] The publication of this work gave a great impetus to the Thomsonian movement. And a movement it was—religious, political, and social. Thomson, who came from a religious background, acquired an apostle in the person of Elias Smith. The two men, both suspicious of the legal, medical, and theological professions, spread the word of Thomsonianism, a cause they equated with that of the common man. Following the publication of his book, Thomson and his agents sold it for twenty dollars, bestowing upon the buyer the right to practice medicine in his own family. As soon as a few individuals in a given town or area had purchased the book, Thomson organized them into what became known as Friendly Botanic Societies.

As noted earlier, Thomsonianism was an aspect of Jacksonian democracy, and in advocating that medicine be taken from professionals and returned to layman, the proponents of Thomsonianism found a receptive audience. The drive by medical societies for licensing laws led to accusations that the profession was trying to achieve a privileged status by means of monopolies. In reaction to these attacks, physicians did their best to harass Thomsonian practitioners, but public sentiment was not on the side of the regulars. Licensure laws were seldom enforced, and local judges and juries usually dismissed criminal and civil actions against irregular practitioners.

As the historian Joseph Kett has pointed out, Thomsonians supported a wide range of social movements in the 1830s and 1840s, including drives against alcohol, tobacco, coffee, and tea, and in favor of dietary reform.[3] The many-faceted appeal of Thomsonianism enabled the movement to sweep through rural areas in all sections of the country. Thomson claimed that he had sold 100,000 copies of his book by 1839. Whether or not this claim is true — and it well may be — his influence over medical practice was far greater than even these figures would indicate. The very success of the movement proved self-defeating. Individuals and companies seized on Thomson's name and cashed in on it. Even more ironic, his later disciples organized medical schools and began institutionalizing Thomsonian medicine, a development contrary to one of the fundamental principles of Thomsonianism.[4]

The Homeopaths and Eclectics

The second major irregular medical sect to make deep inroads into orthodox practice was homeopathy, a medical system propounded by a German physician, Samuel Christian Hahnemann (1755–1843). Hahnemann, who in contrast to Thomson was well educated, had studied medicine in Leipzig and Vienna before finally taking a medical degree in 1779 from the University of Erlangen. He was an intelligent individual, capable of sound judgments, yet he occasionally wandered out in the wild blue yonder. He was a strong advocate of public and personal hygiene, and he recognized the value of moderate exercise, good diet, and fresh air. As a physician Hahnemann deplored the excessive drugging and bloodletting of his day and in particular the use of polypharmacy, complicated prescriptions calling for the inclusion of several drugs. Deciding that each drug should be tested individually, he swallowed doses of cinchona bark for several days and experienced what he thought were symptoms of fever. Since this same bark cured fever (in malaria), he reasoned that a drug that could induce a condition resembling a disease in a healthy person would cure the same disease in a sick one.

Similar experiments with other drugs led Hahnemann to the first of the two basic principles of homeopathy, *similia similibus curantur*, "like cures like." Subsequently his experiences in treating patients convinced him that he had made another equally significant discovery, the law of infinitesimals: the more minute the dosage the more efficacious the remedy. By 1810 Hahnemann had formulated his medical concepts, and he published them in his *Organon of Rational Healing*, a work that was translated into every major European language. Hahnemann's second principle, involving minute doses, virtually negated the effect of homeopathic drugs. The highly diluted homeopathic medicines were so weak as to leave the cure largely to nature—a course of action that was far better than the rigorous treatment of most orthodox physicians. Suffice to say, Hahnemann gradually gained a following and achieved a measure of international recognition.

Homeopathy arrived fairly late in the United States in the person of Hans Gram, an American of Danish parentage who studied medicine in Copenhagen and became a disciple of Hahnemann. Gram returned from Denmark in 1825 and settled in New York, where he gradually began making converts. Meanwhile a number of German physicians were migrating to Pennsylvania, one of whom, Constantine Hering, was both a distinguished physician and a scientist. An enthusiastic homeopath, Hering gained a following and in 1835 established the first homeopathic college in America, the Allentown Academy.

The third major group of irregulars to appear on the scene was the Eclectic School of Medicine founded by Wooster Beach (1794–1859). Beach had received an orthodox medical education, but he shared much in common with the Thomsonians, including their use of botanical remedies and general distrust of professional classes and political authorities. The eclectics differed from the Thomsonians in offering professional medical care rather than advocating a form of domestic medicine. As their name implies, the eclectics freely borrowed any form of therapy that they felt was practical or effective, and this attitude made them receptive to homeopathy. As eclectic medical schools began springing up in the 1830s and 1840s, they helped to spread the homeopathic doctrine. The Eclectic Medical Institute of Cincinnati had a chair in homeopathic medicine until it was abolished in 1850; the professor was converting both students and faculty. Homeopaths frequently mingled eclectic remedies with their own, and both groups benefited from the spread of Thomsonian doctrines. By offering more sophisticated versions of botanic medicine the two medical sects gradually replaced Thomsonianism.[5]

The immediate reaction of organized medicine to homeopathy was not unfavorable. Unlike the Thomsonians, the homeopathic physicians were well educated and operated from what was apparently a sound rationale. The homeopaths claimed their methods were based on research or "provings." These provings consisted of individual physicians testing drugs upon themselves to determine what "diseases" or symptoms they caused in a healthy person. While far removed from the blind and double-blind testing methods of today, they were as valid as much of the research carried on by orthodox medical doctors in the early nineteenth century. Reviews of Hahnemann's *Organon* in medical journals were not too critical, and it is evident that the medical profession was reserving judgment. With the profession still in considerable disarray, new medical concepts or regimens could scarcely be rejected out of hand; even phrenology was accepted as a legitimate aspect of medicine for a few years. Indicative of the profession's open-minded approach, in 1832 the Medical Society of the County of New York voted to bestow an honorary membership on Dr. Hahnemann.

By about 1840, however, the attitude of many regulars had begun to change, and individual physicians and medical journals started ridiculing homeopathy and castigating its followers. One of the first to sound a note of alarm against homeopaths was Dr. Oliver Wendell Holmes. Addressing the Massachusetts Medical Society in 1842 on the subject of homeopathy, he warned that the doctrine represented a serious threat to organized medicine by denying the validity of existing medical knowledge and by rejecting all accepted forms of medical therapy. Holmes—whose remark, "If all the medicines were thrown into the ocean, it would be so much the better for mankind and so much worse for the fishes," is often quoted—was no blind supporter of contemporary medical practice. But he recognized that homeopathy would distract medicine from the pursuit of objective scientific information, and in his address he systematically demolished its philosophic basis.

Logic was on the side of Holmes, but while he and other regular physicians could see the fallacies in the homeopathic principles, in terms of medical practice, they had little better to offer. Whatever the merits of Hahnemann's theory, homeopathic medicine appeared to do far less harm than the rigorous treatment of orthodox medicine. This fact was not lost on observant physicians and laypeople, and so homeopathy continued to flourish. Although not as great a threat as Thomsonianism in its popular appeal, homeopathy constituted a much more serious menace to the medical profession. In the first place, it attracted most of its early membership from the ranks of orthodox physicians; hence homeopaths could not be ignored as unlettered folk practitioners. In the second, homeopathy appealed to the middle and upper classes, the main source of income for the regular practitioners—and nothing can arouse an individual's moral indignation more than the prospect of an economic loss. Finally, homeopaths could not be dismissed as empirics since they offered a rationale for their practice.

By 1844 the homeopaths were strong enough to organize the American Institute of Homeopathy, the first national medical organization. Their success in winning converts among the regulars was greatly aided by the two major American epidemic diseases of the nineteenth century, yellow fever and Asiatic cholera. Since little could be done for the patients other than keeping them comfortable, the homeopathic method, which left the cure largely to nature, was far better than the bleeding, purging, and blistering regimen of the regulars. As might be expected, homeopathy was particularly successful in gaining ground among the orthodox physicians in the southern states where yellow fever was a constant threat. When the second wave of cholera swept through the United States from 1848–53, the success of homeopathic methods over the depletory orthodox treatment converted hundreds of regulars to Hahnemann's doctrines.

With the formation of the American Medical Association in 1847 the battle lines between the regulars and homeopaths became more sharply drawn, and the ensuing hostilities lasted into the twentieth century. The need for physicians to organize on a national basis was becoming more apparent by the 1840s, and the threat from homeopaths and other irregulars was a major factor in stimulating the initial meetings. In drawing up its code of ethics in 1847, the AMA struck the first blow at the homeopaths. The consultation clause stated that no regular physician could consult with any practitioner "whose practice is based upon an exclusive dogma, to the rejection of accumulated experience of the profession." In effect, no physician could consult with a homeopath even at the patient's request. Moreover, a regular physician could not attend any patient, regardless of his condition, unless the homeopath attending the case was first dismissed.[6]

While the intent of the consultation clause was clear, its enforcement was not easy. The AMA itself was a fledgling organization, and the fight against the homeopaths had to be conducted at the state and local level. The problem here was complicated in some cases by the friendly, personal relationships between a number of regulars and homeopaths. Furthermore, refusing help to a desperately ill patient because of a clash between rival medical groups went against one of the most fundamental principles of medical ethics. Nonetheless, state and local societies began excluding homeopaths from membership, and in some instances they rigidly insisted upon adherence to the consultation clause. Fortunately for the homeopaths, exclusion from the relatively weak state and local medical societies of that era was no major blow. In New York, for example, where homeopathy was quite strong and where the state society in 1882 rejected the AMA's code of ethics, the homeopaths more than held their ground.

The regulars won the first battle against the homeopaths at the beginning of the Civil War when they persuaded the Army Medical Board to deny homeopaths admission into the Army Medical Corps. The homeopaths turned to Congress but were unable to reverse the decision. The most successful tactic used by the regular physicians was to deny hospital appointments to homeopaths. The rise of urban areas with crowded slums forced civic authorities to expand existing municipal hospitals and to build new ones. As homeopaths organized their own colleges and medical societies, they began demanding equal privileges in state and municipal hospitals. As might be expected, the orthodox profession flatly refused to make any concession. When Chicago prepared to open its municipal hospital in 1857, the homeopaths applied for the right to participate in staffing the institution. Not only was their petition rejected, but they were even denied the use of hospital facilities. The same fight occurred in connection with Bellevue Hospital in New York from 1856 to 1858 and Boston City Hospital a few years later. Despite strong public support for the homeopaths in both cities, including that of Horace Greeley, editor of the New York *Tribune*, the regulars emerged victorious.[7]

The success of the orthodox physicians in keeping homeopaths out of the major hospitals led the latter to establish their own institutions, many of which compared favorably with those operated by the regulars. In the last decades of the century both groups began raising their educational standards, and in the process they started drawing together. A major factor bringing an end to the conflict between the two groups was the willingness of the homeopaths to accept the tenets of the new scientific medicine. Moreover, both groups shared a mutual concern over professional standards and a common desire to rid the profession of quacks and unqualified practitioners.

While Thomsonianism and homeopathy were the major irregular sects, they were only part of a general health reform movement in this period, one that, according to Richard H. Shryock, was "dedicated to the proposition that all men could stay well, if they would but stay away from their doctors." The eclectics, mentioned earlier, were a medical sect that relied extensively upon botanicals but that believed in formal medical education and even established their own colleges. The better eclectic schools followed the path of homeopathy and eventually either merged into orthodox medicine or simply disappeared. Arising directly out of Thomsonianism were the botanical medical schools founded by Alva Curtis, schools that heralded a movement Alex Berman has called Neo-Thomsonianism. Curtis, a chief disciple of Thomson, broke with him in 1836, and in 1839 chartered his own Botanico-Medical School in Columbus, Ohio. By the Civil War some eight of these schools were churning out students. As Thomsonianism began fading from the scene, Neo-Thomsonian medicine took its place, and Curtis's Reformed Medical Association gradually supplanted Thomson's Friendly Botanical Societies. Although the Neo-Thomsonians attempted to define their medical doctrine, it was at best pseudoscientific; and, with the advance of scientific medicine, it soon fell by the wayside. This same fate befell the other fourteen or fifteen botanic schools founded in the pre–Civil War years.[8]

A common feature of all irregular medical sects, and one shared by a good part of the public, was a strong distrust of orthodox medicine, and this widespread attitude contributed to stimulating the drives for personal hygiene during the years 1830–70. The same period witnessed a wide range of social movements affecting all aspects of society—temperance, abolition, women's rights, and health and hygiene. Although leaders in each of these reform groups tended to ride their own hobbyhorses, they and their followers gave each other mutual support. A key figure in the popular health movement was Sylvester Graham (1794–1851), whose name has since been immortalized by the Graham cracker. Graham, the son and grandson of minister-physicians, was a minister with little interest in medicine until he took up the cause of temperance. In the course of preparing a series of temperance lectures he began studying physiology, diet, personal hygiene, and other matters relating to health. Before long he became the leading exponent of a moderate way of life, one that included exercise, fresh air, cold showers, and a diet marked by coarsely ground whole wheat bread, vegetables, and fruits.[9]

Graham appeared on the scene at the right time. Excessive eating and drinking was a form of conspicuous consumption in his day, and in the rapidly growing urban slums, alcohol rather than religion was the opiate of the masses. In his call for personal hygiene, Graham was again in tune with his times. The downfall of the Roman Empire had led to a decline in both public and personal hygiene. Although public baths were revived during the Renaissance, their appearance, unfortunately, coincided with a virulent wave of syphilis that swept through Europe in the sixteenth century. To the public the connection seemed all too obvious, and the practice of bathing fell into abeyance. In the nineteenth century it was widely believed that getting wet all over was positively dangerous.

The early nineteenth-century reform movements were crusades, and Sylvester Graham preached his gospel of whole wheat grain, moderation, exercise, and hygiene with the fervor of an evangelist. He believed that personal hygiene required a sound understanding of physiological principles, and he and his disciples were staunch advocates of teaching physiology in schools and public forums. To the Grahamites cleanliness, or physiological reform, was literally equated with godliness. One adherent wrote that it was "peculiarly suited to raise man from a state of sensual degradation" to "a rational and immortal being."[10]

One last irregular medical group deserves mention, the hydropaths. Treatment of the sick or ailing by means of internal or external applications of either "pure" or mineral water is an age-old method. After a long period of desuetude, it enjoyed a revival in the eighteenth century and by the mid-nineteenth had achieved a measure of scientific status.

The water cure, as a formal medical practice, first reached America in 1843 when Joseph Shew and his wife began treating patients in their home in Manhattan. The following year Russell T. Hall opened Manhattan's second water-cure establishment, and within a few years hydropathic practitioners and institutes spread throughout the United States. Between 1843 and 1870 over two hundred hydropathic institutes were established in the United States.[11]

The reactions of two Mississippi sisters, Kitty and Penelope Hamilton, to the hydropathic treatment explains its rapid acceptance. One of them wrote of her treatment in a hydropathic institute: "It is a happy change indeed from poisonous drugs to pure cold water. Would to heaven I had come here when I was first taken sick; instead of being butchered by Pill givers. How many hours of pain and anguish I might have been spared. . . ." Both sisters mentioned that they had been given light exercises with dumbbells and skipping ropes. The restricted life of supposedly delicate upper-class females brought on many minor complaints that were often compounded by bloodletting, harsh medications, and enforced bed rest. Bathing, mild exercise, and a moderate diet in a hydropathic institute must have been a welcome change. Small wonder, as Jane B. Donegan notes, that hydropathy had a strong appeal to women. In New York City, Dr. Russell T. Trall broadened the concept of hydropathy to include the ideas of Graham and others, and by the second half of the century hydropathy, under the name of the hygienic system, had come to embrace most of the ideas of the popular health reformers.[12]

Irregular physicians and health reformers often were looked upon askance by conservative laymen, and they encountered strong opposition from the regular medical profession. They were guilty of excesses, exaggerations, and false attributions of disease. And some of their practices, such as the excessive use of enemas, were dangerous. Yet in the long run, with the assistance of science, many of the health reformers' ideas carried the day. While continuing to denounce the irregulars and health faddists, the medical profession gradually accepted some of their principles. Medical practice was moderated and preventive medicine in the form of exercise and sound diet became a principle of orthodox medicine. The public too has accepted the basic ideas of the health reformers. Over twenty years ago Richard Shryock wrote that "the bathroom has become the very symbol of American civilization."[13] And today the thousands of Americans patronizing natural food stores, faithfully performing their daily jogging, or doggedly exercising in health clubs, schools, or in their homes to televised instructions all bear testimony to the success of the health reformers.

A fact frequently overlooked is that in any day and age a good part of medical practice falls into the categories of folk medicine, self-medication, and quackery. For the vast majority of people, sickness represents a serious economic threat, and the first impulse is to try a folk or proprietary medicine or some home remedy. In rural areas individuals with a knowledge of local herbals have always found their services in demand and their prestige increased by any minor successes in dealing with human or animal ailments. Men with a degree of tactile sensitivity and manual dexterity often acquired a reputation for their skill in bonesetting, and older women with a little practical experience established themselves as midwives. Since childbirth is a natural process and most illnesses are self-limiting, purported healers of all types had little difficulty in gaining credibility. As with physicians, those whom they cured remained to praise them, and their failures were in no condition to complain.

For much of American history midwives handled far more than obstetrical services. Midwives landed with the first settlers and handled nearly all obstetrical work. In addition they served as nurses and pediatricians, treated their friends and neighbors for medical problems, and helped lay out the dead. Such training as they had was largely folklore, passed on from generation to generation, and the quality of care provided depended largely on the intelligence and common sense of the individual midwife. The first formal training for midwives was a course offered by William Shippen, who had spent three years in London working with the celebrated English obstetrician William Hunter. In the early 1760s Shippen offered a course in midwifery for medical students and prospective midwives. As medical education became formalized and as women were excluded from medical schools, no subsequent provision was made for training midwives.[14]

Typical of one of the better midwives was the career of Martha Ballard, a midwife who recorded 814 deliveries between 1785 and 1812. During three weeks of August 1787, she performed three deliveries, made sixteen medical calls, prepared three bodies for burial, dispensed pills and herbs, and doctored her husband's throat. As Laurel T. Ulrich points out, individuals such as Ballard, who were much more than midwives, defy all customary classifications. They were part of the network of women who gave caring support during childbirth, but they also served as physicians, pharmacists, and morticians. By the late eighteenth century, upper-class women began using the services of male physicians, although they were typically called only when complications developed. As the reliance on physicians became more common, midwives lost their middle- and upper-class patients, and the failure of efforts to provide midwives with formal training insured a victory for man-midwifery.[15]

In Europe most midwives, herbalists, and bonesetters were the product of generations of folk practitioners. Many of these folk doctors crossed the Atlantic, but mobility, social fluidity, and the newness of the American frontier opened the way for anyone interested in medicine to claim a special proficiency in the field. The early newspapers abound with notices from a wide variety of empirics. Among the announcements in the *Daily Pittsburgh Gazette* in the late 1830s was one for Waterman Sweet, a "Natural Bonesetter," and another for E. Warner, described as an "Old Indian Physician" who had practiced in the city for ten years.[16] Indian medicine shows selling nature's remedies were a common feature of state fairs and other gatherings, and the theme of nature's remedy still survives in modern advertising for proprietary medicines.

From folk remedies to proprietary drugs was a fairly easy step once newspapers and magazines became common and advertising relatively cheap. In the colonial period Widow Read, the mother-in-law of Benjamin Franklin, advertised her ointment for the itch that cured quickly and was safe to use even on sucking infants. In Charleston certain "Dutch Ladies" publicized their "Choice Cure for the Flux, Fevers, Worms, and bad Stomach, [and] Pains in the Head."[17] A number of individuals sought to capitalize on family remedies; others were more interested in exploiting human suffering. In the nineteenth century the state of medicine permitted drug manufacturers to secure the endorsement of their product by physicians or clergymen, and proprietary tonics and other remedies constituted a major source of advertising revenue for newspapers and periodicals.

The line between the makers of proprietary drugs and outright quacks is always a fine one. If we define a quack as someone seeking easy money through chicanery, then we stigmatize many sincere purveyors of preposterous instruments, techniques, and remedies. America's first significant quack was Dr. Elisha Perkins of Connecticut, whose interest in electricity and magnetism led him to devise his "Patent Metallic Tractor." The tractor consisted of two rods, one of brass and one of iron, with which the afflicted part of the body was stroked. Although the device brought considerable wealth to Perkins and his son, it may have led to his death. Convinced of the efficacy of his tractor, Perkins took it to New York City during a yellow fever epidemic in 1799 only to die of the fever shortly after his arrival. If chicanery be the test, then Perkins was no quack.[18] Even individuals with ignoble motives often became persuaded that their cure-all was effective because of the response of the users: their own faith; the placebo effect; the healing power of nature; and the fact that the disease was not as serious as the quack asserted.

As with proprietary drugs, quackery flourished in direct ratio to the availability of cheap newspapers and magazines. A large percentage of quack advertising related to venereal or what was termed "secret diseases." The notices usually promised an easy, painless cure and not infrequently assured husbands that they could continue to perform their marital duties without any danger to the wife. The extent to which quackery and proprietary drugs dominated advertising was made evident by a study of one 1858 New England newspaper that showed that almost a quarter of the entire paper and half of the advertising space was filled with quack advertisements.[19] The story of quackery and proprietary drugs in America is both comic and tragic, and it has been well told by James Harvey Young in his three books, *The Toadstool Millionaires*, *The Medical Messiahs*, and *American Health Quackery*.[20]

Another major source of self-medication was the multitude of medical works aimed at the large market provided by laypeople. The first few pamphlets and books were based on a genuine effort to provide useful medical information. For example, the minister-physician Thomas Thacher published his *Brief Rule* for dealing with the "Small Pocks, or Measles" in 1677 with the laudable intent of disseminating vital information. The same can be said of Cotton Mather's pamphlet on measles, which he published in 1739, and John Wesley's *Primitive Physick*, the first domestic medical book published in America and one that went through literally dozens of editions in the late eighteenth and early nineteenth centuries.[21]

Both antedating and occurring alongside the domestic medical works were the commonplace books in which husbands and wives carefully inscribed recipes for soapmaking, preserving, tanning, and curing the ailments of man and beast. Almanacs usually included medical information along with their jambalaya of miscellaneous facts, and plantation account books also recorded lists of medications. Added to these were the newspapers whose columns carried many items about purported cures and treatments. Many readers faithfully clipped these stories and pasted them in their commonplace books.

By the nineteenth century the publication of domestic medical books was a profitable business, and these publications were a major source for home treatment. A few were openly intended for laypersons, but many were ostensibly designed for the medical profession, although it is clear that their authors had a larger readership in mind. The need for simple and explicit medical books was great, since physicians whose education consisted primarily of attending one or two brief courses of lectures at a medical school were scarcely prepared to deal with patients. Most neophyte doctors had served a brief apprenticeship, but it was a rare physician who did not rely on one or more medical books until he had acquired considerable experience.[22]

James Ewell's *The Medical Companion, or Family Physician*, which was widely used in the southern states, is typical of domestic medical works. Published in 1807, it was dedicated to President Thomas Jefferson, a dedication that the president graciously acknowledged. In his preface Ewell appealed first to patriotism, declaring that most comparable books treat diseases "existing in very *foreign climates and constitutions*, which must widely differ from ours." Having disposed of his British competition, he declared the book had been written by a native of America who had practiced successfully for years in the southern states. He thought the work would be "exceedingly useful to all, but especially to those who live in the country, or who go to sea, where regular and timely assistance cannot always be obtained." The medical student, too, "whose theoretical knowledge has only prepared him to commence the arduous duties of his profession," would also benefit from it. An important section, he pointed out, was the "Materia Medica," which described "those precious simples wherewith God has graciously stored our meadows, fields, and woods, for the healing of our diseases, and rendering us happily independent of foreign medicines."[23]

The chief medical aid in the West was *Gunn's Domestic Medicine, or Poor Man's Friend*, first published in 1830, and written for the average reader. On his title page, Dr. Gunn proclaimed that his book discusses "in plain language, free from doctor's terms, the diseases of men, women, and children" and "contains descriptions of the medical herbs and roots of the United States." Since all aspects of medicine were covered, Gunn confidently assured his readers they need have no qualms about undertaking medicine or surgery. The section on the amputation of arms and legs best illustrates his direct approach. He asserted that the only difficulty is to know when to amputate—a problem, he said, that even the most skillful surgeons frequently cannot handle. Once the decision had been reached, the rest was simple; all that was needed to perform the operation was "firmness and common dexterity." The few essential instruments consisted of a large, sharp carving knife, a penknife, a carpenter's tenon, a shoemaker's crooked awl, a pair of slender pincers, and a dozen or more ligatures made of waxed thread or fine twine. With these, plus "a piece of old linen, large enough to cover the end of the stump, spread with simple ointment or lard," adhesive plaster, bandages, a sponge, and some warm water, Dr. Gunn declared, "You are now prepared fully to perform amputation; which I will so plainly explain that any man, unless he be an idiot or an absolute fool, can perform this operation." The first step consisted of laying the patient on a table covered with a blanket "with as many persons as may be necessary to hold him." The rest of the instructions are equally explicit.[24]

A third medical book worth mentioning is Dr. J. Cam Massie's *Treatise on the Eclectic Southern Practice of Medicine*, published in 1854. Massie's work reflects the rise of southern nationalist or states' rights medicine. As the South closed ranks, its physicians began asserting that southern medicine was unique, basing their arguments on the grounds that blacks were anatomically and physiologically different from whites and that the climate and environment of the South modified diseases. In consequence, physicians trained in the North and medical books written by northerners were not to be trusted in dealing with southern disorders. In his introduction, Dr. Massie printed a letter from a group of Texas physicians pointing out the need for a book "presenting the various modifications which diseases assume in Texas." Massie stressed that his book was "purely scientific" but that it was at the same time "composed in that SIMPLE and POPULAR style which renders subjects, however abstruse, comprehensible and even entertaining to the general reader."[25] He was obviously aiming for the best of both worlds, professional recognition and mass sales.

CHAPTER 7

The Foundations of American Surgery

IN SURGERY AS IN MEDICINE, America made few significant contributions in the antebellum years. At the same time it produced many first-rate surgeons, most of whom practiced in the major urban centers. Surgery in the early nineteenth century was still considered part of the doctor's work, although as the century advanced physicians with the talent and inclination began to concentrate on surgical procedures. In Boston, New York, Philadelphia, and New Orleans, where ample hospital facilities and an abundance of clinical material existed, the level of surgery was equal to, or not far behind, that of the British and Continental centers. American students visiting Paris and London observed the work of such great French surgeons as A.-A.-L.-M. Velpeau and G. Dupuytren and the English surgeons John Hunter and Astley Cooper, and they brought their innovations and techniques to America. Thus American surgery benefited from both European developments and its own contributions.

In the opening years of the American nation surgery was still concerned primarily with ulcers and abscesses, gunshot wounds, injuries of all types, the treatment of fractures and hernias, extracting teeth, amputations, and difficult obstetrical cases. The more able operators cut for the stone, removed cancerous breasts and other more obvious cancers, and ligated aneurysms. Pain was inevitable, and operations were performed with little regard for hygienic considerations. If shock and hemorrhage did not kill the patient, the individual's chances of developing septicemia or gangrene were extremely high. Surgery was always a grim and bloody business, and the dread of surgery carried over to the image of the surgeon. Of necessity he had to be a strong, fast, forceful operator, relatively inured to the screams and struggles of the patient. In the early nineteenth century, surgeons took a measure of pride in their coats stiff with blood and pus, considering them evidence of their experience. The catlin, scalpel, or other instrument was often wiped on the surgeon's coat sleeve before and after cutting into the patient, and sutures were frequently wrapped around a coat button or occasionally held between the teeth of the operator. Lacking an understanding of germs or infection, surgeons used any convenient method for solving emergencies. Reporting in the *Boston Medical and Surgical Journal* in 1833, a surgeon described his difficulty in removing a uterine tumor. Having cut away a section of it, "the remaining part could not be separated from the uterus as a distinct substance; still as it was not supplied with nerves, the great part was torn off by the finger nail."[1] Regrettably, the patient died.

During the first two centuries of American history, surgery was performed in the patient's home or physician's office. The first surgical amphitheater in America was constructed by the New York Hospital in 1803 and the second by the Pennsylvania Hospital in 1804. The name "amphitheater" was well chosen, since operations were invariably public spectacles. Medical students and the public used to fill the surgical amphitheaters when popular surgeons were performing, often crowding around the operating table itself. When surgery was done at home or in the doctor's office, relatives and friends gathered round to help hold the patient or merely to watch. Considering the number of individuals in street clothing jamming into the operating area and the lack of hygienic precautions by the surgeons, the wonder is not that so many patients died in the pre-aseptic era, but that so many survived.

Major surgical procedures were invariably a last resort, and only acute pain, discomfort, and fear could force patients to place themselves in the hands of the surgeon. Some of the prominent surgeons who operated before large crowds required the patient to commit himself to surgery the night before, and then kept him locked in his room until time for the operation. One can only imagine the fears of a candidate for surgery as he listened to the screams coming from the operating room and was then hustled from his room into the amphitheater by two husky attendants. Here his first glimpse would be the glowing brazier heating up the cauterizing irons, and the bloodstained surgeon and his assistants. Small wonder that many patients were too terrified to move or utter a sound, a few bolted for safety, often with the surgeon and his crew in hot pursuit, and others begged to be allowed to forego the operation. In 1847 Valentine Mott, a famous New York surgeon, commented upon the inevitable relationship between pain and surgery. It was commonplace, he wrote, to see "individuals praying in mercy that we would stop, that we would finish, thus imploring and menacing us, and who would not fail to escape if they were not firmly secured." He concluded that "*to avoid pain* in operation is a chimera that we can no longer pursue in our times."[2] Ironically, even as Dr. Mott was despairing of relieving the agony caused by surgery, the introduction of chemical anesthesia was soon to eliminate the grim picture he had drawn.

Before moving to the discovery of anesthesia, it might be well to look briefly at some of the more important American surgeons. Despite what appears to be the relative crudeness of operating conditions and techniques, intelligent and able men were performing innovative and occasionally delicate procedures. The results were not always favorable, for few patients would submit to the knife until their diseases were well along. Nonetheless, lives were saved, and the experience gained helped pave the way for restoring to health countless other individuals.

Surgery in America as a specialized area dates back to Dr. Philip Syng Physick (1768–1837), a professor in the University of Pennsylvania who was appointed to the chair of surgery in 1805, the first such position in an American medical school. Physick was no Antyllus or Paré, but he was a first-rate teacher, a fine operator, and the best-known American surgeon of his day. He was famous for his lithotomies (removal of bladder stones), and his success in removing over a thousand of them from Chief Justice John Marshall firmly established his reputation. Physick is also known for his introduction of buckskin sutures, and for his improvements in the design of surgical instruments. He devised an instrument for tonsillectomies, another for paracentesis (surgical puncture of a body cavity for drainage), and a precursor of the stomach pump.[3]

Insofar as vascular surgery was concerned, aneurysms, caused by syphilis, trauma, or cancer, were the major occasions for surgical intervention, and the operations consisted largely of ligating or tying off major arteries. Here again there are dozens of "firsts," but several outstanding surgeons deserve to be mentioned. Dr. Wright Post (1766–

1822) of Long Island, New York, was one of the earliest American surgeons to tackle vascular problems. He was probably the first to ligate the femoral artery successfully (1796) and the second American to ligate the external iliac (1814). Valentine Mott (1785–1865) of New York City was a student of the famous English surgeon Astley Cooper and, like his mentor, ranks as one of the great pioneers in vascular surgery. In the course of his long career he performed literally dozens of operations involving nearly all the major arteries. His boldness and daring and the degree of success he obtained are all the more remarkable since most of his surgery was performed in the days before anesthesia and antisepsis. A third major figure in vascular surgery was Dr. Warren Stone of New Orleans (1808–72), possibly the top-ranking surgeon in the South. In the 1850s Stone treated two cases of gluteal aneurysms by open incision, a procedure that was both bold and risky at that time. He was also the first to use silver wire for ligating arteries and to insist that the ligature should be tied only tight enough to stop the flow of blood. This latter procedure was designed to avoid the secondary hemorrhage that occurred when the usual ligatures cut their way through the artery. Stone, as with other surgeons of his day, performed a wide range of surgical procedures and was also considered an outstanding physician.

A simple listing of names and surgical accomplishments fails to re-create the milieu in which this work was done, and for this one must turn to contemporary accounts. A newspaper description of an operation performed in New Orleans during the mid-1830s by Dr. Charles A. Luzenberg, a highly skilled surgeon, presents a good picture of American surgery. Luzenberg had just returned from observing surgery in Europe during 1832 and was putting his newly acquired knowledge to work. The operation consisted of "tying the carotid artery and extirpating a sarcomatous parotid gland, involving the ear and a large portion of the integuments of the cheek and neck" on a sixty-two-year-old male. A number of local physicians witnessed the procedure, and the patient "sustained the operation, which was unavoidably painful and tedious, with great fortitude."[4] Here we have the classic picture of an American surgeon trained in Europe performing a long and complicated operation without benefit of anesthesia upon a patient for whom surgery was obviously a dire necessity.

A more vivid account was written by a correspondent for *Harper's Weekly* in 1859. At that time New Orleans had two medical schools with a combined enrollment of over six hundred students, and the surgical amphitheater in Charity Hospital was always crowded when a popular professor was operating. The journalist wrote:

> One of the most exciting spectacles to be witnessed in the institution [Charity] is seen when fifty or a hundred students crowd the couch of some patient who is about to undergo an important surgical operation. The trembling expectancy of the terrified subject, the nervous pallor of the medical tyros, who are about to see a man's leg or arm whipped off for the first time; the careless nonchalance of the hospital habitués; the giant form of that veteran man of the knife, Dr. Stone, as with cuffs thrown back, eyes all ablaze, his lips firmly clenched, he prepares to make the adroit thrust; the quick prefatory whirl of the well-grasped blade; the sudden flash of polished steel; the dull, muffled sound of the yielding flesh, the spirt [*sic*] of blood, the scrape of the keen edge upon the solid bone, the sharp cry of the patient, followed by the heavy moan of pain — these are the outlines of a picture that thrills and terrifies the uninitiated beholder.[5]

Stone, a powerfully built individual, possessed the physical strength, audacity, and dexterity that were so essential to a surgeon, and he may well stand as a symbol of surgery in the first half of the nineteenth century.

Obstetrics and Gynecology

The operative field in which America made its greatest contribution was obstetrics and gynecology. Unlike developments in general surgery, which were associated with hospitals and medical centers, the innovations in this field were made by bold, resolute individuals impelled by circumstances to make grave decisions. Nearly all of them practiced in relative isolation — either on the frontier or in rural areas. It is possible that their isolation was an advantage, since they were less likely to have been deterred by traditional beliefs as to what was and was not possible or to have been restrained by the advice of older, more experienced and more cautious heads. Yet the men who made the greatest contributions were in no sense apprentice-trained empirics with little knowledge of medicine. As will be seen, both Ephraim McDowell and J. Marion Sims received excellent medical training for their day, McDowell in America and Great Britain and Sims in the United States.

Although surgical invasion of the peritoneal cavity was considered a virtual death warrant for the patient, American physicians successfully ventured into this area quite early. Dr. John Bard of New Jersey reported three cases of laparotomies for extrauterine pregnancy in 1759, and this same operation was performed by Dr. Charles McKnight of New York in 1790. William Baynham of Virginia also operated for extrauterine pregnancy in 1791 and 1799.[6] While these operations speak well for the courage and ability of American surgeons, they were in no sense landmarks. The making of gynecological history was left for Ephraim McDowell.

Ephraim McDowell (1771–1830) was born in Virginia but moved with his family to Kentucky in 1784, settling in the small frontier town of Danville. After finishing secondary school, Ephraim elected to study medicine, first under the preceptorship of Dr. Alexander Humphreys, and later by attending lectures at the University of Edinburgh. While attending the university in the years 1793–94, he was influenced by one of the outstanding professors, Dr. John Bell. Returning to Danville in 1795, McDowell quickly established a reputation as the best surgeon west of Philadelphia, but his opportunity to gain fame did not come until 1809 when he was called as a consultant by two physicians attending a patient they thought was slow in delivering twins.

According to McDowell's own account, on examining the patient he discovered immediately that she had a large tumor. He explained the situation, warning her that four of the best surgeons in England and Scotland had asserted that the danger from peritoneal inflammation was so great "that opening the abdomen to extract the tumor was inevitable death." If she was prepared to die and was willing to come to Danville, he would remove the tumor. The patient, Mrs. Jane Todd Crawford, demonstrating even greater courage than her surgeon, unhesitatingly made the sixty-mile journey on horseback in the middle of winter, resting the enormous tumor on the pommel of the saddle. With a minimum of preparation and assisted by his nephew, who had studied medicine in Philadelphia, and by a young apprentice, McDowell began the operation. While the patient lay on a table reciting psalms, the abdomen was laid open, the tube ligated, and the diseased ovary, weighing almost twenty pounds, was removed. As soon as the incision was made, the intestines fell out on the table, remaining there for about thirty minutes. It was Christmas Day, McDowell wrote, and "they became so cold that I thought proper to bathe them in tepid water previous to my replacement." He then pushed the intestines back into the abdomen, sutured the incision, and put the patient to bed. Five days later, on looking in on her, he found Mrs. Crawford making her own bed. Twenty-five days after the operation, she drove home, to live for another thirty-one years.

In 1813 and 1816 McDowell again successfully removed ovarian cysts. Following the third operation, he published an account of the three cases, but his article encountered disbelief and was dismissed. In 1819 he described two more successful cases, and this time his work began to achieve some notice. It was not, however, until a letter he had sent to Dr. John Bell in 1817 was finally published in the *Edinburgh Medical and Surgical Journal* in 1824 that McDowell finally achieved the recognition he deserved. By the end of his career, he had performed twelve or thirteen ovariotomies with the loss of only one patient—a remarkable record for that date. In 1830 he suffered an attack of what was called inflammatory fever. The onset was characterized by an acute attack of pain and nausea followed by fever. Ironically, it is not unlikely that this pioneer in abdominal surgery died of acute appendicitis.[7]

An intriguing sequel to McDowell's success, and one that may have been far more typical of early nineteenth-century surgery, was the first ovariotomy attempted in Tennessee. In 1818 Dr. James Overton diagnosed a case of ovarian tumor and gained the patient's consent to operate. Delighted at the opportunity to demonstrate his skill, Dr. Overton decided to operate on a pillowed table out in the open in front of the patient's home. In full view of a large crowd, he made his incision, exposing the smooth surface of an unusually large tumor. Before he could make a further incision, some irregular movements in the tumor caused him and his assistant to quickly close the abdomen. A few days later the patient gave birth to a healthy child. Although the case cost Dr. Overton his medical career, he apparently did not lose his sense of humor. He subsequently informed a colleague: "I did not retire from the practice of medicine, I was victorious in defeat. The practice retired from me and left me in triumphant possession of the field."[8]

The second American to achieve international fame in the area of gynecology and obstetrics was another small-town southern practitioner, J. Marion Sims (1813–83). Sims's father was a minor local official in Lancaster County, South Carolina, who had visions of his son's becoming a lawyer. But Marion decided to study medicine, and his father, in reluctantly agreeing, made a most revealing comment upon the status of the medical profession: "Well, I suppose I can not control you; but it is a profession for which I have the utmost contempt. There is no science in it. There is no honor to be achieved in it; no reputation to be made. . . ." He then concluded: "and to think that *my* son should be going around from house to house through this country, with a box of pills in one hand and a squirt in the other . . . is a thought I never supposed I should have to contemplate."[9]

As was the case with McDowell, Sims's medical education compared favorably with that of most of his colleagues. It consisted of a brief stint as an apprentice, a session as a student at the Charleston Medical School, and another one at the Jefferson Medical College in Philadelphia, an institution that attracted students from all over the South. Upon graduation from the latter, Sims still felt incompetent to start a practice, and he consequently enrolled in a month's course of private lectures offered by one of the professors. The lectures turned out to be on the subject of regional and surgical anatomy. Commenting upon them, Sims later wrote that he knew a great deal about dissection but absolutely nothing about the practice of medicine. After a shaky start, he managed to acquire a good reputation as a physician in the little town of Mt. Meigs, Alabama. Just as he was becoming well established and his practice was flourishing, a severe attack of malaria forced him to move to Montgomery, the capital of the state. Here he quickly gained recognition as an excellent physician and an outstanding surgeon. Discovering he had an unusual aptitude for surgery, he began concentrating in this area, and successfully treated a wide variety of conditions, including clubfoot, strabismus, and harelip.

After about ten years of practice, he was called in consultation to help with a seventeen-year-old slave girl who had been in labor for seventy-two hours. The child's head was impacted in the pelvis, and, although Sims successfully delivered the child with forceps, so much damage was done that the patient, named Anarcha, was left with complete urinary and rectal incontinence. Touched by her tragic condition, he went home and explored the literature, only to find that the condition was considered hopeless. Shortly thereafter he encountered two similar cases of vesicovaginal fistula in slave women, and in both instances informed their masters he could do nothing. While he was still pondering about these unfortunate women, he was summoned to attend a large white woman who had fallen from a pony and suffered a retroversion of the uterus. In trying to correct the situation, he placed the patient on her knees and elbows. While trying to push the uterus into place manually, he turned his hand in the vagina, and the uterus suddenly disappeared from his touch. The patient expressed immediate relief, but as she lay down, there was a sudden sound caused by the passage of air. The patient was embarrassed, but Sims quickly realized what had happened. In moving his hand, he had allowed air to enter the vagina, and the normal atmospheric pressure had pushed the uterus back into position.

He realized that if he could place one of his vesicovaginal patients in a knee-elbow position, dilate her vagina with normal air pressure, and use some type of speculum, it would be possible to see the extent of the damage and to devise some means for correcting it. One of the patients was still in Sims's small eight-bed clinic waiting to be sent home. Calling on his two medical students to help him, Sims placed her in position and tried the experiment. "Introducing the bent handle of a spoon," he wrote, "I saw everything, as no man has ever seen before. The fistula was as plain as the nose on a man's face."

For the next four years, Sims was to devote most of his energy, effort, and income to a long series of operations on women — all of them slaves — suffering from this condition. The first almost led to the death of the patient, but Sims persisted, gradually gaining more and more experience. Finally, after four years of experimentation, he operated for the thirtieth time on Anarcha, and successfully closed the fistula. Sims then operated on the other two women and quickly restored them to health, demonstrating conclusively that he had devised an effective method for treating this horrible condition. In order to win his victory during the four-year battle, Sims had had to discover the knee-elbow position, devise a special curved speculum (Sims's speculum), make a new catheter to keep the bladder empty while the fistula was healing, and, finally, learn to avoid sepsis by the use of silver sutures. In the process he had to develop new techniques and improve his own skill as a surgeon.[10]

Dr. Sims was a man of perseverance, dedication, and remarkable ingenuity, and he deserves great credit. In his zeal to solve this particular medical problem, he sacrificed a good part of his medical practice, maintained six or seven stricken women slaves at his own expense, and devoted several years to the project. His neglect of private practice caused problems with his family, but he resolutely continued along his chosen course. Note, however, that had Sims not lived in the South where slaves were available to him, his "experiments" would not have been undertaken. These repeated operations were performed for the large part without anesthesia and must have caused considerable suffering. It is highly unlikely that any surgeon, northern or southern, would have experimented on white women in such a way, nor that the patients themselves would have submitted to such a lengthy ordeal, one extending over several years.

Sims's major breakthrough in gynecology did not bring him immediate fame. A few weeks after his first successful operations, a severe attack of diarrhea prostrated him, and the disorder continued to flare up. Despairing of a cure and feeling his life was in danger from the climate, he once again broke up his home and practice, and in 1852 moved his family to New York City. About this time, convinced that he was dying from his disease, he published an account of his operation in the *American Journal of Medical Sciences.* In ill health and with only limited funds, Sims had difficulty establishing his practice in New York. His career took a turn for the better when in 1855, with the aid of friends, he established the Women's Hospital of the State of New York. As head physician, he was given ample opportunity to operate and soon earned an outstanding reputation as a surgeon and gynecologist.

The rest of Sims's career was a happy and productive one. The honors he received in Europe, where he lived during the Civil War, strengthened his position in America, and henceforth he divided his time between the two continents. While the operative procedure for vesicovaginal fistulas was his major contribution, in later years he devised methods for amputating the cervix uteri, clearly described the symptom complex of vaginitis, pioneered in gallbladder surgery, and published a classic work on the problems of abdominal surgery.

The Cesarean Section

The cesarean section, as its name implies, has a long history, but it was still a rare operation until well into the nineteenth century. During the medieval period it was occasionally used as a postmortem method for saving the child. The idea of operating on the live mother was revived in the seventeenth century, although only the boldest and most skillful of operators were willing to attempt it. In the late eighteenth century a bitter quarrel developed between Jean Louis Baudelocque, the elder, the inventor of the pelvimeter and the father of obstetric pelvimetry, and the supporters of the symphyseotomy, an operation that consisted of enlarging the diameter of the pelvis by dividing the cartilage connecting the pelvic bones. The latter was, and still is, a complicated and dangerous operation. Fortunately a number of successful cesarean sections by French surgeons during this period swung the tide in favor of the cesarean.

While all this seems a little far removed from American medicine, these events had a direct bearing on developments in early nineteenth-century Louisiana, where French-trained surgeons performed a series of cesarean sections. The man who introduced this operation into Louisiana was François Marie Prevost (1771–1842), who was born in France and studied medicine in Paris during the French Revolution. His student days in Paris coincided with the clash between Baudelocque, who was elected professor and chief surgeon-accoucheur at the Maternité in 1794, and his rivals, and Prevost may well have heard the arguments put forward as to the relative merits of the two obstetrical procedures. We know little of Prevost's earliest medical career, but by 1800 he was serving as an Officier de Santé in Haiti. The great slave insurrection there forced him to flee to Louisiana, where he settled near Donaldsonville. Although a small town in rural Ascension Parish, Donaldsonville had several French surgeons, all of whom had been trained in France, and at least two of whom had served for many years in Napoleon's armies. Hence Prevost was familiar with contemporary developments in medicine and surgery and had the encouragement of able colleagues.

Reflecting inadequate diet and other conditions, cases of pelvic deformity were not uncommon in the nineteenth century, and slave women in the South were particularly affected. While midwives handled most normal obstetrical cases, in difficult deliveries physicians and surgeons were usually called in, and Prevost, along with his colleagues, must have seen many young mothers labor in suffering and agony for days before succumbing to pain and exhaustion. Sometime between 1820 and 1825 Prevost was faced with the decision of what to do with a slave woman who was unable to deliver normally. We might even wonder how many of these cases he had already seen and what it was that led him on this occasion to accept the radical step of performing a cesarean section. Whatever the case, he performed the operation and saved both mother and child. When the mother became pregnant once more, Prevost again delivered the child by a cesarean section. In

1825 he performed a third cesarean section upon another slave, but on this occasion, although he saved the child, the mother died.

It is possible that some other Louisiana surgeon may have preceded Prevost in delivering by cesarean section. Early in 1824 a St. Francisville, Louisiana, newspaper published a medical fee bill signed by fifteen physicians and surgeons, all of whose names indicate a British origin. The lengthy fee bill included some 160 items. Of the several fees relating to parturition, the most expensive one was simply listed as "Cesarean." [11] Presumably at least some of these surgeons were prepared to perform a cesarean section if necessary. Yet physicians and surgeons in those days frequently sought to build their reputations by offering to do far more than they intended (or were capable of), and there is no evidence that the cesarean section was ever performed in the St. Francisville area.

Stimulated by Prevost's success, a number of physicians performed cesarean sections in Louisiana in the ensuing years. A compilation of all such surgical procedures in the United States between 1822 and 1877 made by Dr. Robert P. Harris showed a total of 79. Of these, 15 were performed in Louisiana between 1822 and 1861. Both Dr. Harris, who published his findings in 1878, and Dr. Rudolph Matas, who confirmed them over sixty years later, commented on the relatively high degree of success obtained by Louisiana physicians. The 15 Louisiana operations resulted in saving 11 mothers and 8 children, a high recovery rate that is all the more surprising since the evidence indicates that none of these early operators practiced uterine suture. As Dr. Matas wrote, they followed the traditional practice and left the healing of the uterine incision to the unaided "efforts of Nature." [12]

It is worth noting, as was true of Sims's attempts to deal with vesicovaginal fistulas, that all the early cesarean sections in Louisiana were performed on slave women. The usual practice in cases where the pelvis was deformed or too small was to resort to craniotomy, destroying the head of the baby in order to facilitate delivery. The fear of abdominal incisions was so great that it was generally considered better to kill the child than risk the life of the mother. Since opening the abdomen amounted to a death warrant, it is more than a coincidence that so many of these early patients were slaves, and clearly indicates that surgeons and physicians were far more willing to try new procedures on slaves than on white women.

The second American physician to perform a cesarean section was

Dr. John Lambert Richmond. A typical product of the West, Richmond had worked at various jobs before becoming a Baptist minister and then a janitor in the Medical College of Ohio. Taking advantage of the opportunity, he enrolled in the school and was graduated as a physician. With this degree, he was, like the colonial preachers, able to minister to both the physical and spiritual wants of his congregation. While preaching in a small town not far from Cincinnati in April 1827, he learned that a woman across the Little Miami River had been in labor for thirty hours and was about to die from repeated convulsions. A storm was in progress with gusting high winds, but he crossed the river, examined the patient, a large black woman pregnant with her first child, and decided to take the baby by cesarean section. In his report on the operation three years later he stated that he began operating at one o'clock at night with "only a case of common pocket instruments." The wind was blowing directly through the unchinked walls of the log cabin so that his assistants had to hold up blankets to stop the drafts from blowing out the candles. Despite these handicaps, he was able to save the mother, but not the child.[13]

The circumstances that led Prevost and Richmond to resort to a cesarean section must have recurred many times on the American frontier. One can only wonder how many other American physicians confronted with similar emergency obstetrical situations dealt with the crisis in the same fashion. Each of the early operators waited several years before informing his colleagues or publishing a report of his surgical procedures. America was primarily rural, and a good part of it was still frontier. Moreover, isolation and the relatively low educational standards among American doctors were scarcely conducive to reporting case histories. In any event, by 1830 the American medical profession was beginning to learn that the cesarean section could be performed successfully. Yet while the work of Prevost and Richmond may have inaugurated a new era for the cesarean section, the operation remained a rarity until well past the Civil War. Most physicians, when faced with the decision, preferred the safer course of craniotomy.

William Beaumont and the Physiology of Digestion

In terms of international recognition as an original contributor to medical science, the American who ranks with J. Marion Sims in the nineteenth century was an obscure army surgeon who, when a remarkable opportunity was presented to him, had the initiative and intelligence to seize upon it. William Beaumont (1785–1853) was born in Connecticut, acquired a medical education through an apprenticeship, and, after gaining a medical license in Vermont, enlisted as a surgeon in the army in 1812. After serving honorably during the War of 1812, he returned to private practice and business until 1819 when a former comrade persuaded him to reenlist. Beaumont was ordered to Fort Michilimackinac, located on an island between Lake Huron and Lake Michigan.

In June 1822 Beaumont was summoned to attend a French-Canadian trapper who had been hit in the side by an accidental shotgun blast at close range. The victim, Alexis St. Martin, was horribly mangled; his chest was torn open; the left lower lung, the diaphragm, and the stomach badly lacerated; and the flesh burned to a crisp. Mixed in with blood, bone splinters, lead shot, wadding, and bits of clothing were the contents of the stomach. Serious stomach wounds were invariably considered fatal, and to Beaumont the case was clearly hopeless. Nonetheless, he cleaned and dressed the wound as best he could and tried to make the patient comfortable. Almost miraculously, St. Martin survived, but his recovery was long and slow. After a year under military care the wound was still open and a gastric fistula refused to close. The military authorities felt they had done enough for him and decided to ship him back to Canada. Beaumont, realizing that the journey would probably be fatal for a man in St. Martin's condition, remonstrated, and when this failed he took the man into his own home. Here for two years he nursed and cared for his patient, who slowly gained strength. Although the wound healed, St. Martin was left with a permanent gastric fistula.

The nature of digestion at that time was only vaguely understood. The seventeenth century had produced two schools of thought about it. One, the iatrophysical group, argued that digestion was a mechanical process in which the churning action of the stomach broke down food. Another, the iatrochemical school, maintained that the process was essentially a chemical one. By the eighteenth century it was recognized that the stomach produced some type of fluid that prevented fermentation and was capable of dissolving food. In the early nineteenth century, experimental physiologists were beginning to feed sample foods to animals, and, after a short period, kill and dissect them to see what had happened to the food. In other experiments animals were forced or induced to swallow sponges on a string in order to retrieve some of the gastric juice. Beaumont saw that the gastric fistula gave him easy access to St. Martin's stomach, and he realized that here was an opportunity to determine precisely how the stomach functioned.

The fistula opened just below the left nipple, making it possible for Beaumont to look directly into the stomach. In giving St. Martin the usual purges that were basic to nearly all medical treatment, Beaumont wrote that he gave them "as never medicine was before administered to man since the creation of the world—to wit, by pouring it through the ribs at the puncture of the stomach." He found that he could pour water directly into the stomach with a funnel, or spoon in food and then draw the contents of the stomach back out with a syphon. He began experimenting with pieces of meat and other food items that he would tie on a string and suspend in the stomach for varying time periods. He was thus able to ascertain precisely how long it took to digest a particular food item and to determine what the gastric juice did to each of them.[14] St. Martin obviously derived little intellectual pleasure from the experiments, and understandably he was a most unenthusiastic human guinea pig. He constantly objected to the experiments and occasionally disappeared. In 1825 he apparently left for good, leaving Beaumont with a great many questions unanswered.

Almost four years later Beaumont learned that St. Martin had returned to Canada and married. Even though the former patient now had two children, Beaumont persuaded him to return, paying all transportation costs and other expenses. The experiments were renewed in August 1829 and continued to the spring of 1831. By this time St. Martin had two more children, and Beaumont permitted him and his family to go home on condition that they would return when asked. In the fall of 1832 St. Martin reported back to Beaumont, who signed him to a contract. Early in 1834 family pressure and a strong personal distaste for his role led St. Martin to return to Canada, and nothing could be done to persuade him to resume his position as a human laboratory. The experiments apparently did him no harm, since he lived to the age of eighty-three, outliving Beaumont by well over twenty years.

By the time St. Martin returned to Canada for good, Beaumont had completed his major research, and although he would have liked to continue the experiments, he had acquired enough knowledge to provide an explanation of the basic digestive process. He had been in contact with Dr. Robley Dunglison of the University of Virginia, who made

some valuable suggestions. Dunglison, along with a colleague, also analyzed a sample of gastric juice and identified it as free hydrochloric acid.
The two men also suggested the presence of a second digestive substance, which was subsequently identified as pepsin. Chemical analysis
at this date was not capable of identifying the various substances in the
stomach juices but a start had been made. And when in 1833 Beaumont
published his classic work, *Experiments and Observations on the Gastric
Juice and the Physiology of Digestion*, the basis was laid for our present
understanding of the digestive process.[15]

Beaumont began by surveying the existing knowledge of digestion
and then gave a detailed account of some 238 experiments. He described
accurately the appearance of the mucous membrane, both normal and
pathologic, noted the movements of the stomach through the digestive process, showed that the gastric juice is secreted only when food
is present and that it contained free hydrochloric acid. His remarkable
experiments concerning the effects of gastric juice upon various foods
helped lay the basis for future dietetic studies. The work was hailed
in scientific circles and received excellent reviews, although the book
was privately published and the author received no financial benefit.
Only a thousand copies were printed, and Beaumont had difficulty in
disposing them. A subsequent German edition and one published in
England showed that European scientists appreciated his findings, but
these editions, too, provided no financial assistance to enable Beaumont
to continue his research.[16]

Beaumont had been fortunate in his army appointment since Surgeon General Joseph Lovell had given him every assistance in his
research. This happy state of affairs ended when Lovell died and was replaced by Colonel Thomas Lawson. A surgeon general with a long and
undistinguished career, Lawson saw little value in Beaumont's research
and virtually forced Beaumont out of the army in 1839.

The Discovery of Anesthesia

The greatest boon America gave to medicine was chemical
anesthesia, and its discovery clearly fits within the American empirical tradition. From earliest days mankind had sought to alleviate pain
and in the process had learned about a great many analgesics. Willow
bark, which contains salicylic acid, and a great many other herbals were
widely used for this purpose, and opium and alcohol were in common

use by the early nineteenth century. Traveling quacks and dentists knew the value of distracting the patient's mind from what was happening to him, and on a more scientific basis a few dentists and surgeons were experimenting with hypnotism, a popular fad in this period. Hypnosis, or mesmerism as it was called, was still in its infancy, and it required amenable patients and time and effort on the part of the physician or surgeon. Had chemical anesthesia not been introduced for a few more years, it is quite possible that the history of hypnotism might have been quite different. As it was, hypnotism was pushed into the background.

Inventions and discoveries usually follow when two elements exist: one, the proper technology, and two, a significant demand. On this basis anesthesia should have appeared somewhere around the beginning of the nineteenth century. By 1800 two of the three basic chemical agents had been known for many years. Although not given its present name until the eighteenth century, ether was discovered by Paracelsus in the sixteenth century, and, under the name of "sweet vitriol," may go back as far as the thirteenth century. The second agent, nitrous oxide, was discovered by Joseph Priestly in 1772. In the 1790s a series of experiments with these gases showed that both of them had the potential for relieving pain during surgery. The famous chemist Humphrey Davy began experimenting with nitrous oxide as a young surgeon's assistant, and in 1800 he published his classic work, *Researches, Chemical and Philosophical; Chiefly concerning Nitrous Oxide. . . .* In it he described how he had relieved the pain caused by an erupting wisdom tooth through inhaling nitrous oxide. Later on he wrote that since the gas "appears capable of destroying physical pain, it may probably be used with advantage during surgical operations in which no great effusion of blood takes place." A few years after this, one of Davy's students, Michael Faraday, made a number of experiments with sulfuric ether and suggested that it too might be used to ease the pain in surgery.[17]

The third of the anesthetic agents was discovered by an American chemist, physician, and farmer, Samuel Guthrie (1782–1848). Guthrie learned his medicine through an apprenticeship with his father and by attending two terms of lectures, one at the College of Physicians and Surgeons in New York City in 1810–11 and another one at the University of Pennsylvania in 1815. He settled in New York, spending most of his life in Sacketts Harbor, at that time a frontier area in the northern part of the state. He was one of those rare individuals with an inventive and practical mind. He dabbled in many areas but was intrigued by chemistry, and in the process of one of his experiments he produced what he called "chloric ether," or chloroform. Shortly thereafter the substance was discovered independently in both Germany and France.

By 1831, then, there were three chemicals available for anesthetic purposes; in effect, the technological problem had been solved. At the same time, the demands for some means to relieve pain were steadily increasing. Developments in gross and pathological anatomy and the rise of localism in medicine—the assumption that diseases were localized—were encouraging surgeons to operate more frequently and to perform longer and more complicated surgery. As surgeons became more venturesome, they naturally encountered a greater reluctance by patients to face the almost unendurable agony of a long operation. Moreover, a patient struggling and writhing in torment was scarcely a suitable subject for delicate surgical excision or repair. Hence surgeons were casting about in search of some way to ease the dreadful pain caused by the knife and the cauterizing iron. At the same time, however, surgery traditionally had been associated with pain and suffering, and any surgeon who did not quickly adapt himself to it could scarcely expect to remain in the profession. In consequence the older and experienced surgeons, as indicated by an earlier quotation from Valentine Mott, accepted pain as inevitable.

While surgical patients often submitted to the knife under the threat of death, that is, either die in pain from their disease or take a chance that the surgeon could effect a cure, the dentists were in an entirely different position. Other than babies who were often assumed to have died from "teething," nobody was believed to die from toothache. If one bore the ache long enough, the tooth would eventually rot out, and the problem would be solved. The gums and teeth are extremely sensitive, and as dentists made the transition from itinerant tooth-pullers to a professional class, the need to ease pain was even more important than in surgery. The aching tooth could be borne, whereas the spreading cancer, the growing pulsating aneurysm, and the urinary calculi blocking the urethra forced their victims to turn to the surgeon. An equally important consideration was that the dentist hoped to see his patient many times, whereas the surgeon rarely expected to see his patient again.

In the eighteenth century France and England held leadership in dentistry, but by the next century American technical skill and mechanical ingenuity enabled the United States to forge ahead. At first training was largely empirical or gained through an apprenticeship, and it was not until 1825 that the first formal lectures in dentistry were offered in the medical school of the University of Baltimore by Professor Horace H. Hayden. In 1840 Hayden joined with several other dentists to organize the first American dental school, the Baltimore College of Dental Surgery. This same year saw the establishment of the American Society of Dental Surgeons, the first attempt by a professional group to create a national organization. By more than a coincidence it was about this time that a number of dentists began experimenting with methods to eliminate or reduce pain during dental surgery.[18]

Precisely at the time when surgeons and dentists were becoming more concerned over the problem of pain, nitrous oxide and ether were becoming easy to obtain, and one of the fads that swept the country in the second quarter of the century was the so-called "laughing gas" party. Medical and chemistry students first began inhaling ether or nitrous oxide at social gatherings, and as news of the euphoric effects spread, "laughing gas" parties or "ether frolics" became quite popular among middle- and upper-class groups. On many occasions individuals hurt themselves stumbling around under the influence of one of the gases and were not aware of it until the effects wore off. Considering how frequently this fact was reported, it is surprising that it took so long to apply this observation to the relief of surgical patients.

Beginning in the early 1840s a number of dentists and one surgeon began experimenting with ether and nitrous oxide. As with many advances, it is impossible to give exclusive credit to any one individual for discovering anesthesia. Possibly the first man to administer ether as an anesthetic was William E. Clarke. In January 1842 he gave ether to a patient while her tooth was being extracted by a dentist, Dr. Elijah Pope.[19] Unfortunately, neither Clarke nor Pope realized the significance of what they had done, and so they receive only brief mention by historians.

Without question the first individual to use ether as a surgical anesthetic was Dr. Crawford W. Long (1815–78) of Jefferson, Georgia. Long was a relatively well educated physician. He had graduated with honor from Franklin Academy, the forerunner of the University of Georgia, had attended the Medical Department of Transylvania University in Lexington, Kentucky, and then had transferred to the University of Pennsylvania, where he took his medical degree in 1839. Following this he spent some eighteen months "walking the hospitals" in New York City. He returned to Georgia in 1841 and settled in the small town of Jefferson. As a medical student he had participated in the ether and "laughing gas" parties and, stimulated by the appearance of an itinerant showman who demonstrated ether's properties in his performance, he introduced ether parties to the town of Jefferson. During these parties, Long observed how individuals became insensitive to pain while under the influence of the gas, and he decided to apply this observation to his surgical practice. On March 30, 1842, he removed a small wen or tumor from the neck of one James Venable while the patient was under the influence of ether. A month or two later he excised a second tumor from Venable's neck under similar circumstances. In July of that same year he amputated the toe of a young black boy using the same painless method. In the next three years he performed three more operations using ether as an anesthetic.

Unfortunately for Dr. Long's fame as an innovator, he did not report any of his operations until 1849, over three years after the first public demonstration of surgical anesthesia by Morton and Warren. As a well-educated physician, Long should have realized the significance of his discovery. On the other hand, he lived in a relatively isolated area, and he may well have felt that reports of minor surgery performed by a rural physician would received little credence in sophisticated medical circles. Furthermore, as a physician in a sparsely settled area, his opportunities to perform surgery were limited, and he may have been waiting to compile more evidence before publicizing his work. Long himself made this argument, when he wrote later that mesmerism was gaining advocates in Georgia at the time of his experiments with ether and that he wanted to perform enough experiments to be sure that his success with ether was not the result of the patients' imagination. It is clear that he used ether for anesthetic purposes at least six times before Morton's demonstration in 1846. With this much experience, why he did not report his work to one of the medical journals is difficult to say, but his failure to do so places him in a category with Clarke and Pope.[20]

The next character in what was to become a tragic quest for the credit of discovering anesthesia was Dr. Horace Wells, a leading dentist in Hartford, Connecticut. Wells may have become interested in the effects of nitrous oxide as early as 1840, but he was stirred to action on witnessing a demonstration in December 1844 by a popular lecturer, Gardner Q. Colton. Wells noted that a member of the audience who volunteered to take the gas injured his leg while jumping around, yet showed no evidence of having felt pain. Wells, who needed one of his own teeth extracted, talked to Colton after the performance and asked about the possibility of using gas in the procedure. The upshot was that Colton came to Wells's office and administered nitrous oxide while an associate of Wells, Dr. John M. Riggs, removed the molar. Wells was delighted that he felt no pain and had Colton show him how to manufacture and administer the gas. After successfully using anesthesia to extract several teeth, early in 1845 Wells went to Boston and through his former partner, Dr. William Thomas Green Morton, was given an opportunity to demonstrate his method before Dr. John C. Warren's medical class. For one reason or another, the patient yelled when the tooth was extracted, and the medical students booed and hissed, causing Wells to retire in mortification. Wells returned to Hartford where he continued to experiment with gas in his dental practice.

The third major figure in the anesthesia controversy was the aforementioned Dr. William T. G. Morton (1819–68), Wells's friend and former partner. As a student at Harvard Medical School, Morton's preceptor had been Dr. Charles A. Jackson, a physician, chemist, and geologist. Jackson, an intelligent and controversial figure, in 1844 suggested to Morton that he might reduce the pain from dental work by applying drops of sulfuric ether to the gums. The method proved of only limited benefit, and Morton turned to the use of ether as an inhalant. When he administered the gas to two of his dental assistants, they became too excited for him to work on them. He again consulted Jackson, who recommended that he use pure sulfuric ether. After experimenting on himself, Morton was eager to try ether on a dental patient. On September 1846 he painlessly extracted a decayed tooth from a patient using sulfuric ether. Wisely, he saw to it that an account was published in the following day's newspaper.

Convinced that he had found the answer to surgery without pain, Morton contacted Dr. John C. Warren, Boston's foremost surgeon, to arrange for a demonstration. Suffice to say, arrangements were made for Morton to test his anesthetic on a young man, Gilbert Abbot, who was to have a tumor removed from the left side of his neck. On October 16, 1846, Dr. Warren, with Morton serving as the anesthetist, gave the first successful public demonstration of surgical anesthesia. The following day Morton again successfully anesthetized a surgical patient, proving that his initial success was no accident. In the meantime the medical community in Boston was searching for a name for the condition produced by "Letheon," Morton's name for the gas. The answer was supplied by Dr. Oliver Wendell Holmes, who wrote to Morton in November suggesting that the name of the condition be called "anaesthesia" and that the adjective be "anaesthetic." [21]

News of Morton's discovery spread rapidly, and, with a few minor exceptions, it was generally hailed as a major advance. Before the end of 1846 ether had been administered in both Paris and London, and within a year its use had spread throughout the entire United States. The first application of anesthesia to childbirth came in 1847. In that year an American woman, Fannie Appleton Longfellow, gave birth to a child while anesthetized, and a famous British physician, Dr. James Young Simpson, introduced chloroform into his obstetrical practice. [22] Since chloroform was easier to handle, it quickly became the anesthetic agent of choice in the United States.

Although it was recognized as a significant breakthrough, over thirty years elapsed before anesthesia came into general use in America. Many American physicians refused to use it, fearing that anesthesia brought patients too close to death. Even those who did administer it often did so selectively, restricting its use to the upper classes, women, and children. Others rejected anesthesia on the grounds that pain was an essential part of the healing process. Homeopaths and other irregulars often objected to it in the belief that it was not a natural form of treatment. Nonetheless, in part as a result of patient demand, its use steadily increased.

Objections to surgical anesthesia were minor compared to those against the use of anesthetics in obstetrical cases. Although a few clergymen and theologians opposed obstetrical anesthesia on religious grounds, the attack from this front was never too serious despite a continued sniping for many years by some of the more fundamentalist clergymen. As late as 1888, the Reverend Henry Hayman denounced anesthesia on the grounds that pain is a "fountain of human affection." The birth pangs, he said, provided a physical basis for maternal love and helped to cement "more closely conjugal affection." [23] Surprisingly enough, the real threat to obstetrical anesthesia came from within the ranks of the medical profession itself. Few physicians openly supported the theological arguments against obstetrical anesthesia, but it is obvious that many were seeking in physiology a means for rationalizing their religious convictions. The opposition of a second group of doctors seems to have been based on an instinctive resistance to anything new, while still another group was comprised of conservative physicians who were reluctant to endorse a radical innovation before it had been adequately tested.

Dr. Charles D. Meigs, a prominent Philadelphia obstetrician, was one of the leaders in the fight against obstetrical anesthesia. The pains of childbirth, he wrote, were part "of those natural and physiological forces that the Divinity has ordained us to enjoy or suffer." He argued that the nature of labor pains had been exaggerated and cheerfully stated that few women "lose their health or their lives in labor." As late as 1887 an Iowa physician proclaimed: "I do not use any anesthetic of any kind, especially in forceps cases. I want the patient to know what is going on." [24]

Although the main battle for obstetrical anesthesia had been won by 1860, the great lag between medical developments and medical practice in the nineteenth century meant that the use of anesthesia was not as widespread as might have been expected. Relatively few doctors read medical journals, and many others opposed innovations on principle. Midwives, few of whom, at least in the United States, had any training, continued to attend the majority of deliveries. Thus it was that the use of anesthesia in normal deliveries continued to be debated in lay and medical journals until the twentieth century. After 1860, however, the chief discussions in medical publications centered more on the relative values of the various anesthetic agents and on the methods for administering them. [25]

Whatever may have been the reaction of doctors and clergymen, there was never any question of the patients' views on anesthesia, for parturient women seem to have been little concerned with abstract questions of morality when an anesthetic agent was available. In England Queen Victoria placed the stamp of approval upon anesthesia in 1853 by taking chloroform during the birth of her eighth child, but this royal approval merely confirmed what thousands of British and American women had accepted. The reaction of parturient women to the use of chloroform was the subject of a paper read before the Massachusetts Medical Society in 1856. The author, Dr. John G. Metcalf, stated, "in every case, if I am called to a succeeding labor, the first question has invariably been, 'Have you brought the chloroform?'" Three years later a Philadelphia physician expressed a similar view, declaring that he had never found "a single instance where a patient would consent to its discontinuance after commencing its inhalations." The universal cry, he added, "has been, 'give me more!' "[26]

The immediate and widespread recognition accorded the introduction of anesthesia should have brought prestige and rewards to those who pioneered in it, but such was not the case. Within a few months a violent quarrel broke out among the various claimants to the honor of having discovered it, one that contributed to the tragic deaths of at least three of them. Up to this point three major figures have been discussed: Crawford W. Long, Horace Wells, and William T. G. Morton. The fourth individual to assert priority in the discovery was Charles Thomas Jackson (1805–80), the Harvard professor who suggested the use of ether to Morton. Shortly after Morton's demonstration Jackson wrote to the French Academy of Sciences claiming full credit for discovering anesthesia, and early in March 1847 he made a similar statement before the American Academy of Arts and Sciences. Morton indignantly responded, and the clash between the two men widened into a four-way battle when Morton, having gained nothing from his patent, pressured the United States Congress to give him a suitable reward. Bills were introduced into Congress to award $100,000 to the discoverer of anesthesia. This brought Horace Wells into the fray, and in 1854 Senator W. C. Dawson of Georgia introduced the name of Crawford Long. The debates over the claims and counterclaims of these four individuals continued in Congress until 1863 when the unresolved issue was finally dropped.

Wells, the most unfortunate of the four claimants, was barely embroiled in the controversy before he took his own life. After seeking to prove his pioneering work, he opened an office in New York. However, while experimenting with chloroform, he was arrested in January 1848 while under its influence and placed in prison. Embarrassed, ashamed, and depressed, Wells committed suicide by cutting his thigh with a razor. Morton continued his legal battle, much of it against Jackson, for another twenty years, impoverishing and frustrating himself in the process. According to John F. Fulton, in 1868 Morton died of a stroke brought on by reading one of Jackson's attempts to undermine his position.[27] Jackson himself was no more fortunate. This able but erratic individual spent much of his later life embroiled in various controversies. These did not end until his mind gave way in 1873, causing him to spend the last seven years of his life in a mental institution. His overweening desire for fame deprived him of the satisfactions that should have come from some real accomplishments. The life of the fourth claimant, Crawford Long, ended on a much happier note. While he assiduously gathered evidence to justify his priority, he maintained his successful medical practice, lived a normal life, and died suddenly in 1878 while aiding in the delivery of a baby.[28]

Of the four conflicting claims, those of Jackson can be dismissed. Crawford Long undoubtedly was the first to perform surgery on an anesthetized patient, but his failure, for whatever reason, to inform the medical world until three years after the Morton-Warren demonstration—and seven years after his first use of ether—deprives him of primary honor. Horace Wells deserves far more credit, and but for a mischance might well stand alone as the discoverer of anesthesia. In any event, his work paved the way for his former partner, William T. G. Morton, to carry on the experiments and bring the project to fruition. While Morton deserves the major credit, there is no question that the time was ripe, that the technology available, and that even without Wells or Morton chemical anesthesia would have appeared on the scene within less than a decade.

CHAPTER 8

Early Leaders in Medicine and Surgery

ONE CAN SCARCELY WRITE about medicine in the years between the Revolution and the Civil War without discussing such outstanding medical figures as Rush, McDowell, Beaumont, and Sims, but a great many more physicians left a permanent imprint upon American medicine, and several of them are worthy of special notice. In Boston the Warren family has been associated with medicine—and Harvard University Medical School in particular—since before the Revolution. Joseph Warren (1741–75), a Boston medical practitioner, was killed at Bunker Hill. His brother, John Warren (1753–1815), helped establish the Harvard Medical School, where he served as the first professor of anatomy and surgery and was one of the founders of the Massachusetts Medical Society.

His son, John Collins Warren (1778–1856), succeeded to his father's professorship at Harvard and taught surgery for forty years. When the Harvard Medical School moved from Cambridge to Boston in 1810, Dr. Warren, along with Dr. James Jackson, took the initiative that led to the founding of the Massachusetts General Hospital. In their appeal to wealthy Bostonians, the two physicians pointed out that the hospital would "afford relief and comfort to thousands of the sick and miserable" and asked: "On what other objects can the superfluities of the rich be so well bestowed?" Dr. Warren was active in medical journalism and was one of the leaders in establishing the *Boston Medical and Surgical Journal* in 1828, a journal that resulted from a merger of the *New England Journal of Medicine and Surgery* and the *Medical Intelligencer*. Close to the end of his teaching career he performed the classic operation with Morton that introduced anesthesia. Warren's prominence and prestige as a surgeon undoubtedly helped to establish anesthesia as a legitimate surgical technique.[1]

New York was the home of many able physicians, and a fine representative of these was David Hosack (1769–1835). His medical education was typical of the best-trained physicians—an apprenticeship, courses at two American medical schools, and two years of study in Edinburgh and London. He had just started his medical practice in New York in 1795 when a series of yellow fever outbreaks began. In opposition to Benjamin Rush, Hosack argued that the disease was imported and that bloodletting and drastic purging were fruitless. In 1796 he was appointed professor of materia medica at Columbia and continued to teach throughout his career, subsequently holding positions at the College of Physicians and Surgeons and later at the short-lived Rutgers Medical School.

While serving as resident physician for the New York Board of Health in 1820, one of many temporary health boards appointed before the establishment of the Metropolitan Board of Health in 1866, Hosack lectured to medical students on the subject of medical police, a term that encompassed sanitation and public health. To protect the residents from yellow fever, which was threatening the city, he recommended major sanitary reforms and large-scale city planning. His proposals were too far ahead of his time, but they reveal him as a humane, perceptive, and intelligent citizen.[2]

Hosack's active social life may have been responsible for his selection as Alexander Hamilton's surgeon on the occasion of the tragic Burr-Hamilton duel. In the days of formal dueling, each participant brought his own physician, one of whose duties was to examine any wounds to determine whether or not his principal was too badly injured to continue the fray. In Hamilton's case, Hosack immediately recognized that the wound was fatal. All he could do was to make his patient as comfortable as possible during the "almost intolerable" suffering Hamilton endured for the remaining thirty hours of his life.

The career of Dr. Daniel Drake (1785–1852) presents a sharp contrast to that of the two sophisticated easterners just described. Drake was essentially a product of the frontier. He was raised under typical frontier conditions in Mays Lick, Kentucky. At the age of fifteen his father took him to Cincinnati and apprenticed him to Dr. William

Goforth. When Drake completed his four-year apprenticeship, Goforth took him in as a partner. Realizing his medical shortcomings, Drake headed for the Medical College of the University of Pennsylvania late in 1805, a journey of eighteen days by horseback. Here he attended the lectures of Benjamin Rush, Philip Syng Physick, William Shippen, and Caspar Wistar. When the semester ended early in March 1806, Drake returned to his home in Kentucky and began practicing. Anxious to advance, he went back to Cincinnati in 1807.

While in Cincinnati he wrote the earliest description of milk sickness, a disease caused by drinking the milk or eating the flesh of cows that had ingested white snakeroot or rayless goldenrod, and one that was to become a major problem in the Midwest. In 1815 he returned to Philadelphia to take his medical degree at the University of Pennsylvania. His growing reputation soon led to an invitation to become professor of materia medica and botany in the Medical Department of Transylvania University, Lexington, Kentucky.

Realizing the desperate need for trained physicians and having positive ideas about medical education, in 1819 Drake returned to Cincinnati and secured a charter for the Medical College of Ohio, the forerunner of the Medical School of the University of Cincinnati. There, as president, he spent a stormy three years embroiled in quarrels with faculty members. A contemporary book dealer and author wrote that the early history of the college could aptly be styled "a history of the Thirty Years War." Quarrels among the professors and the town's medical faculty became quite bitter. On one occasion, after a Dr. Oliver B. Baldwin had published a caustic attack on Drake, the latter entered Baldwin's house early in the morning purportedly armed with a club to force the owner to retract his statement. Baldwin claimed that Drake seized him by the throat and threatened to beat him. In the ensuing struggle, Baldwin's shirt was torn and he fled into the street. Drake, while denying Baldwin's version, admitted he entered the house "to remonstrate against the publication," and, when Baldwin became alarmed and left in haste, Drake said: "I ran a few steps after him to get him fairly under way." A local jury, on the testimony of bystanders, convicted Drake of assault and fined him ten dollars.

To add to Drake's troubles, in January 1820 Dr. Coleman Rogers, the college's vice-president and professor of surgery, challenged him to a duel after Drake dismissed him from the college faculty. Drake wisely refused. After further wrangling, the faculty expelled Drake. Although pressure from local citizens forced his reinstatement, Drake was ready to give up. He resigned in 1822 and accepted a position at his former school, Transylvania University. His stay in Lexington was more or less uneventful, but for some reason he elected to return to Cincinnati in 1827. Here he helped found *The Western Medical and Physical Journal* and was the prime mover in establishing the Cincinnati Eye Infirmary. Always restless, he accepted an appointment in 1830 to the Jefferson Medical College in Philadelphia.

In the meantime Drake had been mulling over the problems of medical education and setting forth his ideas in essay form in his medical journal. In 1823 he collected these articles and issued them in book form under the title *Practical Essays on Medical Education and the Medical Profession.* In this work Drake urged the need for a solid background in Greek and Latin, required attendance at lectures, a four-year period of medical training, and stricter examination of candidates for graduation. Few intelligent medical professors questioned Drake's ideas, but the colleges were dependent upon student fees and most students merely wanted easy degrees. Drake's hopes of being able to put his ideas on medical education into effect led him to leave Jefferson in 1831 to found a new medical college associated with Miami University in Oxford, Ohio. Insurmountable difficulties soon caused the college's dissolution, and the following year Drake was again on the faculty of the Medical College of Ohio. For the next twenty years he moved back and forth between Louisville, Lexington, and Cincinnati, finally returning once more to the Medical College of Ohio, only to die shortly after the opening of the school year in 1852.

Notable as his other accomplishments may have been, Drake's chief claim to fame lies in his great two-volume work *A Systematic Treatise, Historical, Etiological and Practical, on the Principal Diseases of the Interior Valley of North America, as They Appear in the Caucasian, African, Indian and Esquimaux Varieties of Its Population.* This study was the result of a lifelong interest in the subject. As early as 1808 he had published *Some Account of the Epidemic Diseases which Prevail in Mays-Lick in Kentucky*, and his two following studies, *Notices Concerning Cincinnati* (1810) and *Picture of Cincinnati* (1816), show how he was broadening his interest to include the population and environment.

To appreciate Drake's interest in this subject, we must remember that virtually nothing was known about epidemic diseases. As it became evident in the eighteenth and nineteenth centuries that distinct and separate disease entities did exist, the search for a causal factor or factors turned to meteorological phenomena and the physical environment. The quest was not new, for Hippocrates had suggested such a relationship in his *Airs, Waters, Places* many centuries earlier. Two eighteenth-century American books showing the revival of interest in the Hippocratic thesis are Lionel Chalmer's two-volume work *An Account of the Weather and Diseases in South Carolina* (London, 1776) and William Currie's *An Historical Account of the Climates and Diseases of the United States of America* . . . (Philadelphia, 1792). Public health in the nineteenth century to a large extent was equated with sanitation, and the sanitary movement was profoundly influenced by the various attempts to explain disease in terms of climate and geography. Hence, Drake's study of the people and diseases in the Mississippi Valley was in a well-established tradition.

Throughout his career Drake seized every opportunity to travel in what he termed the great central valley of North America, observing every conceivable phenomenon, and in 1844 he began writing his comprehensive study. The first section was a detailed account of the topographical and hydrographical features of the valley. The second dealt with climatic conditions and included tables showing such phenomena as winds, rainfall, snow, and humidity. The third section described the people—diet, housing, occupations, clothing, and so forth. The final section was a thorough account of the diseases. The first volume appeared in 1850 and the second was published posthumously in 1854. Reviewers were unanimous in their praise, and the book was hailed as a major work in the field of medical topography. Researchers may no longer scan Drake's work searching for clues as to the nature of febrile diseases, but the descriptions of the topography, climate, people, and diseases of the Mississippi Valley make it an invaluable historical source.[3]

It is fitting that the next physician and surgeon discussed was closely associated with Drake in the field of medical education. Dr. Samuel David Gross (1805–84) began his study of medicine as an apprentice but quickly realized the need for more formal medical training. He left his preceptor and, after finishing at an academy, entered the newly established Jefferson Medical College in Philadelphia. Upon graduating in 1828 he began private practice in Philadelphia. With only a few patients and a great deal of time on his hands, he busied himself translating various French and German medical books, a project that was educational but not particularly remunerative. Unable to build a decent practice, he returned to his home in Easton, Pennsylvania, where he continued his research and publication. In 1833 he was offered the post of demonstrator in anatomy at the Medical College of Ohio. His success as a teacher and his growing medical reputation led to an invitation two years later to move to the Cincinnati Medical College as professor of pathological anatomy. While there he published his classic study *Elements of Pathological Anatomy*, the first comprehensive work on the subject in the English language. This book, published in 1839, established Gross's reputation in America and Europe. The following year he was appointed professor of surgery at the University of Louisville, where he remained for the next sixteen years save for a brief interlude in New York. In 1856 he returned to his old school, Jefferson Medical College, and spent the rest of his long life in Philadelphia.

Gross was an indefatigable worker, maintaining a large surgical practice, teaching, and pouring out a stream of articles and books. While at the University of Louisville he wrote three major works: one on intestinal lesions; a second on diseases of the bladder, prostate, and urethra; and a third entitled *Foreign Bodies in the Air-Passages*. In 1859 he brought out his two-volume textbook, *A System of Surgery: Pathological, Diagnostic, Therapeutic and Operative*, a work that remained standard for many years. As with all great surgeons, he was keenly interested in the history of his field and the work of his predecessors, and in 1861 he edited *The Lives of Eminent Physicians and Surgeons of the Nineteenth Century*. He was a founder of the American Medical Association and was active in establishing several pathological and surgical organizations. Most of Gross's career antedated the emergence of the era of abdominal surgery, but he was a pioneer in the field and his work helped lay the basis for subsequent developments.[4]

One of the more able nineteenth-century physicians, Dr. Oliver Wendell Holmes (1809–94), is best known as a poet and essayist. Yet Holmes was an outstanding teacher of anatomy and made one of the few significant American contributions to nineteenth-century medicine. Holmes, born in Cambridge, Massachusetts, came from an old New England family. After graduating from Harvard, he briefly studied law and then switched to medicine, beginning his studies at a private medical institution and enrolling in courses at the Harvard University Medical School. He then headed for Paris, the mecca for American medical students, where he spent two years observing Pierre Louis,

Baron Larrey, Dupuytren, and the other outstanding French clinicians. He returned to Boston, took his medical degree from Harvard, and began practicing. He had already contributed literary essays to the *New England Magazine* and in 1836 he published his first book, *Poems.* As he moved into his medical career, he wrote several prize-winning medical papers. In 1838 he was appointed professor of anatomy at Dartmouth, a position that required only three months a year of his time.

Holmes gave up the Dartmouth professorship in 1840 and devoted himself to literature and his medical practice until his appointment in 1847 as Parkman Professor of Anatomy and Physiology at the Harvard Medical School. It was in this position that his graceful use of English, his wit, and his skepticism endeared him to the students. His reputation as a lecturer was such that he was assigned the last of five morning lectures. Anatomy is a subject that can be deadly to unruly medical students already worn out by a grueling schedule, but Holmes successfully kept their attention for the entire hour from one to two o'clock in the afternoon. Holmes held his chair for thirty-five years, retiring in 1882.

Holmes's intellectual interests resulted in his appointment to the American Medical Association's Committee on Medical Literature. Reporting for the committee in 1848 he castigated American medical writers, noting sarcastically that the great forte of American scholarship was editing British works. He then accused editors of medical journals of borrowing most of their material from foreign publications and of neglecting the American scene. The number of American medical journals, he wrote, had increased to approximately twenty, a fact he attributed to the profitability of advertising. Driving his point home, he commented sardonically: "The advertising portion of the journals seem to be considered by some editors as beyond the jurisdiction of medical ethics."[5]

In all likelihood Holmes would have been remembered primarily as a literary figure who was incidentally a great medical teacher had it not been for the publication in 1843 of an article in the *New England Quarterly Journal of Medicine* entitled "The Contagiousness of Puerperal Fever." In the prebacterial era, puerperal fever was a mysterious disease that periodically swept through maternity wards or struck at parturient women immediately after they had given birth in their homes. The medical profession was at a loss to account for it and was equally at sea as to the means for curing it. Holmes's attention was drawn to this disease when a local physician who had dissected a victim of puerperal fever fell sick and died with symptoms closely resembling those of the fever. After reflecting on this case, Holmes became convinced that the disease was a specific contagious infection that could be passed by direct contact. Since maternity patients had little or no contact with each other, he surmised that physicians were responsible for carrying the disease. Working on this assumption, he urged physicians with patients about to deliver to avoid participating in autopsies of puerperal fever victims or, if they did so, to wash themselves completely, change all clothes, and wait at least twenty-four hours before attending an obstetrical case. If any patient developed the disease, he warned, her physician should take extreme sanitary precautions before visiting another obstetrical case. If two cases of puerperal fever develop under his care, the physician should give up practice for at least a month. Holmes also advised physicians to insist that all nurses and attendants take the same precautions.[6]

Holmes's article was printed as a pamphlet and was reprinted in many medical journals. Although some readers expressed skepticism, the article was quite influential in encouraging American physicians to practice elementary sanitary precautions in dealing with parturient women. Holmes never doubted the validity of his advice, and when his ideas were attacked early in the 1850s by Drs. H. L. Hodge and C. D. Meigs, two prominent obstetricians, Holmes republished his article with an introduction reaffirming his position. The significance of Holmes's article is that it preceded the work of Ignatz Philipp Semmelweis by four years. The latter, who is generally credited with discovering the contagious nature of puerperal fever, arrived at his discovery in a manner similar to that of Holmes. Semmelweis, however, met considerable opposition, was hounded from his position, and eventually died in an asylum in Vienna. The stark tragedy of Semmelweis's life has caused him to loom larger than Holmes in medical history, but Holmes was the first to recognize the role of the physician as a carrier of puerperal fever.

One of the more intriguing of early American physicians was Dr. Benjamin Waterhouse (1754–1846). Although generally credited with introducing vaccination into the United States and being its chief advocate, Waterhouse did not make a favorable impression upon his contemporaries. It was not until the closing years of the nineteenth century that Waterhouse began to assume a place among the near greats in American medical history. His star shone ever brighter until 1957 when Dr. John Blake reappraised his work and firmly relegated him to a very minor role.[7] Waterhouse was a well-educated physician, having served an apprenticeship, spent three years studying in London and Edinburgh, and taken a medical degree in Leyden. Incidentally, it is a commentary upon the day that Waterhouse, an outspoken American patriot, should have spent the years from 1775 to 1778 in London and Edinburgh.

Few American physicians had the academic credentials possessed by Waterhouse by the time he returned to America, and in 1783 he was offered the professorship of the theory and practice of physic in the newly organized Harvard Medical School. He might have fallen into obscurity had he not received a copy of Edward Jenner's book in 1799 describing his discovery of "variolae vaccinae," or cowpox. Waterhouse published a summary of Jenner's work in the *Columbian Centinal*, a Boston newspaper. In 1800, along with several other physicians, Waterhouse acquired some cowpox virus and inoculated his son and several other persons. The traditional account states that he was besieged with requests for the vaccine but refused on the grounds that he wanted to be sure it would be administered properly. Blake has shown that he was far more concerned with establishing a monopoly, for he soon began offering it to select physicians in return for a guarantee of one-quarter or more of the revenue derived from it. Other American physicians soon began receiving vaccine matter from England, and Waterhouse was unable to control the supply.

Throughout his life Waterhouse constantly promoted his claim to have been the first to administer vaccination in the United States. In doing so he disregarded the many other physicians who had imported vaccine matter themselves and who had not hesitated to share it with their colleagues. His attempt to make money out of the vaccine did little to endear him to his fellow physicians, and his relations with the Massachusetts Medical Society soon became embittered. He also fell to quarreling with his colleagues on the Harvard medical faculty, resulting in his dismissal in 1812.

In contrast to Waterhouse was Dr. John L. Riddell, a student and friend of Daniel Drake. Riddell, who served as professor of chemistry at the Medical College of Louisiana (Tulane) from 1836 to 1861, dabbled in many areas of science, ranging from natural history, an early interest, to physics. In the course of his long career he drew up a proposed bill providing for a geological survey of Louisiana, analyzed the local drinking water, designed a method for filtering and softening it, and then turned his attention to the construction of microscopes. Early in the 1850s he designed the first binocular microscope, publishing a detailed description of it in the *New Orleans Medical and Surgical Journal* in November 1853. The following spring he informed members of the Physico-Medical Society that he was constructing a new kind of objective for the microscope. By making the objective "in two vertical halves," Riddell explained, he anticipated that with "ordinary (not erecting) eye-pieces, the binocular image produced [would] be both erect and orthoscopic." Riddell has generally been overlooked by medical historians, but he was one of the better physicians-scientists of the early nineteenth century.[8]

CHAPTER 9

The Education, Licensing, and Status of Physicians

A<small>LTHOUGH MEDICAL SCHOOLS</small> began to appear in large numbers in the nineteenth century, the apprenticeship system still remained an integral part of the doctor's training. Ordinarily the student paid a fee of one hundred dollars per year and agreed to remain with his mentor for a period of from one to five years. Daniel Drake's father, for example, apprenticed his son for four years, agreeing to pay Dr. William Goforth the standard annual fee. Apprentices lived with the physician, and their duties varied widely, ranging from currying his horse to compounding medicine. Frequently prominent physicians accepted several young trainees. Dr. Benjamin Rush, for example, had seven apprentices at one time.[1]

Medical school professors, who lectured and carried on an extensive practice, usually referred to their apprentices as private students. During the year 1807–8 Dr. David Hosack had four private students in addition to those pupils enrolled in his course. The regulations he prescribed for his private students clearly indicate that they were in effect apprentices. The students were expected to be in his office from 9 A.M. to 9 P.M. except when at the hospitals, attending lectures, or eating meals, and they could not leave the city or be absent from the office without permission. Their duties involved taking care of the office, preparing and dispensing medicines, and keeping a register of the weather. Dr. Hosack, recognizing that the devil finds work for idle hands, also required the students to restrict their conversations and reading to medicine during office hours.[2]

Physicians strongly supported the training of apprentices, since they provided both an added income and a measure of cheap labor. The apprentice system and the medical colleges, as William G. Rothstein has pointed out, worked harmoniously until the colleges began offering clinical training, a development that did not occur on any appreciable scale until after the Civil War.[3] One consequence of the continued existence of an apprentice training program was a relatively high percentage of physicians without any formal medical training as late as 1900.

The most remarkable development in the years from the Revolution to 1820 was the phenomenal growth of medical schools. The two pre-Revolutionary institutions survived the war years, but not without considerable difficulty. The Medical College of Philadelphia managed to reopen, but it was threatened by competition from the newly created University of Pennsylvania. The problem was solved in 1791 when the Medical College merged with the university. Columbia Medical School (King's College) had even greater problems when it was revived in 1792. Part of the trouble was a personality clash between Dr. Samuel Bard and Dr. Nicholas Romayne, the "stormy petrel" of New York medical politics. Romayne resigned from Columbia and established a private school in the late 1780s, making arrangements for his students to receive medical degrees at Queen's College (Rutgers) in New Jersey. In 1807, assisted by David Hosack, Samuel Latham Mitchell, and several other doctors, Romayne established the College of Physicians and Surgeons under the auspices of the University of the State of New York. In the meantime Columbia was struggling to survive, granting only thirty-four medical degrees between 1792 and 1811. By 1810 both schools were in trouble, and the following year the Regents of the State University decided to merge Columbia into the College of Physicians and Surgeons.[4]

While the schools in Philadelphia and New York were trying to solve their problems, new medical colleges began appearing. In 1782 Harvard established a medical department with three professors, and in 1798 Dartmouth formally established a medical school. It should be noted that the latter school consisted of only one professor, Dr. Nathan Smith, and an assistant, Lyman Spalding. It was not until 1810 that the Dartmouth trustees appointed a second professor.[5] Transylvania University in Kentucky created a Medical Department in 1799, but it was 1817 before any official courses in medicine were given.[6]

Medical education received a notable setback in 1788 as a result of what was termed the Doctors' Riot. A brash young medical student engaged in dissection in New York City reportedly waved a dissected arm at a group of young boys. One of them peeped into the window and was told that it was his mother's arm. Since his mother had died recently, the boy was horrified and ran to tell his father. The father visited the grave and discovered it had been robbed. He gathered a group of fellow laborers and literally tore the dissecting rooms apart, destroying an anatomical museum that Drs. Richard Bayley and Samuel Clossy had been in the process of creating. The mob then started looking for medical students and doctors, some of whom took refuge in the jail. Their anger and frustration intensified by social problems arising from the transition from a colonial town to a major city, the members of the mob rampaged through the city for over two days before being brought under control.[7]

The destruction of the anatomical museum was a major loss because of the difficulty of securing subjects for dissection. Out of necessity, physicians and their pupils in the antebellum period resorted to grave-robbing, a practice that did not endear them to the public. In some cases medical students were responsible for acquiring their own subjects, but most medical schools relied upon professional "resurrectionists," "sack-'em-up men," or "body-snatchers," who charged a standard fee according to the age of the subject and the condition of the body. Since any medical school of consequence had to give its students a chance to dissect, the public justifiably viewed medical schools with suspicion and resentment. People's reaction to grave-robbing varied from area to area, with the consequences ranging from relatively mild fines and prison sentences to violent mob action. Accusations of grave-robbing led an unruly mob in Baltimore to burn down what would have become the University of Maryland's first medical building in 1807.[8]

The shortage of subjects made medical students quick to seize any opportunity that came their way. When news of John Brown's raid was first heard, the entire student body of Winchester Medical College in Virginia boarded the next train for Harper's Ferry. On leaving the train shortly before it reached the station, they chanced on a dead body. Acting on the moment, they shipped it back to the college. There, papers on the body revealed it was John Brown's son Owen. Undeterred by this fact, a dried preparation was made of the body, and it was added to the other anatomical specimens used for demonstrations. A Union commander, learning about this on entering Winchester in 1862, recovered the body, and burned the college buildings to the ground in retaliation.[9]

The first state to pass an anatomy act was Massachusetts, where public outrage over body-snatching in 1830 led the state assembly to legalize the granting of bodies to medical schools. Unfortunately, Massachusetts was an exception to the rule, for it was not until the mid-century that other states began following suit. Some legislatures did not act until near the end of the century. Pennsylvania, for example, did not pass an anatomy act until June 1883.[10]

The one place where the medical profession had no difficulty procuring subjects was New Orleans. As mentioned earlier, the city's Charity Hospital, opened as a private institution in 1736 and taken over by the state in 1811, was designed primarily to provide medical care for the poor. Since New Orleans was a major seaport, the vast majority of patients were outsiders. By 1849 the hospital was admitting over eighteen thousand patients annually at a time when hospitals were largely places of last resort and when a case fatality rate of from 10 to 12 percent was considered quite satisfactory. The majority of those who died were poor and homeless, or else poor and away from home, and their bodies were usually consigned to the potter's field; consequently, there was no one to object when the bodies were assigned to physicians or medical schools for dissection. The notices and advertisements sent forth by the New Orleans medical schools invariably stressed the ample clinical material at Charity Hospital and the unlimited number of subjects for dissection.

The vast majority of medical schools organized during the nineteenth century were proprietary institutions, a term that needs explanation. As of 1800 it was obvious that the number of graduates from the existing medical colleges was hopelessly inadequate for America's burgeoning population. As noted earlier, the vacuum in medical education was filled by small groups of ambitious physicians who took it upon themselves to establish schools. Under these conditions, the traditional concept of professional medical training as an academic discipline simply had no validity. Entrance requirements were virtually eliminated, and the emphasis was placed upon practical skills and knowledge. Many of the professors were themselves products of the apprentice system, and they could see little value in laboratories or libraries.

The caliber of these schools varied widely, depending upon the educational background and conscientiousness of the professors, but, as already indicated, even in the best schools it was possible to acquire an easy degree. From a professional and economic standpoint, physicians had much to gain by an attachment to a medical college. The students paid a matriculation fee usually ranging from $5 to $10 and a graduation fee of from $25 to $35. In addition, they purchased a ticket at a cost of about $20 from each professor whose class they wished to attend. A popular professor could also expect to attract the public to some of his lectures; hence a professorship could mean a substantial addition to a physician's income. The matriculation and graduation fees were generally applied to overhead costs, and the professors paid any extra expenses out of their lecture fees. More important than the income from teaching was the prestige attached to it. A physician's standing in the community was enhanced by a professorship, and consultation fees from former students tended to grow during long teaching careers.

As of 1800 the United States had only four small medical colleges to serve a fast-growing population of over five million. Two more schools were added in 1807 when the College of Physicians and Surgeons was established by Romayne and the College of Medicine of Maryland was chartered. The latter institution was largely the work of John Beale Davidge, a Baltimore physician who had been giving private lectures in obstetrics and surgery. The state legislature left the operation of the school largely to the professors, except for authorizing a series of lotteries in 1808 to help with the construction of the school building. The new building was not ready until 1813, and in the meantime, Dr. Davidge's original anatomical laboratory having been destroyed by a mob, the professors lectured successively in an old warehouse, a church, and a theater.[11]

While medical schools had been slow in appearing during the first thirty years of the new nation's history, their numbers increased rapidly after 1810. No less than twenty-six were founded between 1810 and 1840, and another forty-seven between 1840 and 1875.[12] Since neither clinical training nor laboratory work was considered necessary for a medical degree, all that was required to start a medical college were several physicians willing to lecture and a classroom or hall. Many medical schools obtained a charter first and then started looking for quarters. The promoters of these schools usually consisted of a group of from four to seven young physicians. Once a charter was obtained, they would borrow, hire, or rent a lecture hall until they could raise enough money to buy or erect a building. Most of the building funds were usually contributed by the founding professors, and for the rest they usually appealed to state legislatures and private subscribers.

Tulane University School of Medicine is a fine example of how the early proprietary medical schools began. The originators were three young men, not one of whom was older than twenty-six. In 1833 Dr. Warren Stone, the product of a poor Vermont family, and Dr. Thomas Hunt, a well-to-do Charlestonian, arrived in New Orleans where they met Dr. John Harrison, a recent arrival from Maryland. Hunt, the best educated of the three, was elected as spokesman for the group and later was named the first dean. Four other physicians were quickly recruited, and in 1834 the Medical College of Louisiana was chartered. A notice that the school would open in January 1835 was sharply criticized by the French-language newspapers. The French-speaking physicians, many of whom held university degrees from France, argued that a medical school was impossible for New Orleans since the city did not have a university.[13]

Untroubled by these arguments, Dean Hunt gave his inaugural lecture on January 5 in a local church.[14] Lectures were first given in borrowed rooms until the faculty was able to rent a hall for twenty-five dollars a month. The legislature was unresponsive to appeals for help, and for several years the school struggled along in temporary quarters. Finally, in 1843 the medical professors offered to provide all medical care in Charity Hospital and to admit one poor student free of tuition from each parish (county) in the state in return for a building site for their school. The legislature acquiesced, and by the end of 1843 the college was housed in a three-story building designed in the typical classical style of the day. The first floor contained a large lecture hall, a chemical laboratory, and a small library; the second was occupied by a surgical amphitheater, a museum, and two small classrooms; and the third was used as a dissecting room.

Two years later, in 1845, the legislature chartered a state university and specified that the Medical College of Louisiana would become the Medical Department of the University. Subsequently this same body appropriated funds to erect a new and larger building for the Medical Department. Although the legislature continued to give some financial support, the medical school remained under control of the professors and was to all intents and purposes a proprietary institution.[15]

In this respect, and in others, the medical school was typical of the day. Despite a rising enrollment, which exceeded four hundred in 1860, the number of professors remained at seven. The school term ran from November 1 to the end of March, and students seeking a degree were expected to attend the same lectures for two successive sessions. An additional year's experience in a physician's office was also required, but the certificates attesting to this were often worthless. For conscientious students it was possible to acquire the rudiments of a medical education, but for those content to get a medical degree life was much simpler. Dr. Stanford E. Chaillé, an 1853 graduate who subsequently became dean of the school, wrote that "students could enter very late and leave very early, [and] there were instances of cases in which little more was required than one's presence, payment of the entrance fees, and attendance at the final examinations." Even the examinations were nominal, since the students visited the seven professors for an oral quiz within the space of an hour and a half, and it was customary for each professor to spend a few minutes inquiring about the student's family and his plans. Chaillé added that he himself graduated with a unanimous vote of the faculty only seventeen months after he had first entered the study of medicine.[16] Significantly, the University of Louisiana was the leading medical college in the Deep South and ranked as one of the better ones in the country.

In his classic study of American medical education in 1910 Abraham Flexner blamed the University of Maryland for the introduction of proprietary schools, a system, he wrote, that divorced American medical schools from universities and led to a progressive lowering of educational standards. Flexner's criticism was too harsh, since it is clear to anyone who studies conditions in early nineteenth-century America that the universities to which medical schools might have been grafted did not exist. When the Maryland legislature established the College of Medicine of Maryland, there was no university within the state. The same was true in 1845 when Louisiana transformed the Medical College of Louisiana into the Medical Department of the University of Louisiana. The university existed only in name. Moreover, even in the case of schools such as Harvard and the University of Pennsylvania the medical school professors collected their own fees and remained virtually autonomous for much of their universities' history.[17]

Yet Flexner was right in attributing the decline in standards to the rise of these schools. The ease with which medical colleges could be established and the fact that many professors were more concerned with collecting fees than with providing a medical education led to keen competition for students. As this competition sharpened, there was a tendency to lower standards, both for entrance and graduation. Yale presents a good illustration of this point. When medicine was first offered in 1813, the course was six months long. After losing students to schools offering much shorter courses, Yale gradually reduced the academic year to four months.[18]

Several other attempts were made to raise the standards of medical schools in the pre–Civil War years, but they proved equally fruitless. In 1825 the Vermont State Medical Society circularized a number of state societies and medical colleges urging higher requirements for medical degrees and licenses. The result was a meeting in Northampton, Massachusetts, that included representatives of five New England medical societies and four medical schools in five New England states. Apparently only Yale sought to conform to the recommendations agreed upon at the meeting, but it was forced to back down when its enrollment began to decrease. In the succeeding years a number of other abortive attempts were made by medical societies in Ohio, New Hampshire, and New York. The most persistent efforts were those of the New York State Medical Society, and although the society did not achieve its aim, its fight for reform did lead to the formation of the American Medical Association in 1847.[19]

At the first National Medical Convention (the forerunner of the AMA), held in New York in 1846, a committee was appointed to study medical education and to recommend any needed changes. After having made contact with about half of the existing schools, the committee recommended lengthening the academic year to six months, requiring students to attend lectures for two six-month terms, and insisting that the students must present clear evidence of having served an apprenticeship with a qualified physician. College faculties were to have seven professors, each of whom was to be capable of providing instruction in one of the seven branches of medicine: medicine, surgery, anatomy, physiology and pathology, materia medica and pharmacy, midwifery and gynecology, and chemistry and medical jurisprudence. The committee further recommended that the students spend three months dissecting and that the college provide clinical instruction and hospital practice.[20]

Carried away by the enthusiasm displayed at the second national convention, held in Philadelphia in 1847, that year two schools lengthened their courses to six months, the University of Pennsylvania and the College of Physicians and Surgeons in New York. The net effect in Philadelphia was to increase the enrollment of the Jefferson Medical College at the expense of the University of Pennsylvania. The latter school continued the experiment for several years, but eventually was forced to return to the four-month term.[21] The experiences of these two schools illustrate that, while most medical colleges favored reform in principle, they had no intention of raising standards at the cost of student enrollment, or more specifically, student fees. Dr. Richard Arnold of Savannah in 1857 denounced "the growing abuse" of "taking a winter student, hurrying him through a Summer Course and turning him out a Doctor in less than a year."[22] During the 1850s the rise of sectarian or irregular colleges may have aggravated the situation. Whether or not the level of medical education declined in the antebellum years, clearly the movement to reform medical schools came to nought. It might be noted that the Medical Department of the University of Louisiana (Tulane) met all of the recommendations of the AMA educational committee except for the six-month course of instruction. Yet, as Dr. Chaillé had observed, it was still possible to slide through to a degree with a minimum of medical knowledge.

The New Orleans School of Medicine was the only medical college to make any significant advance in the late antebellum period. Established in 1856 under the leadership of Dean E. D. Fenner, it was the first school to emphasize clinical teaching. Instead of a straight lecture course with an occasional patient brought before the class to illustrate a point, the clinical professors conducted their students through the hospital wards each day. Medical students were assigned individual patients and were expected to keep a complete case history, closely observing all symptoms and the effects of the treatment. The school term was expanded from the usual four months to five, and a new professorship on the diseases of women and children was created. From its opening the school flourished, the enrollment growing from 76 to 236 within four years. With two large medical schools New Orleans had become the leading medical center in the South. The outbreak of the war in 1861, however, closed both medical schools. The New Orleans Medical School reopened in 1865, but, handicapped by the death of Dean Fenner in the spring of 1866, it struggled along only to close for good in 1870.[23]

Although the general picture of medical education was rather discouraging, the situation was not without its redeeming qualities. In the first place, these schools supplied America with doctors and surgeons whose empirical skills were not too far behind those of their European contemporaries. Conscientious students learned a great deal from their preceptors, broadened their medical knowledge by reading, and, if they could afford it, supplemented their training abroad. In the second place, these proprietary medical colleges established the principle that medicine was a profession that required formal academic education. While the caliber of these schools remained low during the antebellum period, they laid the base for an effective system of medical education.

The Decline of Medical Licensure

Influenced in part by the relative shortage of physicians, American colonial officials made few efforts to require the licensing of physicians. The early and unsuccessful efforts in this direction by New York City and the colony of New Jersey have already been discussed.[24] The 1760 New York law was reenacted in 1792 and five years later made applicable to the entire state. It was justified on the grounds that "many ignorant and unskilful persons presumed to administer physic and surgery."[25] As state and local medical societies blossomed in the early nationalist period, state legislatures tended to turn licensing over to them. New Jersey adopted this policy in 1790 and was followed by New York and most other states. Louisiana, where the French and Spanish regimes had consistently maintained strict controls over physicians and surgeons, reenacted and eventually broadened a licensure law shortly after coming under American control. In 1816, four years after gaining statehood, the legislature established a state board consisting of four physicians and one apothecary. The following year the act was amended to create two separate boards, an Eastern Board and a Western Board. The Eastern Board, which served the New Orleans area, continued to grant medical licenses until 1854. The Louisiana licensing boards survived much longer than their counterparts in other states, but even so the acquisition of a license was more a matter of prestige than a legal requirement, for there is little evidence to show the prosecution of unlicensed practitioners.[26]

The emergence of state medical societies as licensing agents brought them into conflict with the medical colleges, which assumed that possession of a degree automatically gave their graduates the right to practice. The issue first came to a head in connection with Harvard University. In a public examination of candidates for licenses, the Harvard medical graduates were so much better prepared than other candidates that the Massachusetts Medical Society, which had insisted on examining all prospective physicians, was forced to retreat. In 1803 it agreed to accept a Harvard degree in lieu of an examination. The dual system established by the Massachusetts Medical Society, a medical degree or an examination, was soon followed by most state societies and licensing boards. While virtually all of the older states passed licensure laws of one type or another, few of them prescribed penalties for noncompliance. In most cases an unlicensed practitioner was simply denied the legal right to collect fees, a dubious punitive measure, since the licensed physicians themselves were constantly protesting their inability to collect from their patients.

Even in those states where licensing boards existed, it was still relatively easy to obtain a license. Licensing agencies collected a fee only if they granted a license, a situation likely to discourage them from rejecting candidates; all the more so, since an individual rejected by one board could often apply to another. License fees proved a substantial source of income for a few medical societies. For example, the fees constituted 27 percent of the Maryland State Medical Society's income during the year 1827, a fact of life that undoubtedly encouraged its licensing board to be lenient.[27]

By 1820 the public was becoming increasingly skeptical of the medical profession and equally suspicious of what it referred to as "monopolies." In part this attitude was a reflection of the Jacksonian spirit of egalitarianism, with its distrust of intellectuals and learning. This democratic spirit also implied the right of any American to choose his own doctor or lawyer—and the right, too, to practice medicine and law himself. In the newly created states west of the Appalachians the legislatures rejected all attempts at professional licensing, and, in the older states where licensure laws existed, they were repealed. As of 1845 ten states had repealed their licensure laws and another eight states in the West had never enacted any. In the early 1850s only Louisiana, New Jersey, and the District of Columbia were making any effort to regulate medicine, but these areas, too, were not immune to the laissez-faire movement. In 1852 the Louisiana legislature repealed all existing licensure laws and by 1864 New Jersey took away the authority of the state medical society to license physicians. In so doing it joined the rest of the states in opening the practice of medicine to anyone. Thus by the end of the Civil War not a single state was attempting to regulate the practice of medicine.[28]

The Income of Physicians

While prominent physicians in urban centers could make a substantial income from teaching and medical practice, the vast majority of doctors who lived in rural areas either eked out a bare living from medicine or else used it as a supplement to farming or business. Dr. Goforth of Cincinnati, to whom Daniel Drake was apprenticed, was considered an excellent physician, but he could scarcely have accumulated any substantial capital. According to Drake, he charged 25 cents for bleeding, 25 to 50 cents per visit, and $1 for sitting up all night with the patient. For country calls an added charge of 25 cents per mile was added to the bill. A fee bill drawn up by seven Nashville physicians in 1821 showed the following charges: visit in town, $1; obstetrical case, $20; prescription at shop, $1; amputation of thigh, leg, or arm, $50; vaccination, $2; and blister, $1. Fee bills issued by Louisiana doctors show rates roughly comparable to those throughout the other southern and western states.[29]

Charges by physicians in the small towns and rural areas in the East varied little from those in the West and South. Dr. Lyman Spalding of Portsmouth, New Hampshire, charged an average of 60 cents per patient visit from 1800 to 1807. After seven Portsmouth physicians agreed on a fee bill in 1806, Spalding's average bill increased to 82 cents. The fees established by the Portsmouth physicians ranged from 25 to 100 percent higher than those set by the Southern District of New Hampshire Medical Society, an area that was largely rural. At the same time, the Portsmouth fees were only about a half to two-thirds of those set forth in a fee bill adopted by Boston physicians in the same year.[30] An 1817 Boston fee bill listed an initial home visit at $2.00 to $5.00 and each succeeding visit at $1.50. Vaccination cost $5.00. A New York fee list about this same time showed a charge of $5.00 per home visit plus extra charges for any distance traveled. Bleeding by cupping glasses or the jugular vein was listed at $5.00, although bleeding from the arm, probably the most common form, was only $2.00. A number of major surgical procedures were listed in the New York fee bill with charges generally ranging from $50 to $150. Lithotomy, for example, cost $150, while surgery for aneurysms, depending upon the type and location, could run as high as $200.[31]

Few medical associations were able to maintain their published fees. In many cases adverse public reaction forced the doctors to rescind the fee bill, and in others so many physicians refused to subscribe that the fee bill became inoperative. The failure of most efforts to establish standard fees was only one of the financial problems besetting physicians. In small towns and rural areas cash was always in short supply, and doctors often had to accept produce and personal services. What was much worse was the even greater difficulty of collecting bills in any form. Since farm income depended upon the annual sale of crops, in rural areas the doctor's bill was often paid on an annual basis. In the South and certain other areas, too, it was not unusual to let a medical bill run for years, often until the death of the patient.

The bare living eked out by the majority of physicians led to the growth of the contract system of medical practice. It gained its greatest foothold in the South, where it was helped by the growth of plantations. Unless a young physician could find work with an established practitioner, he frequently found it difficult to get started. By contracting with one or more plantations he was assured of a minimum income and a chance to gain needed experience. In urban areas these same inducements led neophyte practitioners into agreeing to treat members of labor unions and social organizations on a flat per capita basis. Since the medical profession always has claimed an interest in patient well-being, the contract system, which at least in theory emphasizes keeping patients well, should have appealed to it. Preventive medicine, however, traditionally has been a stepchild of medicine. The fee system is a far more profitable — and for many physicians a more congenial — form of employment than working on a salary basis. For these and other reasons, virtually every medical society in the last two hundred years has fought the contract system.

During the antebellum era medical professors and practitioners alike agreed that there was little money to be made in medicine. They also agreed that the root of the problem lay in the excessive number of doctors. *The Western Journal of the Medical and Physical Sciences* asserted in the late 1820s that wherever one went he would find twice as many lawyers or doctors as were needed. A survey of New York State in 1831 showed that it had 2,549 physicians, 1,742 lawyers, and 1,300 clergymen. Cincinnati in 1839 with a population of 50,000 had 100 physicians, or one for every 500 residents.[32] As long as the profession remained overcrowded and disorganized, medical degrees easy to obtain, and entrance to medical practice open to anyone, little could be done to improve the average physician's income. While serious attempts were made to solve all of these problems in the second half of the nineteenth century, it was the twentieth century before any significant improvement came about.

The Social Status of Physicians

Since social status is determined by many variables, any generalizations about the medical profession can scarcely apply to individual doctors. Two of the most important determinants of social position are education and money. In the nineteenth century those who could afford to go to college and medical school, and then on to Europe to complete their medical training, were usually those who held the best positions as medical professors and enjoyed the most lucrative practices. Between fees from medical students, consultation fees from former students, and their own practice, physicians in this category could make in excess of ten thousand dollars a year, a substantial sum in the early nineteenth century.

Below this top group were those physicians with medical degrees from reputable American medical colleges who practiced in towns and cities. They usually made a comfortable living, since the role of physician guaranteed them a certain respect in the community, and, once they had achieved a successful practice, this respect was reinforced by their educational background and economic position. Still further down the social and economic scale was the large number of physicians whose training was derived from an apprenticeship or from one of the many second- and third-rate medical schools. While able individuals could rise from this group and reach the top rank, they were exceptions. Many of the doctors in the lower echelon were barely literate, a situation that did little to enhance the reputation of the medical profession, and they supplemented their income by farming or business — one might almost say they supplemented their business income by practicing medicine.

The majority of those who depended upon medical practice exclusively lived in towns and cities. Although the University of Pennsylvania ranked among the top medical schools, Benjamin Rush advised students planning to practice in a rural area to purchase a farm to keep them busy during slack periods. Even students from reputable schools often had great difficulty establishing a practice, since the ratio of doctors to the population was quite high and competition was always keen.[33] In 1847 a survey of physicians practicing in Virginia showed that about one quarter had neither a medical degree nor a license. In the new states west of the Appalachians where life was even more freewheeling, it was estimated that half of the practitioners had no formal qualifications.[34] Illustrative of this, in 1850 a cursory survey of 201 practicing physicians in east Tennessee showed that only 35 had medical degrees, 42 had attended one course of lectures but had not graduated, 95 claimed to be orthodox physicians but had never received any formal training, and another 29 professed to be Thomsonians or homeopaths.[35]

The many untrained individuals professing to be doctors added to the number of semiliterate practitioners and further lowered the popular image of the medical profession. Far too many physicians fitted the description given by Daniel Drake of one of his colleagues in a small town: ". . . his medicines unlabelled, and thrown into a chaos . . . bundles untied and bottles left uncorked, or stopped with plugs of paper; dead flies in the ointment within his jars, . . . his spatulas, foul and rusty; . . . his surgical instruments oxidating and rusting away, like his mind; . . . his walls overspread with a tapestry of cobwebs; . . . and his floor spotted over with the blood of his surgical patients, and his own tobacco juice."[36] Small wonder that J. Marion Sims's father was almost in despair when he discovered his son wanted to enter the medical profession.

To make matters worse, it was axiomatic that medical students, even in the better schools, were a coarse, crude, uncouth lot. A medical student at Dartmouth in 1808 wrote of his fellow students: "Such a motley collection I am sure I never set eyes on before," although he conceded that a few of them appeared "the complete gentleman."[37] The classic description of medical students was Daniel Drake's characterization of them as too stupid for classics, too immoral for the pulpit, and too dishonest for the bar. The low cost of medical education undoubtedly opened the field to individuals from all social levels. For example, students attending the Vermont Academy of Medicine in 1827 paid $1.50 a week for room and board and a total of $63.00 for tuition. Whatever the reason, medical students were considered in a class by themselves for much of the nineteenth century. Charles W. Eliot, president of

Harvard University, wrote of the medical school in one of his annual reports that "until the reformation of the School in 1870–71, the medical students were noticeably inferior in bearing, manners, and discipline to the students of other departments."[38]

As if the handicap of having a large mass of semiliterates practicing medicine was not enough, the profession faced a great many other difficulties, some of which it created for itself. The major handicap for the profession arose from the sheer lack of medical knowledge. Although, as John Harley Warner has noted, the assumptions about disease shared by doctors and patients alike were in the process of changing, medical practice remained much the same.[39] Despite great strides in anatomy and other areas, physicians still had little comprehension of the cause of most diseases, and out of necessity they continued to rely on traditional methods. When these proved inadequate to deal with the great fever epidemics, in desperation they applied their therapeutics even more rigorously.

Heroic medical practices have already been described and little further need be said, other than that the wholesale bloodletting and dosing finally reached a point in the 1820s and 1830s where it not only gave pause to sensible physicians but brought a strong public reaction. Medical journals, newspapers, and private diaries and correspondence are replete with horror stories of repeated bloodletting and the disastrous results of excessive and prolonged administration of mercurials, arsenicals, and other dangerous drugs. Thomsonians, hydropaths, and other irregulars all seized upon this issue and based their appeal to the public on the grounds that they did not resort to drastic therapeutics. One could say that the rise of the irregular medical sects bore a direct ratio to the administration of drugs by orthodox physicians.

A second major disadvantage suffered by the medical profession was the constant quarreling and bickering among orthodox physicians. This too resulted in part from the increasing doubts about the existing medical rationale for treating patients. While the nineteenth century saw a rising skepticism with respect to all medical theories, intelligent physicians were fully aware of the need for some basic principles. Unfortunately discovering them was not all that simple. As the various medical theories, including Rush's concept of the unity of diseases, were gradually discarded and the realization dawned that all medical questions were not be solved by the discovery of some grand principle, doctors fell to disputing over the cause and treatment of particular disorders.

Physicians of strong convictions soon gained disciples, and the profession found itself divided into warring groups, each one passionately affirming a particular medical viewpoint or course of treatment. Aside from the element of ego involvement in these clashes, the work of the physician was no abstract intellectual endeavor. He was dealing with suffering and dying human beings and was desperately seeking some way to provide relief and save lives. Understandably those doctors who thought—as did Benjamin Rush, for example—they had found a way to save lives enthusiastically promoted their particular form of therapy. State and local medical societies, which generally included only the more educated physicians, were constantly rent by bitter arguments or by personal quarrels. In addition to denouncing each other's medical views, the arguments frequently degenerated into violent personal quarrels. Opposing individuals wrote letters to newspapers, printed pamphlets, and on occasion resorted to fisticuffs, knives, and duels.

It will be recalled that when Dr. Benjamin Waterhouse quarreled with the Massachusetts Medical Society in 1806 he began by attacking his colleagues in a letter to one of the local newspapers. An even more flagrant example of these public quarrels involved Dr. Charles A. Luzenberg of New Orleans. In 1838 he was accused of professional misconduct by the Physico-Medical Society of Louisiana for permitting an embellished account of one of his operations to be published. After an exchange of correspondence, the society expelled Luzenberg, published a pamphlet defending its position and scathingly denounced him as "abrupt in speech, uncouth in manners, irritable and petulant in temper, and arrogant and overbearing in his demeanor."[40]

Not content with this denunciation, the society printed a statement by Dr. John J. Ker that before fighting a duel with Dr. J. S. McFarlane, Luzenberg was "in the habit of suspending bodies of persons who had died under his care whilst House Surgeon of Charity Hospital, and shooting at them as marks with pistols, in order to improve his skill as a marksman in his expected contest with Dr. McFarlane." Astonishingly, although an exchange of correspondence in the New Orleans newspapers continued for some time, alternating testimonials published by the society with retaliations by Luzenberg, the latter did not deny the charge. The New Orleans medical faculty split wide open over the Luzenberg case, with prominent physicians on both sides. In the midst of it all, Luzenberg issued challenges to two members of the medical society, both of whom declined. Luzenberg's seconds promptly placed a paid notice in one of the newspapers proclaiming one of the men who had refused the challenge to be "a most consummate coward, and a dastardly poltroon." He replied the following day: "The infamy which has been stamped upon Dr. Luzenberg's character cannot and shall not be wasted away in my blood." The upshot of this long and bitter controversy was the dissolution of the Physico-Medical Society, and a general lowering of public esteem for the medical profession.[41]

The clashes that disrupted medical societies were only one part of the violent public quarrels between members of the medical profession. Keen competition among physicians led to many accusations of stealing patients. In the South, where dueling persisted until the Civil War, a number of duels were fought over this issue. Louisiana was notorious for dueling, and its physicians fought at least their share. In 1856 one of Dr. Samuel Choppin's students was injured in a brawl and taken to Charity Hospital. He asked for Dr. Choppin, who came and dressed his wound. When Dr. John Foster, the house surgeon, heard of this, he indignantly ordered the nurse to throw out Choppin's prescription and redress the injury. The result was a shotgun duel between the two physicians. Fortunately both principals missed, and the affair seemed settled. Three years later they quarreled over a patient suffering from an aneurysm in the right external clavicle who was admitted to Foster's ward. Choppin wanted to operate, but Foster refused to release the patient. After some troubled relations, the two men met at the gates of Charity, both well armed. Following an exchange of angry words, they drew their weapons. Foster got off the first shot, the bullet entering Choppin's neck cutting the exterior jugular vein in two and causing Choppin's first shot to go wild. Foster fired again, this time hitting Choppin in the iliac region. Bleeding badly from two serious wounds and with his guns empty, Choppin drew his bowie knife and staggered toward Foster; fortunately some of the medical students intervened and separated the two men. Since dueling was illegal within the New Orleans city limits, Foster was arrested. Choppin, who recovered from his wounds, refused to press charges and Foster was released after a night in jail.[42]

One of the most amusing duels, which has a comic-opera touch, occurred between a celebrated French heart specialist, Dr. Joseph Rouanet, who had come to New Orleans, and a Creole physician, Dr. Charles C. Delery. Rouanet, who was given to expounding with great authority, was presented with the heart of a goose that had died of cardiac disease and asked to give his opinion of it. Without hesitation,

Rouanet pronounced it to be the heart of a young baby and spoke of its pathology at some length before learning the truth of the matter. Upon hearing about this incident, Dr. Delery composed a satirical poem in French entitled "The Doctor and the Goose." The Creoles, always irritated by the condescension of the French physicians, gleefully circulated Delery's poem. When Rouanet heard of it, he challenged Delery to a duel. Happily both shots merely grazed the two opponents, and their seconds declared that honor had been satisfied.[43]

In addition to the rivalry between medical schools and the public hostilities among professors, there was a clash between medical schools and medical societies. The first source of irritation was the matter of licensure, a power that many states had given to the state medical societies. The colleges assumed that their degrees were an automatic license to practice, and this assumption eventually carried the day. Another cause of friction was the threat that the colleges posed to the apprenticeship system. As mentioned earlier, apprentices were both a source of income and a form of cheap labor for the physicians. Originally medical school courses were designed to supplement apprentice training, but this situation changed when college professors began offering private clinical instruction and eventually incorporated these private courses into the medical school curriculum. The effect was to cause the traditional apprentice system to wither away.

Since the best general education was offered in eastern schools such as Harvard, Yale, Princeton, and Columbia, the percentage of well-educated physicians was much higher in the East than was true for the West and South. Understandably, educated easterners tended to be condescending to their counterparts in the West, and even more understandably westerners resented this patronizing attitude. As medical centers developed in Cincinnati, Lexington, and Chicago, their medical faculties were critical of the alleged superiority of the eastern schools. Many western physicians reacted by becoming highly nationalistic and accusing easterners of being subservient to foreign science.[44]

The recurrent epidemics and the public disputations between physicians as to the causes and means for preventing these outbreaks brought further discredit to the profession. Without going into details, we may note that the major issue in nineteenth-century public health was whether diseases were specific entities brought into a locality or whether they were spontaneously generated whenever the correct combination of filth, crowding, and meteorological conditions existed. (There were, of course, many variants of these two theses.) Physicians could be found on both sides of the question, although the majority, conditioned by their experience with malaria and yellow fever, were inclined to support the anticontagionist or sanitationist view, one that considered quarantines to be useless. The long series of yellow fever and Asiatic cholera epidemics that ravaged large segments of the population in this century aroused a tremendous furor and helped to focus public attention upon the inability of physicians to agree. A New York physician in 1822 advocated the appointment of a city board of health, but the majority of members, he said, should be laymen since if the board was "exclusively made up of medical gentlemen there is too much reason to fear that their different opinions might lead, as too often happens, to interminable disputes, and to most disastrous consequences." In New Orleans a law creating a board of health in 1848 specified that practicing physicians could not constitute a majority of the members, and, when a sanitary commission was organized the same year, the law excluded practicing physicians and engineers from membership. A commission studying the New Orleans yellow fever epidemic of 1853, which killed eleven thousand people, reported that the medical faculty had not cooperated. The loss was not too great, the report continued, for the few who "deemed the subject worthy of consideration . . . [did] not agree together."[45] The creation of the New York Metropolitan Board of Health in 1866 is a landmark in municipal health, but its membership too was deliberately balanced in favor of lay personnel.

The medical profession had no illusions about the wrangling and discord that characterized its membership. Dr. J. Augustine Smith in 1828 warned the readers of the *New-York Medical and Physical Journal* to beware of speculation and theories. Since speculation was easier than collecting and systematically organizing factual knowledge, he wrote, there had been no change or improvement in medicine for centuries. Frustrated by this lack of progress, most members of the profession had grown querulous. "Let half a dozen medical men be required to give their professional opinions to the public," Dr. Smith asserted, "and they certainly disagree about their facts, and almost as certain fall to calling each other hard names." Dr. H. H. Childs in giving an introductory lecture to the medical class at Willoughby University in 1844 declared: "Need we be surprised that intelligent men extend to the profession a hesitating and doubtful confidence, when educated physicians differ so widely among themselves, avowing the most opposite views, both in

theory and practice . . . that 'Doctors disagree,' has passed into a prov-
erb." A few years later the *Cincinnati Medical Observer* commented: "It
has become fashionable to speak of the Medical Profession as a body of
jealous, quarrelsome men, whose chief delight is in the annoyance and
ridicule of each other." [46]

Newspapers and magazines happily joined in the attack on medicine.
Sarcastic or satirical editorials and stories of malpractice and excessive
bleeding and drugging abound in the journals. When New Orleans
was threatened by yellow fever in 1839 the New Orleans *Courier* advised unacclimated residents to leave town or arrange for good nursing.
"We mention nurses more particularly," the editor added, "inasmuch
as we are convinced that the recovery of the sick depends more on
their attention and discrimination than on the skill of the physician."
Another Louisiana newspaper in deploring the disunity among physicians asserted: "There is just as much uncertainty and confusion among
medical men as among Theologians and Politicians." The Philadelphia,
Pennsylvania, *Item* in 1858 accused the profession of "poisoning and
surgical butchery." One can cite dozens of similar quotations showing
clearly that the public viewed the profession with a mixture of derision
and amused contempt. [47]

The prestige of the medical profession was scarcely high at the end of
the eighteenth century, and if any change occurred during the next fifty
or sixty years, it was probably for the worse. Fortunately, many forces
were at work to remedy the situation. The observations of perceptive
physicians, the impact of the French Clinical School, the pressure from
irregular sects and the public, and developments on the broad front
of advancing science were all helping to modify medical practice and
pave the way for major strides in medicine. In America a rising demand among physicians for improvements in medical education and
for a measure of professional unity led to the formation in 1847 of the
American Medical Association. While the AMA remained compara-
tively ineffective during the nineteenth century, it was one of many
forces that enabled medicine to achieve true professional status by the
beginning of the twentieth century.

CHAPTER 10

Medicine in the Civil War

THE CIVIL WAR inflicted the greatest loss on the United States in its entire two hundred years of history. This bloody, fratricidal struggle caused more casualties than any other military action between the Napoleonic period and World War I and killed more Americans than any war to date. Over 600,000 American soldiers died from battle wounds, disease, or accidents during the four years of fighting. In the course of the war, the Union army enlisted approximately 2,900,000 men and its peak strength stood at 2,100,000. The Confederate enlistments are estimated at between 1,300,000 and 1,400,000. Because of short-term enlistments and thousands of deserters, the strength of the armies varied considerably throughout the war. The records of the Confederacy were destroyed in the burning of Richmond, and any statistics on troops and casualties are at best educated guesses. Dr. Joseph Jones, an indefatigable Confederate medical inspector who kept voluminous but incomplete records, estimated that some 200,000 Confederates either were killed or died of battle wounds and disease. He believed the ratio of battle deaths to those from disease was roughly one to three: 50,000 deaths from battle injuries to 150,000 from sickness. The ratio for the Union forces, which were better fed, clothed, and housed, was approximately one to two: 110,000 battle deaths and 225,000 from sickness.[1]

The bitterness of the fighting can readily be seen from the casualty figures. One North Carolina regiment lost 708 men or 85 percent of its strength at the Battle of Gettysburg, and some 63 Union regiments suffered casualties of more than 50 percent of their strength in single engagements. Neither the celebrated Charge of the Light Brigade nor any single battle in World War I caused losses comparable to these. Grim as these battle statistics are, the troops faced an even greater threat from sickness. Dr. Jones estimated that each of the Confederate soldiers fell ill about six times during the course of the war. Jones's statistics show that during the last two months of the Atlanta campaign, at least half of the Confederate troops were out of action as a result of sickness.[2]

The Union records reveal well over 6,000,000 cases of disease, more than two per soldier. These figures probably underestimate the true number of illnesses, since the widespread distrust of physicians and the incompetence of many army surgeons made soldiers reluctant to report to the medical officer. The common fear of hospitals, and army hospitals in particular, also induced men to take care of their own sick. Moreover, on both sides it was not uncommon for the sick simply to go home, a practice that scarcely contributed to the accuracy of the morbidity and mortality reports.

Despite rising tension, the federal government and the Confederate States were unprepared for war when the final break came — and both sides were handicapped by the confident belief that victory was at most a few months away. The United States began the war with a handful of military surgeons. As of January 1861 the army had a total strength of 16,000 men. The medical staff at the time when hostilities started consisted of 114 surgeons, of whom 24 resigned to join the Confederate forces and 3 more were dismissed for disloyalty.[3] The Confederacy with no previous experience used a handful of former army surgeons to inaugurate its Medical Department. As it turned out, this proved advantageous since its Medical Department was not handicapped by the red tape and inertia engendered in a peacetime army. Neither side had any experience with mobilizing large bodies of men, and the early army camps were characterized by chaos and confusion. Regiments mobilized by various towns and cities were sent to army camps and military centers only to find no provision had been made for housing or food; some regiments arrived with a surgeon but no medical supplies, and others arrived with neither. To make matters worse, the vast majority of those recruited were young men from rural areas where they had experienced little contact with the so-called childhood diseases: measles, mumps, chickenpox, whooping cough, scarlet fever, and diphtheria.

The result was that these disorders—measles in particular—spread like wildfire through the army camps on both sides. Many of the recruits had never been vaccinated, leading to repeated outbreaks of smallpox. Added to these woes were the disorders incident to exposure, poor food, and the incredibly bad sanitary conditions in the camps.

In terms of the quality of army surgeons, one can only say that they represented a cross section of American medicine, ranging from very able individuals to virtual quacks. Most of them had served an apprenticeship and spent some months in a medical school, and sick soldiers received medical attention that was at least as good as the care they would have had in civilian life. The major deficiency was the doctors' lack of experience with gunshot wounds and trauma. Few of the physicians recruited by the army were qualified as surgeons, and many of them gained their first surgical experience under battle conditions.

The Union Medical Department was handicapped during the early war years by a penny-pinching attitude on the part of Congress. The atrocious conditions experienced by the wounded in the first bloody battles were fully reported, but in the early years Congress consistently reduced requests for appropriations to enlarge the medical staff, provide supplies, and establish an ambulance corps. It is difficult to explain this attitude. Undoubtedly the universal distrust of the medical profession played some role, although it does not seem to have affected the Confederate government. The attitude of the federal legislators is all the more surprising in view of the willingness of the Confederate government to comply with requests from its surgeon general. Unfortunately, while the Confederacy was more generous, it simply did not have the vast resources open to the federal government.

Reference has already been made to the conservatism and petty-mindedness that characterized the Army Medical Department. The two first surgeons general could think only in terms of a peacetime army of twelve thousand to sixteen thousand men. Colonel Thomas Lawson, a veteran of the War of 1812 already in his eighties, considered medical books an extravagance. He died shortly after the opening hostilities only to be replaced by another aged veteran, Clement A. Finlay. He too had spent a lifetime in the army making do with as little as possible, and he could not bring himself to ask for the budget and staff necessary to fight a major war. Conditioned to the army's emphasis on seniority and the rituals of peacetime life, he simply could not cope with an emergency situation. More important, as a military professional he was sensitive to civilian interference and consistently opposed the United States Sanitary Commission, a civilian group concerned with the health and welfare of the troops. By December 1861 the disorganization and inadequacies of the Medical Department were all too obvious. The Sanitary Commission, capitalizing on the growing dissatisfaction, pressured Congress into reorganizing the department.[4]

The United States Sanitary Commission originated with two prominent New York reformers, Dr. Elisha Harris, a significant figure in public health, and the Reverend Henry W. Bellows, a well-known Unitarian minister, but the real impulse came from the thousands of women who were anxious to emulate the work of Florence Nightingale and her cohorts in the Crimean War. In countless towns and cities Ladies' Aid Societies and similar groups were springing into existence, and Harris and Bellows sought to coordinate their efforts. Immediately after an organizational meeting in New York, the group offered its help to the surgeon general. Colonel Lawson dismissed the offer, stating that the situation was well in hand and no help was needed. A delegation then went to Washington, where it found the army in a virtual state of chaos. Noting the filthy camps and appalling health condition of the troops, the delegation asked the government to establish an official sanitary commission. Despite strong opposition and considerable skepticism on the part of every official, including President Lincoln, the United States Sanitary Commission came into official existence on June 13, 1861. Three army officers were appointed to the commission, but they were so preoccupied with their army duties that the management of the commission remained in the hands of civilians. The commission's original purpose was to investigate and recommend, but under the leadership of its able secretary, Frederick Law Olmsted, it took a far more active role.[5]

Olmsted was a firm believer in the sanitary movement, and he recognized that the first task of the Sanitary Commission was to educate the officers and men on the need for sanitary measures. The undisciplined troops flooding into Washington were befouling their camps in an incredible fashion, and the poorly organized and understaffed hospitals were often in a similar state. The commission promptly printed and distributed pamphlets on the need for personal and camp hygiene. In general the army cooperated, although the degree of cooperation depended largely upon individual commanders; nonetheless, it took a long educational process before the troops were required to build latrines and forced to use them. Recognizing the inadequacy of army rations, the commission collected tons of fresh meat, fruits, and vegetables. It also distributed thousands of blankets and other supplies, and it was a major agency in improving living conditions for the troops and providing care for the sick and injured. Investigating the Union defeat after the first Battle of Bull Run, Olmsted noted that the best regiments were those that were disciplined and provided with good food, clothing, and housing. Although it seems obvious that healthy troops would fight better, throughout the war Olmsted found many officers and physicians who believed that providing anything more than minimal living conditions pampered the troops and spoiled them as fighting men.[6]

In addition to the work of the Sanitary Commission operating out of Washington, virtually every town and city had its own committee concerned with the welfare of troops from the local area. For example, in June 1862 the Pittsburgh Sanitary Committee sent a delegation of nurses and surgeons to Washington to check on medical care and hospital facilities. Following the Battle of Gettysburg this same committee posted notices calling on surgeons in Pittsburgh and vicinity "to volunteer their services to visit the fields of the late battles in Pennsylvania, to attend to the wounded." According to the local paper, thirty-four physicians and surgeons promptly reported for duty. During the entire war the United States Sanitary Commission continued to receive strong public support and the backing of newspapers. In January 1864 the *New York Times* declared: "No individual — man, woman or child — in all classes of society that have a single luxury, should suffer this winter to pass without contributing something to the great agency for the wants of the army — the Sanitary Commission."[7]

Probably the greatest contribution of the Sanitary Commission was the steady pressure for reform it exerted on the Army Medical Department, the Quartermaster Corps, and other army departments. It had direct contact with the secretary of war, and its members could bring political influence to bear upon Congress. It shares much of the credit for the various congressional measures reorganizing the Medical Department, and the commission was largely responsible for the appointment of Dr. William A. Hammond to replace Surgeon General Finlay on April 25, 1862. Hammond had served as an army surgeon for eleven years and had compiled an outstanding record before resigning his commission to accept a professorship at the University of Maryland. Upon the outbreak of war, he reenlisted and, in accordance with the seniority system, found himself at the bottom of the list of assistant surgeons. Fortunately, he came to the attention of the Sanitary Commission at a time when it was looking for a young man to head the Army Medical Department.

Hammond promptly appointed a number of able medical directors and instructed them to get the job done, disregarding traditional procedures when necessary. He pressed Congress to enlarge the Medical Department, to create a special hospital and ambulance corps, to raise the rank and pay of surgeons, to establish a medical school, and to place ambulances, medical supplies, and hospital construction under the control of the surgeon general's office. Congress, in no mood to waste the taxpayers' money on the Medical Department, contented itself with adding about three hundred surgeons and assistant surgeons. The proposals for a medical school, a hospital, and an ambulance corps were undercut by opposition from within the army and from Secretary of War Stanton. Over and above making drastic changes in the Medical Department, Hammond instituted the pavilion design for army hospitals and introduced the "ridge ventilation" system to provide a continuous flow of fresh air into the wards. A pavilion hospital consisted of a central unit with wings extending in various directions, thus permitting the segregation of patients according to their medical problems.

While Hammond was fighting for major reforms, the medical directors he had appointed were busily straightening out affairs in their respective areas. Jonathon Letterman, one of the most able, reorganized his entire department and created an effective ambulance service for the Army of the Potomac. Unfortunately, Hammond's energetic overhauling of the Army Medical Department outraged too many old hands, and his fight for needed reforms further irritated his relations with Secretary of War Stanton. Moreover, Hammond was a prickly individual who managed to irritate many of his subordinates as well as his superiors. Among his reforms, Hammond had revised the army supply table, but he incurred the wrath of most of his surgeons when he took one further step. In May 1863 he sent out a circular ordering the removal of calomel and tartar emetic from the supply table. Calomel, as noted earlier, was one of the most widely prescribed drugs, and its excessive use was responsible for a vast amount of acute and chronic mercurial poisoning. Tartar emetic was equally dangerous, and Hammond's action was correct from a medical standpoint. Whatever its merit, his circular flew in the face of medical tradition and supplied his enemies with their final weapon. He was removed from office in

November 1863 and subsequently court-martialed for ungentlemanly conduct. Fortunately his major reforms had already taken effect by this date, and the many able men he had appointed carried the Medical Department through the war.

The physicians and surgeons who served in the Medical Department fell into four main categories: regular army surgeons and assistant surgeons who were used primarily for staff work; volunteer surgeons who were given temporary commissions; regimental surgeons commissioned by state governors; and acting assistant surgeons or "contract surgeons," civilians employed by the army largely for general hospital work. With the regular army officers engaged in staff work, medical and surgical care was provided primarily by regimental surgeons in the field and contract surgeons in the general hospitals. Theoretically medical commissions for regimental surgeons were issued by state governors, but in practice most medical officers were chosen by the senior regimental officer. With politics and personal favoritism playing a major role in the selection of surgeons, their quality varied widely. A few states immediately provided examining boards, but they were exceptions. As the war progressed, army medical boards assisted in winnowing the worst of the political appointees, and the caliber of the surgeons improved.[8]

For troops wounded in the early battles the lack of coordination between regimental and regular army surgeons, the want of an ambulance system, and the inadequate field hospitals were sheer disaster. At the Battle of Bull Run in July 1861 regular army surgeons found themselves unable to exercise authority over the regimental surgeons. To make matters worse, many of the latter assumed that their sole responsibility was to care for men of their own regiment. Civilians hired as ambulance drivers led the retreat and left most of the wounded lying on the battlefield, some of whom received no attention for three days. The situation slowly improved, but not before Second Bull Run, when it took a week to clear the field of dead and wounded. Hammond's appeal for an ambulance corps was turned down by Commander in Chief Henry W. Halleck and Secretary of War Stanton. Fortunately, General George B. McClellan of the Army of the Potomac allowed his medical director, Jonathon Letterman, to organize an effective ambulance service that eventually set the pattern for the entire army. His ambulance service and reorganized field hospital system proved its worth at the Battle of Gettysburg, July 1863, where the wounded were removed from the field at the end of each day's fighting. Despite the evident success of Letterman's ambulance service, it was not until early in 1865 that the Army Medical Department was given control over hospital transports—ambulances, ships, and trains.[9]

The Confederate Medical Department had two initial advantages. It was a new organization relatively unhindered by custom, tradition, and deadwood, and almost from the outset it was directed by an intelligent and capable surgeon general, Dr. Samuel Preston Moore. A second advantage came from the southern victories in the early years of the fighting. By remaining in control of the battlefield, the Confederate forces did not feel the lack of ambulances as acutely as did the Union army. The Confederacy was also ahead in organizing a system of field, divisional, and general hospitals, and in 1863 it established a number of "way hospitals" along major railways to help troops furloughed or discharged because of sickness or wounds. In addition the South had interior lines of communication that made possible a greater use of railways for transporting the wounded. The southern railroad system, however, was inadequate for the strains imposed on it, and, as the war progressed, the loss of equipment and the breakdowns due to excessive use nullified this advantage. Not only was the railway system weak, but the South was always short of other forms of transport, both vehicles and animals, and the situation steadily worsened as the war drew on. Moreover, as the northern armies closed in on the South during the last two years, the medical service was forced repeatedly to relocate its hospitals, straining transport to the breaking point.

Surgeon General Moore began building his medical organization immediately upon taking charge. Whereas the Union army relied largely upon state-appointed regimental surgeons, the Confederate government directly commissioned its approximately 5,800 medical officers.[10] Medical examining boards interviewed all candidates from the beginning, thus keeping the number of incompetents to a minimum. Unfortunately, the South had only a few good medical colleges, and the average southern practitioner was not as well educated as his counterpart in the North. The situation was made worse when, in the first wave of enthusiasm for the southern cause, medical colleges were literally depopulated as students and faculty members enlisted in the Confederate service. Only one school, the Medical College of Virginia, managed to keep its doors open after March 1862.

Surgeon General Moore shared with Hammond the ability to pick able subordinates. His best appointment possibly was that of Dr. Samuel H. Stout as superintendent of hospitals in the Department of Tennessee. Stout demonstrated the same initiative and executive ability that characterized his counterpart, Jonathon Letterman, in the Army of the Potomac. Stout carefully chose hospital sites, improved the design of pavilion hospitals, and established a hospital transport system and kept it functioning despite all difficulties.

The South experienced the same problems besetting the Union army during the first years of the war, but, like the North, it learned by experience. Southern troops were plagued with measles and other crowd diseases; they were at least as reluctant as northern soldiers to observe sanitary regulations; and they were probably even less amenable to discipline than those from the North. Yet southerners were fighting on their own soil, and the civilian population rallied to their support. Local residents often flocked to the temporary hospitals to assist in caring for the sick and wounded, and the Medical Department made excellent use of makeshift facilities. There were justifiable complaints against particular surgeons and certain hospitals, but, once the medical service was organized, it provided as good care as might be expected.

As indicated, both sides suffered heavily from diseases, and the first year or so saw widespread outbreaks of disorders associated today with childhood. In 1863 Dr. Joseph J. Woodward of the Union army referred to measles as one "of the most characteristic diseases of the present war." The official returns, he wrote, greatly underestimated the number of cases and fatalities, since many occurred while the regiments were mobilizing in the states, and, even after the regiments became part of the regular army, some months elapsed before the regimental surgeons began submitting reports on the sick and wounded.[11]

Once the ill-disciplined troops were collected in camps, major sanitary problems developed — and with them came diarrhea, dysentery, typhoid fever, and other gastroenteric complaints. With a mean strength of 281,000 men, the Union army recorded 215,214 cases of diarrhea and dysentery during 1861–62. Typhoid, which had been relatively rare in the peacetime army, rose to major proportions in the crowded and unsanitary camps. Approximately 8 percent of all federal troops suffered an attack of what was diagnosed as typhoid during 1861–62, and this figure does not include the thousands of unreported cases or the large number that was listed under the heading of "typho-malarial fever."

As the war progressed and the Union troops pushed further into the

South, the incidence of malaria rose sharply, disabling and debilitating thousands of men; and combined with other diseases, it hastened the deaths of many more. Without laboratories to make positive diagnoses and relying only upon physical symptoms, doctors had great difficulty discriminating among the many fevers, particularly when patients suffered from multiple complaints. Small wonder that the term "typhomalaria" came into general use in this period. This disease was described as one in which "the great majority of cases [show] the well marked enteric symptoms . . . complicated by malarial and scorbutic phenomena." [12] The term "scorbutic phenomena" referred to the widely noted presence of scurvy, both acute and subclinical, among the troops on both sides. With bacillary and amoebic dysentery, typhoid, and malaria widespread, multiple infections were common, and it is easy to see why a syndrome broadly classified as typho-malaria was considered a major disease.

It was inevitable that recruits housed in poorly built army camps or tents and constantly subject to exposure would experience a high percentage of respiratory ailments. Almost half the Union army was affected during the first year, and respiratory disorders continued to plague both sides during the war. Pneumonia was a major killer, with a case fatality rate of about 20 percent. In addition to respiratory complaints, a great many acute and chronic rheumatism and lumbago cases were recorded. While seldom fatal, they were responsible for thousands of medical discharges. It is likely that a large number of these individuals were older men or those whose physical condition should have excluded them from the army.

The diseases that attacked the Union army bore even more heavily upon the Confederate forces. Many more of the Union troops came from urban areas where they had already encountered such diseases as measles and mumps, whereas the South recruited largely from isolated rural areas. Furthermore, the Union forces had the advantage of better clothing, housing, and food. The greater susceptibility of southern troops to communicable diseases was evident from the beginning. Measles, one of the first epidemics to plague northern armies, had a devastating effect upon newly organized southern regiments. One surgeon reported that during a five-month tour of duty in a basic training center he saw four thousand cases of measles among five thousand men. Another southern observer claimed that measles and its sequelae caused more deaths and sickness than any other single cause. [13]

In the warmer climate of the South, enteric infections tended to be both more common and more virulent, and diarrhea and dysentery affected the soldiers from the first mobilization and continued to sicken and debilitate them throughout the entire war. Typhoid, as was true in the North, became more common. Today it is difficult to determine which were the most prevalent enteric disorders, particularly since scurvy and other dietetic complaints contributed to the problems. Significantly, one epidemic of dysentery was stopped when the troops helped themselves to some green corn. Several shrewd observers attributed much of the gastroenteric disorders among southern troops to their almost exclusive use of the frying pan.

Malaria was endemic throughout most of the South and was the most common of the so-called fevers ravaging the troops. Although the value of quinine in remittent and intermittent fevers was recognized, the drug was used largely to alleviate symptoms rather than prevent or cure the disease. Moreover, the abundance of mosquitoes insured constant reinfection. Respiratory infections were normally less of a problem in the South than the North, but the poorly clad and ill-fed southern soldiers may have suffered more than was the case with Union forces.

Since the Civil War was fought before the bacteriological revolution, medical practice varied little from that of the American Revolution. Insofar as surgery was concerned, advances had been made in the prewar years, and the discovery of chemical anesthesia was a major breakthrough. However, aside from dealing with an occasional major injury, the average doctor had had little opportunity to perform surgery. He may have watched a few operations in a surgical amphitheater, but he would have had little hands-on experience. Many physicians literally learned their surgery in the process of treating serious gunshot wounds and performing amputations under wartime conditions.

The vast majority of wounds, 94 percent, were caused by bullets. The widely used minie bullet was made of soft lead and tended to flatten on contact, often lodging in the tissue. By making a large wound and carrying with it bits of skin and clothing, the bullet almost insured infection. Its impact often shattered a section of any bone it encountered, leading to a high percentage of amputations. This was especially true of the first years of the war when few surgeons were skillful enough to do complicated repair work. The almost certainty of infection was another argument for amputation, since hospital statistics showed that cases of primary amputation had a higher survival rate than when the operation was delayed.

The vivid word pictures of surgeons at work following major engagements are almost too painful to recount. Often using makeshift operating tables — the tailgate of a wagon or a door placed over two barrels — surgeons, with their sleeves rolled up and their arms and clothing covered with blood, cut and slashed and sewed. When the pressure was great, amputated legs and arms were simply tossed on a pile close to the operating tables. Surrounding the surgeons were dozens and sometimes hundreds of seriously wounded men, lying on makeshift stretchers or on straw placed on the ground, some still quiet in a state of shock, others moaning with pain.[14]

Although some surgeons were doubtful about anesthesia, it was widely used, with chloroform, because of its ease of handling, being the anesthetic of choice. A folded towel, cloth, or handkerchief was placed over the patient's nose and mouth and the chloroform was dropped on it until loss of consciousness. The deaths from chloroform averaged 5.4 per 1,000 cases, and from ether, 3 per 1,000. These figures are not too bad considering the crudity of the procedure and the weakened condition of so many of the patients.[15]

Antiseptic surgery was still in the future, and it was a common practice for surgeons to probe for bullets with a finger and to wipe their hands on bloody and pus-stained aprons. Bandages and dressings were not sterilized, instruments were frequently washed in a common basin, and dressers repeatedly used the same water to dress several wounds. Infection was so universal that for centuries surgeons had spoken of the "laudable pus," assuming that suppuration was part of the normal healing process. Unless a wound became too inflamed, gangrenous, or showed symptoms of blood poisoning, the infection was allowed to run its course. During the war, hospital gangrene, most likely caused by *Streptococcus pyogenes*, was rampant and led a number of surgeons to anticipate Lister's work by attempting crude antiseptic methods. Among the remedies they applied to gangrenous wounds were iodine, bromine, and chlorine; carbolic and nitric acids; and turpentine. In many cases the infection was too far advanced for the treatment to be effective, and despite a few successes, most surgeons remained doubtful of these antiseptic agents.

Other than these early efforts at antiseptic wound treatment and some innovations in the use of splints, the war brought no major advances in surgery. It did, however, teach several thousand physicians how to deal with serious injuries, help raise their technical skill, and thereby contribute to major surgical advances later in the century. Also, as in previous wars, the ever-present flies hovering around wounds led to the appearance of maggots in the diseased flesh. Whenever possible the maggots were killed with chloroform or one of the disinfectants. Several Confederate surgeons attending southern prisoners in Chattanooga in 1863, lacking dressings and disinfectants, were compelled to leave the wounds alone. They were surprised to discover that the maggots ate the diseased flesh, leaving the tissue clean and healthy. This lesson, which had been learned in earlier wars, was soon forgotten, only to be relearned in the bitter experiences of World War I.[16] Probably the one important lesson taught by the Civil War was the need for cleanliness and sanitation in hospitals and camps.

The value of female nurses was recognized by both sides early in the fighting, and the Civil War saw them used on a relatively large scale for the first time. Shortly after the outbreak of the war, Dorothea Dix, whose activities on behalf of the insane had made her a national figure, volunteered her services and was appointed Superintendent of Female Nurses. A public controversy immediately broke out over whether or not delicate females should be exposed to the horrors, brutality, and moral dangers of war. Acutely aware of these threats to American womanhood, Dix instituted the same rigorous standards for her nurses that had been applied by Florence Nightingale. Nurse candidates had to be over thirty years of age, plain in appearance and dress, and willing to subscribe to a host of regulations dictating almost every waking moment of their lives. Dix's exacting standards hindered recruiting, and, in any case, she turned out to have little administrative skill. The Medical Department solved the problem by simply bypassing her.

Army surgeons generally opposed the introduction of women into hospital wards as a matter of principle, and they believed they had justification for their prejudices. The women volunteers came from diverse backgrounds, few had any experience, and a number of them were more troublesome than helpful. At the same time, most of them were intelligent and capable individuals who quickly made their presence felt. They provided tender care, cleaned up the wards, improved the preparation of food, and did much to improve the morale of the wounded. Officially the Union army enlisted more than three thousand nurses, but this did not include the many women who volunteered following individual battles nor those who helped in general hospitals.

The role of nurses in the South is difficult to assess. Southern women were reluctant to serve as army nurses, since southern traditions did not encourage "ladies" to venture into what was considered a man's world. Yet, since the fighting took place largely in the South, it is probable that a higher percentage of them were involved. A considerable number of women on their own initiative journeyed to the scenes of fighting during the early months and demonstrated that female nurses could play a useful role. Ten days after the first Battle of Manassas (Bull Run), one of the first of these, Sally L. Tompkins, at her own expense organized and began operating the Robertson Hospital in Richmond, one of many hospitals in the South run independently of the military. When the Confederacy brought these voluntary hospitals under military control and ordered that a commissioned officer be placed in charge, Tompkins appealed to President Jefferson Davis, who commissioned her a captain—the only southern woman to hold a commission in the Confederate army.[17]

Another determined woman was Kate Cumming of Mobile, Alabama. Over the objections of her family, she and some other women from the Mobile area headed for the Shiloh battlefield in April 1862. On seeing the desperate need for help, Cumming elected to serve with the troops for the rest of the war.[18] The example of Tompkins, Cumming, Ella K. Newsom, and others led the Confederate Congress in September 1862 to authorize the hiring of women as matrons, nurses, and cooks in army hospitals. In Virginia, where so much of the fighting took place, civilian volunteers, men and women, played an important part in caring for the sick and wounded, and throughout the rest of the South, as injured men were brought into small towns, local people provided food, clothing, shelter and medical care.

The Civil War did not give as much impetus to women's rights as did World War I, but it helped to break down the prejudice against women in the medical area. This prejudice, which applied equally to women whether as nurses, physicians, or technicians, was firmly rooted, and it took over a hundred years of constant struggle before any appreciable gains were made.

One other aspect of Civil War medicine deserves mention—that of medical supplies. Both sides started with virtually nothing, but, whereas the North was producing vast quantities by the end of the war, the South was beginning to face serious shortages. When Hammond took over from the short-sighted Lawson and Finlay and began revising the Army Supply Table, he began stockpiling medical supplies at major depots. When problems arose over the quality of drugs supplied by private manufacturers, Hammond decided the army needed its own laboratories for testing and manufacturing drugs. In January 1863 he established two laboratories in Philadelphia, and between the drugs bought from private manufacturers and those produced in its own laboratories, the Union Medical Department was amply supplied during the last two years of the war.[19]

. The Confederate government recognized from the start that procuring medical supplies was an immediate and pressing need. In the instructions to commercial agents, the purchase of medical supplies ranked third behind arms and clothing, and almost every blockade runner carried some drugs and hospitals supplies. Well before the Union blockade became effective the Confederacy made plans to utilize its native resources. Dr. Francis P. Porcher, an outstanding Charleston physician, was the leading spirit in urging the South to make use of its native flora and to develop its own processing facilities. Surgeon General Moore followed Porcher's appeal by directing his medical officers to search for "indigenous medicinal substances of the vegetable kingdom." He followed up by asking Dr. Porcher to provide a complete manual. The result was Porcher's classic work *Resources of Southern Fields and Forests*, published in 1863, which included descriptions of some four hundred medicinal plants and considerable useful miscellaneous information—a recipe for making soap, for example.[20]

Faced with a growing demand for medicinal supplies, the Confederate government sought to guarantee adequate quantities for the army by prohibiting the sale of items such as calomel, opium, quinine, castor oil, and alum except to government purchasing officers. To meet the growing demand, the Confederacy established manufacturing plants and pharmaceutical laboratories and was able to provide a wide range of pharmaceuticals during the war. Individual states also assisted in the production of medical items. In 1864, for example, Louisiana had two laboratories producing substantial quantities of castor oil, turpentine, and a variety of other medicines.[21]

Two items in short supply in the South were surgical instruments and medical literature. Surgeon General Moore ordered the publication of *A Manual of Military Surgery* in 1863 and encouraged publication of several other works. Unfortunately the South was not equipped to produce surgical instruments on the scale necessary for a major war, but enough were on hand or smuggled in to get by. On the whole, medical supplies were never a serious problem until the last few months of the war, when increasing complaints of shortages appear in the records. Throughout the war supplies were usually available, but the breakdown of the southern transportation system hindered their distribution.

CHAPTER 11

The Emergence of
Modern Medicine

THE CIVIL WAR stimulated both industry and agriculture in the North and provided a major thrust toward
making the United States a ranking industrial nation. One might have
expected that the American penchant for mechanics and technology
would have carried over into science, but Americans were too preoccupied with economic growth and making money to concern themselves
with an abstraction such as basic research. Unless an immediate benefit could be seen, neither business nor government was interested. In
consequence, while European scientists were making major discoveries in chemistry, physiology, and related medical sciences, with a few
exceptions American physicians were content to concentrate on their
medical practices, and, when new viewpoints were set forth, to defend
traditional ideas. As will be seen later, the caliber of medical schools
was only a little better in the immediate postwar years than in the
early nineteenth century, and, with the multiplication of diploma mills
toward the end of the century, it may even have been worse. This fact,
combined with the inability of physicians to deal with the major diseases, guaranteed that while individual physicians were admired, the
profession collectively continued to have little public respect.

Insofar as the low status of physicians was concerned, it should be
borne in mind that in nineteenth-century America no profession was
held in much regard. The dominant profession in the colonial period,
the clergy, had lost government support as a result of the disestab-
lishment of the church during the Revolution. In the succeeding years

ministers had weakened their position by concentrating on individual salvation almost to the exclusion of community affairs, thus limiting their role in society. The third profession, law, was little if any better, since it lagged behind medicine in terms of education and did not gain any real status until the twentieth century.[1]

For various reasons American colleges and universities were not research-minded, and professional schools had little success in raising endowments. Whereas in 1891 theological schools, with their long tradition of education, had a total endowment of $18,000,000, medical schools had been able to attract only $500,000.[2] American medical schools contributed virtually nothing to medical research in the second half of the nineteenth century, and American medical graduates who wished to keep up with the latest in medicine were forced to study abroad. As their predecessors had gone to Great Britain in the seventeenth and eighteenth centuries and to France from 1820 to 1860, American physicians in the post–Civil War period headed for Germany and Austria. Between 1870 and 1914 an estimated fifteen thousand American physicians studied in German universities. Not surprisingly, between one-third and one-half of all leading American physicians in these years had completed their medical education in Germany.[3]

It was not until William H. Welch and other American students returned from Germany filled with enthusiasm for the possibilities inherent in laboratory research that America began to participate in the worldwide explosion of medical knowledge. In the 1890s Welch shaped the newly established Johns Hopkins Medical School into a research center, setting a new pattern for American medical education. He also encouraged General George M. Sternberg to establish the Army Medical School in 1893 and to promote scientific work by Army medical officers. By 1900 dozens of research laboratories had been established in universities and under governmental auspices. By this date, too, American medical researchers were confirming the results of European scientists and making discoveries on their own.[4]

The one major American contribution during these years came in the field of medical literature, an area that earlier had reflected the backwardness of American medicine. In 1876 Dr. John Shaw Billings dismissed the majority of medical theses as hopeless and deplored the fact that medical editing was merely an avocation for busy practitioners and teachers. In writing his student medical thesis Billings had become aware of the need for a first-rate medical library. After service in the

Civil War, he was placed in charge of the Surgeon General's Library and was able to use some $80,000 that had been returned with the closing of army hospitals to build the library's collection. In the 1870s he began work on the *Index Medicus*, the monthly guide to current medical literature, a work still indispensable to medical researchers.[5]

The second half of the nineteenth century saw the beginning of the transformation in medicine and surgery. Of the changes taking place, the bacteriological revolution, which made possible the conquest of the major contagious diseases, was the most significant. Although this revolution occurred in a relatively short period of time, it did not spring full-blown from Pasteur and Koch. Beginning in the 1830s investigations were made of parasites and infusoria, and by the 1850s the causative agents of trichinosis, hookworm, and tapeworm had been identified. Pasteur's work with fermentation in the late 1850s and his demonstrations that settled the question of spontaneous generation had, by 1862, paved the way for the identification of microscopic pathogenic organisms in the latter part of the century.

American medicine remained relatively untouched by these developments. The majority of physicians seldom questioned the traditional theories, and medical journals continued to speak of atmospheric factors, miasmas, predisposing causes, and epidemic constitutions. By 1866 well-educated American physicians generally accepted the evidence of Budd, Snow, and others that cholera was spread by human feces, but many did not realize that the excreta had to come from cholera patients, and other physicians were still convinced that the fecal matter had to undergo decomposition before becoming infectious. A sampling of doctors in 1866 indicates that about half of them still believed that atmospheric causes were the prime factor in the spread of cholera. A few physicians asserted that diseases were caused by fungi or "germs," but even these individuals believed that the pathogenic organisms could be generated spontaneously and that the seeds of infection could be spread atmospherically to germinate under suitable conditions.[6]

The concept of minute pathogenic organisms was given short shrift by the American medical profession, whose members and journals paid little attention to European developments in bacteriology before 1875. When the fungus theory was first set forth in America by John Kearsley Mitchell of Jefferson Medical College in 1849, Austin Flint, whose medical textbook became a standard work in the latter part of the nineteenth century, referred to it as a fanciful hypothesis that would only leave the medical profession open to ridicule. Despite the work of Pasteur and Koch, Flint did not even mention the germ theory until the fifth edition of his medical text in 1881. Even then he thought it applied only to relapsing fever and anthrax. In 1883, a year after Koch had identified the tuberculosis bacillus, a motion was offered in the AMA's annual session to the effect that the profession should have "accurate and disinterested" studies of meteorological conditions at health resorts in order to evaluate their effectiveness in treating "pulmonary affections."[7]

Even though the better physicians were slowly accepting the bacteriological theory, when William Osler worked in the University Hospital in Philadelphia during the 1880s and 1890s, his personal microscope was the only one in use in the hospital. Twenty-five years after Pasteur had laid to rest the theory of spontaneous generation, a Tulane Medical School student based his graduation thesis in 1887 on a series of diphtheria and typhoid cases that seemingly had developed in isolation. The candidate concluded, presumably with the approval of his professors: "From the facts before me, I have been led to the conclusion that both typhoid fever and diphtheria may be spontaneously originated; or, in other words, that there are conditions in which these diseases may arise *de novo* without the transmission of the specific poison from pre-existing causes."[8]

Whatever the medical profession may have thought about the transmissibility of disease, the public never questioned it; hence it is not surprising that laypeople showed more interest in the germ theory than did physicians. *Popular Science Monthly* began writing about the theory in 1874, and the *Atlantic Monthly* and *Harper's Magazine* both stimulated and reflected the growing public interest in the germ theory. Biologists, too, were keeping abreast of the new findings and in 1878 began investigating the role of fungi and bacteria in pear blight, walnut blight, and California vine disease. By the early 1880s, however, the accumulating evidence supporting the germ theory brought a change in the attitude of leading American physicians.[9]

Although a few physicians trained on the Continent had brought back the findings in bacteriology and the new laboratory techniques, America did not move into the mainstream of Western medicine until Welch introduced the principle in the 1890s that laboratory training and research were fundamental to medical education. Welch was not alone in this. He was ably assisted by Dr. T. Mitchell Prudden, who joined Welch in bringing experimental pathology and bacteriology to America; by Dr. George M. Sternberg, another pioneer in bacteriology; by Theobald Smith, first director of the Department of Agriculture's pathological laboratory and organizer of the departments of bacteriology at George Washington and Cornell universities; and by a number of other intelligent and open-minded individuals.

The most important American discoveries in the field of bacteriology during these years came out of the Department of Agriculture. In 1884 Daniel E. Salmon, a veterinarian who had been appointed to organize a Bureau of Animal Industry within the department, employed Dr. Theobald Smith to assist him in studying the diseases of cattle and hogs. By 1891 the two men were able to differentiate hog cholera from swine plague and had identified the microorganisms responsible for both diseases. In the course of their work, they made the important discovery that killed cholera bacteria could provide immunity to the disease and were thus able to provide a vaccination for hog cholera.

Significantly, their success in creating a vaccine from dead bacteria pointed the way to creating vaccines for other diseases. Since hog cholera belongs to a genus of bacteria responsible for a number of disorders, including various forms of food poisoning, the genus was named Salmonella. Theobald Smith then turned to a study of Texas cattle fever. By 1891 Smith and his collaborator, Dr. F. L. Kilborne, had isolated the pathological agent responsible for the disease and were able to demonstrate conclusively that a cattle tick was responsible for its spread. In confirming the role of insect vectors, Smith helped open an entirely new vista for preventive medicine.[10]

The year 1893 was a significant one for American medicine; in addition to the publication of Smith's study on Texas cattle fever, Johns Hopkins School of Medicine opened its doors; George M. Sternberg was made United States Surgeon General; and the New York City Health Department began using its bacteriological laboratory for diagnostic purposes. University, federal, state, and municipal laboratories were springing into existence, and American physicians and scientists were not only beginning to reproduce the experiments and discoveries of their European counterparts but were preparing to make contributions on their own.

The period from 1890 to 1910 has the distinction of clearly marking the start of an era that brought greater changes in medicine and medical practice than at any other time in history. The accumulated impact of bacteriology, pathology, and physiology, and the vast developments in all of the basic sciences that had been taking place in the previous centuries were rapidly applied to medicine in the early 1900s. Since medicine is not a science in itself but rather an art that draws upon the sciences and since the human organism is an exceedingly complex one, scientific knowledge had to reach a critical mass before it could begin to shape medical practice. By the turn of the century this state had been reached, and in no country was its impact greater than in the United States. American medicine had lagged behind that of Western Europe, but within a relatively short period of time major reforms in medical education, combined with a series of other developments, enabled the United States to forge into a leadership role in medicine.

Aside from the zeal and intellectual ability of its scientists, a number of whom had migrated from Europe, this advance was made possible largely through private philanthropy. Led by the Rockefeller and Carnegie foundations, wealthy Americans poured millions of dollars into medical schools and research institutes, and the success of these agencies in turn encouraged both the government and private corporations to follow suit. The Rockefeller Institute for Medical Research established in 1901 — the first of its kind — set an exceptionally high standard and served as a model for many subsequent research institutions. Within a few years the Hooper Institute for Medical Research in San Francisco, Phipps Institute in Philadelphia, Cushing Institute in Cleveland, McCormack Institute for the Study of Infectious Diseases in Chicago, and similar institutions were all making notable contributions.[11]

Meanwhile, following the example of New York City, which established a diagnostic laboratory in 1893, many states and municipalities recognized the practical value of the new laboratory techniques, and researchers in their laboratories began venturing into new areas. One of the ironies of American history is that at the federal level the Department of Agriculture supplied most of the funds for medical research during the latter part of the nineteenth and the early years of the twentieth century. Congress, which evinced little concern for human health, was more than willing to allocate money for sick hogs, cattle, and fowl. Farm animals were valuable property, whereas human life apparently was of little consequence. A few crumbs were doled out to the United States Marine Hospital Service, which, feeling threatened in 1887 by a congressional bill to create a federal bureau of health, had sought to forestall the proposal by establishing a small laboratory on Staten Island, New York. In 1891 the laboratory was moved to Washington, D.C. Ten years later Congress gave official recognition to this Hygienic Laboratory by providing $35,000 for a new building and authorizing it to investigate "infectious and contagious diseases, and matters pertaining to the public health." The following year, 1902, the Biologics Control Act authorized the Hygienic Laboratory to regulate the processing of serums and vaccines, and the service was renamed the United State Public Health and Marine Hospital Service. An important result of these measures was to make research an official function of the health service.[12]

During the regime of Surgeon General Walter Wyman, 1891–1911, the Hygienic Laboratory greatly broadened its scope. The 1902 act changing the name of the Marine Hospital Service enlarged the Hygienic Laboratory to include four divisions, bacteriology and pathology, chemistry, pharmacology, and zoology. The $35,000 congressional appropriation for construction enabled the laboratory to move to a new building overlooking the Potomac in 1904. The next major change came in 1912, when the service was reorganized and given additional responsibilities. Reflecting the broadening of its purpose, the words Marine Hospital were dropped, and it became the United State Public Health Service (USPHS). The law prescribing these changes authorized the service "to study and investigate the diseases of man and propagation and spread thereof, including sanitation and sewage and the pollution either directly or indirectly of the navigable streams and lakes of the United States."

Throughout these years of slow expansion and limited funds, the service performed very creditably. It assisted in the yellow fever work of the Reed Commission and performed notably in connection with the elimination of hookworm and pellagra from the United States. The outbreak of World War I greatly enlarged the operations of the service, as indicated by the increase in its annual budget from $3,000,000 in 1917 to $50,000,000 in 1918. Concern over the rising incidence of venereal disease in the armed forces led Congress to appropriate over $2,200,000 for venereal disease control during 1918. A Venereal Disease Division was established in the USPHS with a budget of $200,000 per year, and another $2,000,000 was appropriated to promote state and municipal venereal disease programs. The Venereal Disease Division managed to survive in the postwar years when governmental activity at all levels was in the doldrums, though its funding was greatly reduced.[13]

With a few exceptions, most breakthroughs in research are the result of a number of small steps taken by many individuals. This has been especially true of the twentieth century, where so many of the discoveries have been team projects. Moreover, advances in communication have enabled researchers in widely separated countries to aid in the steady accumulation of knowledge; thus, to single out a few scientists is to do an injustice to the many. American researchers began by building upon a base established by Europeans, but they were soon engaged in a mutual exchange of information. Possibly as a result of frontier conditions, Americans have always been a practical people with a facility for applied research, a facility that we seem to be sharing with the Japanese. The demonstration in 1900 that yellow fever was carried by a particular mosquito was the first major American medical accomplishment of the twentieth century, and other success stories include the mass production of penicillin and DDT during World War II and that of polio vaccine in the 1950s.

Yellow fever had been a major threat to the United States for well over a hundred years. Following a great epidemic in 1878 that swept far up the Mississippi Valley, the attacks appeared to be lessening, but the Spanish-American War, which involved the occupation of Cuba where yellow fever was endemic, raised the specter of serious losses among the armed forces. Surgeon General George Sternberg, a first-rate bacteriologist, had already done considerable research on yellow fever and had encouraged Dr. Aristides Agramonte, a Cuban bacteriologist and a U.S. Army contract surgeon, to devote his time to the project. In 1900 Sternberg decided that a full-time medical team was needed to work on the problem, and he created a special army board headed by Major Walter Reed and including Agramonte, James Carroll, and Jesse W. Lazear. Reed was an excellent choice; he had studied under Welch at Johns Hopkins and had worked closely with Sternberg.

Some nineteen years earlier, in 1881, a Cuban physician named Carlos Finlay had uncovered strong evidence showing that a particular mosquito, the *Culex* or *Stegomyia fasciata* (presently *Aedes aegypti*), was responsible for transmitting the disease. Other than Rudolph Matas, a New Orleans surgeon, few investigators at that time gave credence to Finlay's findings. Shortly before the Reed Commission began work, Dr. Henry Rose Carter of the Marine Hospital Service, after making an intensive study of a yellow fever outbreak in a small Mississippi town, also became convinced that mosquitoes were the vectors of yellow fever. Reed and his associates, aware of the work of Rose and others, first tested various hypotheses and then centered their efforts on the mosquito thesis. With the help of Finlay, they were able to demonstrate the validity of his original hypothesis.[14]

Based on an intensive study of the writings and correspondence of the individuals involved, François Delaporte argues in a recent book that Finlay believed that the mosquito was merely a carrier and not an intermediate host. Furthermore, Delaporte maintains that the Reed Commission was searching for the yellow fever bacillus purportedly discovered by an Italian, Giuseppe Sanarelli, until a two-man British commission visiting Cuba informed the Yellow Fever Commission members about Sir Ronald Ross's findings on the connection between mosquitoes and malaria. Even then Reed had two staff members continue the bacteriological studies and assigned only Jesse Lazear to investigate the mosquito hypothesis. Delaporte concludes that Walter Reed played only a minor role and that most of the credit should go to Ross and Lazear.[15]

Few medical breakthroughs have had so great an effect as the work of the Reed Commission. Major William Gorgas, the chief sanitary officer in Havana, soon rid the city of yellow fever, a disease that had been endemic at least since the eighteenth century, and his antimosquito campaign in Panama made possible the completion of the Panama Canal, a project that might have been delayed for many more years. The conquest of this dramatic killer disease was of inestimable value in terms of its economic, social, and psychological impact on the southern United States, the Caribbean area, South America, and other tropical and semitropical regions.

An individual American who made a significant discovery on his own was a young American pathologist at the University of Chicago, Howard Taylor Ricketts. In 1902 two pathologists, Louis B. Wilson and William M. Chowning, began studying a mysterious fever in the West and concluded that wood ticks were the source of infection. Responding to requests for assistance, Surgeon General Walter W. Wyman of the Public Health Service sent Charles W. Stiles to aid in the investigation, but Stiles, in a cavalier fashion, dismissed the Wilson-Chowning thesis. Chowning then asked Ricketts for help. Ricketts began work in 1906 and confirmed that the disease was transmitted between animals, and in some cases to man, by infected ticks. He also discovered that infected ticks existed in nature. Finally he was able to identify the pathogenic organism causing the disease in ticks and their eggs and in the blood of infected humans. Since Rocky Mountain spotted fever closely resembled Mexican typhus fever or tabardillo, in 1909 Ricketts went to Mexico City to study the latter disorder. Here he discovered the role of lice in transmitting typhus and was able to identify the pathogenic organism, one belonging to the same family as Rocky Mountain spotted fever. Tragically, in 1910 Ricketts fell victim to typhus. In his honor, the genus he had identified was named rickettsia.[16]

The team approach, which helped Reed and his associates show the way to subdue yellow fever, enabled Americans to make major contributions toward the elimination of two other costly disorders, hookworm and pellagra. Interestingly enough, the three diseases have little in common: yellow fever is a virus infection; hookworm is a parasitic disorder; and pellagra is a deficiency disease. In 1900 Captain Bailey K. Ashford of the United States Army noted the prevalence of hookworm in Puerto Rico, and shortly thereafter the parasite was recognized as a common disorder in the American South. A zoologist, Dr. Charles Wardell Stiles of the USPHS, in 1902 identified the American organism as a new species and began studying methods for attacking it. As the scope of the hookworm problem became evident, in October 1909 the Rockefeller Foundation stepped into the picture and established the Rockefeller Sanitary Commission. Working closely with Stiles and the USPHS, the Rockefeller Commission began a massive educational campaign to awaken southerners to the problem. Utilizing state and local school boards, health boards, medical societies, and journals and newspapers, a two-fold program was undertaken, consisting first of treating those infected and second of developing preventive measures to stop the dissemination of the intestinal parasite. While Stiles was concentrating on the United States, Ashford had launched a massive campaign against hookworm in Puerto Rico. In 1915 the Rockefeller Foundation disbanded the Sanitary Commission on the grounds that hookworm had almost disappeared from the United States. Stiles justifiably criticized the decision, knowing all too well that hookworm was still a major problem. Despite the Rockefeller Foundation's failure to continue the battle against hookworm, it had created a public awareness of the disease and made a major contribution to public health in the rural South.

Since hookworm is a disease of poverty, its elimination from the United States awaited the vast social and economic changes of the late 1930s and early 1940s.[17]

Like hookworm, dietetic disorders are also social diseases, and their control involves both medical science and socioeconomic changes. The first of the dietetic diseases to be recognized was scurvy. Although the association between it and diet had been recognized by a few perceptive individuals as early as the sixteenth century and much more had been learned about it in the succeeding years, as late as the Civil War many physicians were still treating it with mercurials and other dangerous drugs. Physicians generally, however, had no illusions about the cause and cure of scurvy, but the same cannot be said for pellagra and the other deficiency diseases. The bacteriological revolution in the late nineteenth century precipitated a frantic search for the microorganisms assumed to be responsible for virtually every disorder, and pellagra was a fine case in point. When it was first found to be widespread in Europe in the eighteenth century, there was much speculation as to its cause. Hereditary factors, meteorological conditions, diet, and spoiled corn all had their advocates until early in the twentieth century when an Italian bacteriologist triumphantly announced that he had isolated the bacillus causing the disease. Although his claims were soon disproved, the bacteriological origin of pellagra continued to be asserted as late as the 1920s.

In 1902 a case of pellagra was diagnosed in a poor Georgia farmer, and within the next three or four years the disease was found widely dispersed throughout the southern states. By 1908 it was clear that pellagra was a major southern problem, and newspapers and magazines began playing up the more lurid aspects of this strange and mysterious plague, variously depicted as a hereditary, constitutional, insect-borne, bacterial, or dietetic disease. In May 1909 the USPHS, using its limited resources, assigned Dr. C. H. Lavinder to the South Carolina Hospital for the Insane. Lavinder began his research in two bare rooms without water or gas. In 1912 two teams of scientists began an intensive study on the cause of pellagra: one was a USPHS team and the other, the Thompson-McFadden Commission, was a privately endowed study under the auspices of the New York Graduate School of Medicine. Two years later, with congressional backing, the USPHS decided to broaden its assault on pellagra. Consequently, Surgeon General Rupert

Blue assigned a staff of forty-one men, provided a budget of $80,000, and—more significant—appointed Dr. Joseph Goldberger to head the project.

After a quick survey of the studies already made and a field trip into the South, Goldberger was convinced that a food deficiency was the root of the problem. He began a series of experiments in which he first demonstrated that the disease could be cured by a balanced food intake and then culminated his work in 1915 by showing that pellagra could be induced in humans by an inadequate diet. The publication of his findings should have made him a popular hero, but instead he was immediately denounced by southern politicians, newspapers, and physicians for casting aspersions on their region. Despite what would appear to be indisputable evidence, Goldberger's findings continued to be derided or dismissed by many physicians. As late as 1918 the Pellagra Commission of the National Medical Association declared firmly that pellagra was a communicable disease resulting from poor sanitation.

World War I temporarily raised living standards in the South and reduced the incidence of pellagra. When a depression struck in the immediate postwar years, Goldberger warned the USPHS that any decline in southern living standards would cause pellagra to flare up again. On his advice, President Warren G. Harding in a national address mentioned the problem of poverty and famine in the South. Southerners were once again outraged at the suggestion of poverty within their region, and southern politicians and health officers joined together in denying the existence of pellagra. Only Mississippi conceded that it had a problem and requested help from the USPHS. As with hookworm, pellagra remained a serious public health problem until the New Deal and World War II raised economic and educational standards in the South.

By 1921 Goldberger was determined to find the specific cause of pellagra, and he began concentrating on amino acids. He was working on a vitamin theory when cancer cut short his career in 1929. In 1937 Dr. Conrad A. Elvehjem and his colleagues in the agricultural chemistry department of the University of Wisconsin reported the discovery of nicotinic acid as a cure for pellagra. The immediate result was a sharp reduction in the death rate from pellagra, one that had been going down slowly. Within the next few years pellagra was virtually eliminated.[18]

Captain Edward B. Vedder of the Army Medical Corps graduated from the Army Medical School in 1904 and was assigned for a number of years to the Philippine Islands. Here he encountered and began studying beriberi. Beriberi is a deficiency disease that owes its existence to advancing technology. As more efficient machines for milling rice were developed, they turned out a more attractive but far less nutritious product, with the result that a new disease appeared among those populations whose food consisted largely of rice. In 1913 Vedder published his findings in a classic work entitled *Beriberi*. Meanwhile, Casimir Funk, a Polish chemist working in Germany, had discovered a substance in rice hulls that cured beriberi in pigeons fed milled rice, a substance he named *vitamine*. The next step in the discovery of vitamins was taken by a young agricultural chemist working for the University of Wisconsin, Elmer V. McCollum, who developed a technique for feeding rats on highly selective diets in order to determine nutritional values. His work enabled him to discover vitamin A in 1913 and vitamin D in 1922. Having discovered a substance in rice and yeast that cured beriberi, Captain Vedder immediately began working with R. R. Williams, a chemist, trying to identify it, but the prevailing technology and scientific knowledge was not adequate for the task. Since the term "vitamine" had just been coined by Funk, McCollum called this unidentifiable nutritional agent vitamin B. Williams, who continued his research, was able in 1933 to isolate the substance, which he termed thiamin, a part of the B-complex. Subsequently he was able to learn its structure and by so doing was able to synthesize it.

While medical discoveries were being piled one on top of another at an ever-accelerating rate, the average American physician, at least until the later years of the nineteenth century, continued the even tenor of his ways, little concerned with what was happening in laboratories. Aside from a trend toward moderation, medical practice for most of the second half of the century did not differ too greatly from that of earlier days. In 1862 Dr. Flint wrote of the change that had taken place in medicine during the previous twenty-five years. "Formerly," he wrote, "boldness was a distinction coveted by the medical as well as the surgical practitioner. 'Heroic practice' was a favorite expression, consisting in the employment of powerful remedies or in pushing them to an enormous extent. Now," he continued, "conservatism has become a leading principle in medicine." [19]

This is not to say that treatment was no longer active, but bloodletting and other depletory therapeutics were giving way to stimulants such as quinine. As faith in traditional medical theories declined, a more empirical view of medicine emerged, a change that augured well for the trend toward therapeutic moderation. Empiricism, combined with advances in all areas of medicine, led to the gradual discarding of many traditional drugs, and by the early twentieth century many of the elite physicians were tending toward therapeutic nihilism.[20]

Responding to advances in the biological sciences in the later years of the century, educated physicians became less concerned with the patient's family background and home environment and began placing more emphasis on the individual's physical condition as determined by instruments and laboratory tests. Nonetheless, the art of physical diagnosis was limited to the elite physicians, and most practitioners relied largely on quizzing and observing the patient before prescribing. The ability to prescribe was considered the real art of medicine. The thermometer and other diagnostic instruments were slowly making their way into medical practice, but physical diagnosis remained handicapped by the reluctance of patients, particularly females, to bare their skin to probing, palpation, and percussion by physicians.[21]

Nonetheless, while Flint spoke for well-trained, intelligent physicians, thousands of other doctors, particularly in the West and South, continued their vigorous assault upon the ills besetting mankind. The treatment given a parturient patient by a southern physician in 1887 clearly showed that heroic medicine still survived. According to Dr. D. R. Fox's report to the local medical society, within the space of twenty-four hours he cupped and bled the patient of eighty ounces of blood, dosed her with castor oil, gave a purgative enema, and vomited her with tartar emetic every two hours. As a result of his treatment, she was completely "restored to health in about four weeks."[22]

Most physicians had only a hazy notion of etiology, and they prescribed largely for symptoms such as fevers, coughs, diarrheas, consumption, and sore throats. The treatment itself was often hit or miss. While dosage was moderating, quinine, aconite, opium, alcohol, mercury, strychnine, arsenic, and other potentially dangerous drugs still formed the materia medica. Opium, long used for bowel complaints, began to rival calomel as a cure-all. It was sold wholesale as raw gum opium, laudanum, and morphine and as a constituent of dozens of prescriptions and patent medicines. In one form or another it was administered for inflammations, sprains, coughs, colds, sore throats, colics, diarrheas, female complaints, and neuralgia. Its administration for chronic and acute pain and for insomnia was almost automatic, and medical professors and medical textbook authors seldom warned medical students about the danger of addiction. Attesting to its growing popularity, the annual importation of crude opium increased from 24,000 pounds in 1840 to a yearly average in the 1890s of about 500,000 pounds plus another 20,000 ounces of morphine and its salts. While a few physicians blamed the growing number of opium addicts upon quacks and irregulars, by 1900 more and more doctors were recognizing that indiscriminate prescribing by their own profession was largely responsible.[23]

The old standby, alcohol, was used as a tonic, stimulant, preventive, and cure. Usually prescribed in the form of whiskey or brandy, it was cheap, easily available, and readily accepted by the patient. A popular textbook stated: "alcohol in some form should be used in *every* case of typhoid *from the beginning.*" It was considered equally valuable for chronic and acute diseases, and it was freely prescribed for all ages. A usual dose for infants and children was one-half to two teaspoonsful every three hours.[24] Alcohol, often in conjunction with opium in some form or another, was also a basic ingredient of the thousands of proprietary drugs that were promoted by every means possible. For example, a Department of Agriculture chemist found that Hostetter's Bitters, a highly popular nostrum, contained 32 percent alcohol.[25]

Bloodletting, particularly venesection, had begun to fall out of favor by the 1830s, and its use had steadily declined as the century advanced. Many older physicians, however, were reluctant to see phlebotomy (bleeding) fall into disuse, and their plaintive appeals on its behalf can be found in medical journals into the early twentieth century. Dr. Moritz Schuppert insisted in the *New Orleans Medical and Surgical Journal* in 1882 that in many cases a bold and vigorous use of the lancet was still essential.[26] Even Dr. Austin Flint, an early voice of moderation, asserted in 1886 that within fifty years bloodletting would once again take its place among the physicians' armament.[27] In 1893, one of America's best known physicians, Dr. William Osler, declared: "Pneumonia is one of the diseases in which timely venesection saves life," and as late as 1913 Fielding H. Garrison wrote that there is scarcely a physician "who may not suddenly encounter some circumstances in his experience in which venesection would turn out to be his sheet and anchor and his patient's salvation."[28]

Although the public image of the physician was rallying from the low point it had reached in the 1840s and 1850s, the average physician before World War I enjoyed neither money nor social position. The aim of nearly all young physicians was to establish themselves in a comfortable family practice, preferably among the well-to-do, but unfortunately the number of physicians far exceeded the demand, and the majority eked out a bare living, supplementing their income by operating a pharmacy or a small business, or else by farming. The middle and upper classes expected to be treated in their homes, and the physician who cared for the family and their servants was guaranteed a good income and social acceptability. Young doctors without family connections were forced to rely on an office practice or else serve as a dispensary physician or visiting physician to the poor. An office practice itself carried some stigma since an office visit was the resort of those workers who could not afford to have the doctor call on them in their homes. Moreover, the physician with an office practice faced keen competition, not only from his colleagues, but from druggists, who were not averse to prescribing, and from a host of midwives, irregulars, folk practitioners, and quacks. The lowest income groups could not afford to pay any medical fees and were forced to depend on the free medical care offered by dispensaries. For example, in 1900 some 875,000 patients were treated in New York City's dispensaries.[29]

As had been true in the past, a wide gap separated the top physicians from those conducting an ordinary practice. In contrast to the relative poverty and limited status of the average physician, the leading ones enjoyed both social position and wealth. In most cases these affluent physicians came from well-to-do families, had attended college and medical school, and then had completed their medical education by studying abroad. They generally held professorships in the better medical schools and had the additional advantage of an entrée into a middle- or upper-class practice. As the nineteenth century advanced, they also tended to become specialists.

By 1900 basic societal changes were beginning to undermine both the practice of home care and the role of general practitioner. Treating the patient in his or her home was consonant with the belief that the mind and body were closely related, and that hereditary (constitutional), environmental, emotional, and moral factors were all determinants of sickness. Consequently, in order to make a diagnosis, a physician needed to know his patient's family, background, and home environment. In part because they were unable to prevent or cure the major medical problems, nineteenth-century physicians took on the role of moral guardian and family counselor. The advent of bacteriology, medical technology, and a rapidly increasing knowledge of pathology and physiology provided the profession with more effective methods for dealing with medical problems. As "scientific medicine" gained wide acceptance, social factors such as the home environment were no longer considered significant. In addition, a rising standard of living in the twentieth century created a growing demand for medical services precisely at the time when the AMA, through promoting stricter licensing laws and reform of medical schools, was drastically reducing the number of physicians. Under these circumstances, office practice, a far more efficient method of delivering health care, became both more respectable and lucrative.

Over and above these developments, another factor contributing to the reduction of home care was the changing status of hospitals. Traditionally they had been charitable institutions operated by laypersons and supplying limited medical care for the poor. In colonial America the sick poor usually were cared for in their own or their neighbors' homes. As discussed earlier, in the eighteenth century a few almshouses were built and the first general hospital to care for the sick in the English colonies, the Pennsylvania Hospital, was established. Since sickness was often a cause of poverty, a number of the almshouses evolved during the nineteenth century into public hospitals. This century also saw the appearance of many voluntary hospitals. The impetus for them came first from doctors seeking to promote medical education and their own practices, and second from well-to-do individuals motivated by humanitarianism and a concern for the community welfare. The staff physicians in these hospitals received no fees, but the prestige associated with the positions carried over into their private practice. The majority of patients were charity cases, although, since most hospitals were founded in the major port cities, a few paying patients were accepted.

For much of the nineteenth century, hospitals were considered places where the deserving poor were sent to die, for respectable people expected to be treated and to die in their own homes. Hospital management remained in the hands of the well-to-do trustees, to whom the admission of patients was a form of patronage. While a few institutions provided reasonably good care, conditions in the majority of them were deplorable. The hospital, the bedding, and all facilities were filthy, nursing was performed largely by convalescent patients or disreputable women, and the medical care was minimal.

The sanitary movement in the second half of the century, the Civil War, and the discovery of antiseptic surgery all contributed to improving the condition of hospitals. Antiseptic and aseptic surgery, in conjunction with the earlier development of anesthesia, also made possible an explosive rise in surgery in the last decade of the century. As surgery became more complicated, it became advantageous for both surgeons and patients to utilize hospitals. These advances in surgery, along with those in medicine, began transforming hospitals into effective institutions providing a wide range of medical and surgical services.[30]

Meanwhile urbanization was creating a demand for hospital beds for those patients able to pay. Caring for the sick in their homes was no longer feasible with so many single workers residing in boardinghouses and the middle class beginning to move from spacious homes into smaller apartments. The increasing number of paying patients gradually changed the perception of hospitals from a place for the sick poor to an institution caring for the acutely sick. At the same time technological and other changes in medicine and surgery steadily increased the cost of medical care, forcing an even greater reliance on paying patients.[31]

For much of their history American hospitals had been community institutions controlled and financed by lay trustees, who were as much concerned with the moral welfare of the patients as with their physical well-being. By the end of the nineteenth century, social and economic changes, plus those in medicine, led to a fundamental restructuring of hospitals. By that date hospitals were in the process of being transformed into bureaucratic institutions reflecting the interests and perceptions of physicians. Rising medical costs meant that lay trustees could no longer bear the major burden of hospital costs, and hospital administrators were forced to look to patients for revenue. Since private physicians were responsible for referring patients to hospitals, they gradually assumed the authority formerly held by the trustees. While all of these factors undoubtedly played a role in the development of the modern hospital, Charles Rosenberg argues that the history of American hospitals can best be understood by focusing on the physicians' role in shaping them. And there can be little question that the turn of the century saw the emergence of a strong, well-organized medical profession.[32]

One can scarcely read medical journals in the late nineteenth century without becoming aware of the apprehension with which physicians viewed the rise of specialists. The first of the specialties, ophthalmology, emerged in the first half of the nineteenth century, although its origins go far back in history. It received a major impetus in 1851 from Hermann Helmholtz's invention of the ophthalmoscope, and within the next twenty years medical schools began appointing instructors in diseases of the eyes. The second half of the century saw a rapid increase in the number of medical specialties. In 1875 the International Medical Congress had eight different sessions. By 1900 the number had grown to seventeen, and by 1915 there were an estimated thirty-four specialties. By the 1880s the number of specialized medical publications was growing faster than those of generalists. In the early 1900s the family doctor, who was already complaining about the poor going to dispensaries or hospital outpatient clinics, found the middle class beginning to go directly to specialists. Most specialists in these early years, however, continued as family physicians to their well-to-do patients.[33]

While the more able physicians tended to be preoccupied with their teaching and medical practices, during the second half of the nineteenth century the demands on most doctors were not too great, and they had ample time to engage in political and social affairs. In smaller communities they were often among the best-educated citizens, and they frequently gravitated toward political office. In addition, they occasionally supplemented their income by lecturing. A Pittsburgh newspaper announced on February 19, 1868, that "A. O'Leary, M.D.," would give a course of physiological lectures on the subject "Laws of Life, Health, Strength, and Beauty," the lectures to be illustrated by French manikins, models, pathological specimens, and skeletons.[34] Judging by Dr. O'Leary's title, his lectures were clearly designed to appeal to the general public.

The role of family doctor in Protestant America had always carried with it certain aspects of a father confessor and moral arbitrator. Many physicians happily accepted their moral obligations and used the authority of medicine to support the accepted middle-class moral values. They cited anatomical and physiological reasons to explain why females were delicate, sensitive, and dominated by their emotions, and most of them agreed that normal, decent females derived no satisfaction from sex other than giving pleasure to their husbands and enabling them to bear children. Paradoxically, while holding this latter view, a number of them were uncommonly concerned with both male and female masturbation, considering it a specific disease entity. There is scarcely a symptom, syndrome, disease, or pathological condition that was not ascribed to masturbation—dyspepsia, urethral constriction, epilepsy, blindness, deafness, vertigo, headache, loss of memory, and irregular action of the heart, to name a few. Chronic masturbation led to moist, clammy hands and feet, stooped shoulders, pale or sallow skin, dark circles under the eyes, acne, and a hangdog look. Any individual who was nervous, tired, or rundown was automatically suspect.[35] On the basis of any of these symptoms, it was a simple matter for a physician to interrogate closely—or browbeat—any patient suspected of masturbation and, since few could deny ever having masturbated, confirm the diagnosis.

As the subject of race became a popular study in the late nineteenth century, the old arguments of southern physicians about the innate anatomical and physiological differences between whites and blacks were revived, and doctors in all areas raised their voices in support of Anglo-Saxon superiority. Whereas in the 1850s Dr. Samuel A. Cartwright had cited his own research to show that blacks' inferiority resulted in part from their use of 20 percent less air than whites, a medical editorial in 1909 solemnly declared: "Medicine . . . showed that the white man's brain is capable of more development because his skull does not harden or ossify as early as the black man's"—a hypothesis at least as valid as the early one.[36]

The demand for women's rights was met by scientific medical proof of female inferiority and dire warnings of the disastrous impact of education upon the delicate and sensitive female mind and body. Members of the Medical and Chirurgical Faculty of Maryland in 1881 were alerted by their annual orator to the dangers from the decay of home life and the rise of divorce and abortion. To stop these abuses, the members were exhorted to "redeem woman from the bondage of her education and restore her to wifehood and motherhood; to uplift the sexual conscience of the community; . . . and to fill our homes with prattling children—these be the great missions of the physician, missions which he must cheerfully and manfully accept as his Duty of the Hour."[37]

Fortunately, medicine has always had its iconoclasts, and there were many physicians who objected to this nonsense. The entire profession was agreed about the danger from tightly laced corsets and the many layers of clothing worn by middle- and upper-class women. When the bicycle fad developed at the turn of the century and ministers railed against its moral impact upon young girls (it freed them from adult supervision and supposedly turned them into tomboys and regular hoydens), the medical profession was more sanguine. A few physicians felt the exercise was too violent for females and a few others worried about the effect of the bicycle saddle upon young girls, but most of them welcomed cycling as a healthy form of exercise.[38] Clearly physicians at the turn of the century, as with those of today, were products of their time; they accepted the prevailing moral and ethical standards and saw nothing wrong in rationalizing them in terms of their professional knowledge.

The first two decades of the twentieth century saw the revolutionary changes in medicine gradually filter down to the average practitioner. In 1964 Professor Lawrence J. Henderson of Harvard wrote that somewhere in America between 1910 and 1912 "a random patient, with a random disease, consulting a doctor chosen at random had, for the first time in the history of mankind, a better than fifty-fifty chance of profiting from the encounter."[39] The statement may well be valid insofar as physical factors are concerned, but medical care also involves comfort, reassurance, and emotional support. Moreover, a number of effective drugs had been discovered in the nineteenth century and early physicians were able to alleviate or cure many medical problems. While medical practice was greatly improved, as of 1912 many medical diploma mills were still operating, and the licensure laws, which were a relatively new development, had blanketed many poorly trained practitioners into the profession. Nonetheless, medical practice by World War I was vastly different from what it had been at the end of the Civil War.

CHAPTER 12

The Flowering of Surgery

By the end of the Civil War, anesthesia, the first of two discoveries that revolutionized surgery, had already gained wide acceptance. No longer under the pressure from dealing with agonized struggling patients, surgeons were much more willing to resort to radical measures and to perform longer and more complex procedures. The consequence was a sharp rise in the death rate from postoperative infections, the traditional septicemias and gangrenes. In 1865 an English surgeon, Joseph Lister, deduced from a study of Pasteur's work that microorganisms derived from the air or some other source must cause the septic poisoning of wounds. In 1865 he began experimenting with an operative technique involving cleanliness and the use of a weak carbolic acid solution as an antiseptic. His hope was to kill any pathogenic organisms in the wound and to prevent the entrance of any others. He first published an account of his method in 1867 and thereby precipitated a heated controversy. The elaborate precautions required by the Listerian method seemed ridiculous to traditional surgeons, and even under the best of circumstances the system did not always work. The few skeptical surgeons willing to attempt antiseptic procedures often applied them in so perfunctory a manner as to render them ineffective.

In America, Oliver Wendell Holmes's earlier plea for cleanliness and antiseptic procedures in connection with obstetrics had won many converts, but even so the cumbersome Lister method found no immediate support. Whereas anesthesia had won almost instant acceptance, antiseptic surgery took over twenty years to gain respectability. In 1877 Dr. Robert F. Weir, a well-known New York surgeon, declared that only recently had the teachings of Lister received any attention in American surgical practice. "In fact," he went on, "aside from an article by Schuppert in the *New Orleans Medical and Surgical Journal* little or nothing has appeared in our medical journals relative to the result of the so-called antiseptic method."[1]

Dr. Moritz Schuppert, a German physician who had settled in New Orleans in the 1850s, heard of the remarkable results achieved by German surgeons using the Listerian technique and decided to visit Germany and see for himself. On his return to New Orleans in 1875, he immediately began using the antiseptic method in Charity Hospital. In January 1878 he reported that he had performed 120 operations in the previous two and a half years using Lister's method, and that the mortality rate had been only four percent, an astonishing figure for this period. Shortly thereafter Schuppert retired, and the antiseptic method fell into disuse in Charity Hospital. It was not revived until a flare-up of puerperal fever in 1887 led the assistant house surgeon, Dr. Frederick W. Parham, to reinstitute rigorous antiseptic procedures. The success of these measures with obstetrical patients encouraged him to reintroduce the antiseptic method into the surgical service.[2]

Even after Lister went to Philadelphia to address the International Medical Congress in 1876 the medical profession remained skeptical of his procedure. The first completely antiseptic operation was not performed in Boston until 1879. Growing interest in the subject led to great debates over the issue in the American Surgical Association's meetings. In the course of a discussion in 1883 a New York physician declared: "I do not think Listerism is going to die—it is dead." Dr. Claudius H. Maston of Alabama stated that not a surgeon in Alabama used Lister's method, and he was followed by physician after physician echoing his assertion.[3]

As indicated, cleanliness in dealing with open wounds had already won some converts even before Lister, and the value of carbolic acid, along with other antiseptic agents, had been recognized during the Civil War. Consequently, some aspects of Listerism were accepted almost immediately, but it was the 1890s before the Lister principles carried the day. Their relatively late introduction into America meant that the aseptic procedures developed by the Germans quickly won out over the antiseptic methods. Rather than kill microorganisms with antiseptics, the aseptic procedure sought to create a sterile operating field in order to prevent the entrance of pathogenic organisms. It involved sterilizing all instruments, dressings, sponges, gowns, and other items used in the operating room. A major item that did not lend itself to sterilization was the surgeon's hands, but this problem was solved almost inadvertently. In 1889 Dr. William S. Halsted of Johns Hopkins suggested that his surgical nurse, Caroline Hampton, use rubber gloves to protect her hands from the antiseptics to which she was allergic. It was not until six years later that Dr. Joseph C. Bloodgood, one of Halsted's assistants, began using them routinely for surgery.[4] The value of rubber gloves was not immediately grasped, but in 1906, eleven years after Bloodgood made them his standard practice, a New York hospital administrator spoke of what he called "a craze for the use of rubber gloves."[5]

Before discussing the remarkable advances that characterized surgery in the late nineteenth century, it is well to realize that surgery had still not cast off its former reputation as a callous and bloody business. Nor were physicians — and surgery was still in the hands of physicians — willing to operate except in cases of dire emergency. Dr. Rudolph Matas, probably the best southern surgeon of his day, wrote that "even in the eighties, *noli me tangere* was written large on the head, chest and abdomen, and their contained organs were still held as in sanctuaries which no one dared to open with unhallowed hands. Surgery," he continued, "was still largely restricted to such interventions in the visceral cavities . . . made compulsory by accidental injuries or imperative vital indications."[6]

Probably no better illustration of Dr. Matas's point can be found than the case of President James A. Garfield. He was shot on the morning of July 2, 1881, by a single bullet that entered his body above the third rib. Other than probing the wound with their fingers to look for the bullet — a procedure almost guaranteeing infection — his attending physicians followed a policy of watchful waiting. When inflammation was reported on July 5, one of the physicians described it as natural. On July 13 the medical report stated there were indications of a "circumscribed peritonitis in the abdominal region," but it was not considered "alarming." The wound, which was continuing to "discharge healthy pus," was doing quite satisfactorily. As the infection slowly spread, the physicians continued to stand by helplessly. Aside from making incisions to permit the accumulated pus to escape, they gradually watched the president decline until his death on September 19.[7]

As with many medical developments, surgery required hospitals and a large patient population to become a specialty. Hence urban areas were the first to support physicians who could concentrate on surgery. Traditionally specialization had been equated with traveling lithotomists, eye doctors, and venereal disease practitioners and other quacks — and so strong was the distrust of specialism within the medical profession that even the better surgeons maintained a private medical practice into the early twentieth century. Away from major cities, surgery generally did not emerge as a full-time practice until World War II.

The one major exception to this latter statement was the outstanding work of the Mayo family in Minnesota. The father, William W. Mayo, gained recognition in Rochester as an able physician and surgeon. His two sons, William J. and Charles H., following in their father's steps, took medical degrees and returned to practice in Rochester. In 1889 St. Mary's Hospital, the forerunner of the Mayo Clinic, opened with the Mayo family serving as the attending staff. Within fifteen years the surgical accomplishments of the two younger Mayos gained for the clinic an international reputation. Although both of the brothers performed a wide range of operations, their most outstanding work was in the area of abdominal surgery. This latter field was a particular specialty of Dr. William Mayo, while Dr. Charles Mayo was best known for his surgery of the thyroid gland. Both men kept abreast of surgical developments and contributed many new operative procedures. The clinic's growing reputation attracted a number of exceptional young surgeons. With the opening of a new building in 1914, the clinic was reorganized, making it the first example of a cooperative group practice.

In the immediate post–Civil War years American surgeons made relatively few contributions to surgery. The United States was still largely rural, and most surgery was still performed by physicians operating in private homes — either their own or those of their patients. Although a few large hospitals and urban centers provided some opportunity for surgery to develop as a specialty, America had nothing comparable to the great European medical centers. The large crowded European hospitals, however, were plagued with what was termed "hospitalization" — the rampant surgical infections that regularly swept through the wards, nullifying the best efforts of the surgeons. The dread of "hospitalization" was undoubtedly a factor in the European acceptance of the antiseptic principle, and the fact that the danger was not so acute in America may help to explain the reluctance of American surgeons to adopt the Listerian method.

Two outstanding surgeons in the postwar era were Henry Jacob

Bigelow (1816–90) of Boston, the first American to excise the hip joint, and Samuel David Gross (1805–84), professor of surgery at Jefferson Medical College in Philadelphia from 1856 to 1882. As mentioned earlier, Gross made many contributions to surgery but is best known for his writings on pathology, surgery, and medical history. His two-volume works *Elements of Pathological Anatomy* (Boston, 1839) and *A System of Surgery: Pathological, Diagnostic, Therapeutic, and Operative* (Philadelphia, 1859) remained standard for many years. Another out-standing surgeon in this period was Nicholas Senn (1844–1909), a graduate of Chicago Medical College who became professor of surgery at Rush Medical College in Chicago. His major contribution was in the area of intestinal surgery. The 1880s were a transition period in American surgery. Writing in 1885, Dr. Stephen Smith, a prominent New York physician, surgeon, and public health figure, emphasized that surgeons in New York's Bellevue Hospital no longer accepted suppu-ration as an inevitable process but rather expected primary healing: "Cleanliness is the one great object sought . . . in all operations," he wrote, for by this means the surgeon may with "absolute certainty, pro-tect an ordinary open wound from suppuration."[8] The significance of this statement lies in the fact that it was written only four years after President Garfield's wound had been probed by the attending surgeons' fingers.

In the 1890s American surgery came of age. Aseptic techniques gen-erally had been accepted, and a new generation of surgeons appeared on the scene. These men were far better educated than their predecessors, and nearly all of them had studied in Vienna, Paris, and other Euro-pean medical centers. Not all of the prominent surgeons in this period belonged to the new generation, for William W. Keen (1837–1932) had a career spanning the entire latter part of the century. As a young man he had seen Dr. Gross sharpen his scalpel on his boot before making an incision and witnessed surgeons threading needles by moistening the suture with saliva. Keen is best known for his pioneering work in abdominal and cranial surgery and for his medical textbooks. He also helped lead the fight against the early antivivisection movement in the 1880s.[9]

Among the new men coming to the fore at this time was Rudolph Matas (1860–1957) of Tulane University Medical School. His long career, akin to that of Keen, encompassed almost the entire period that has been called the century of the surgeon. He is best known for his innovative surgery on the blood vessels, most notably his endoaneurysmorrhaphy, first performed in 1888. Some of Matas's procedures for dealing with aneurysms continued in use as late as 1951. He also introduced catgut rings for use in enteroanastomosis and, in the field of anesthesia, he was the first to use continuous intravenous infusion and spinal anesthesia.[10] Another of the master surgeons to work on the major blood vessels was William S. Halsted (1852–1922). Like Matas, Halsted performed a wide range of surgical operations, but he is best remembered for his meticulous surgical technique and gentle management of tissues. In 1904 Halsted spoke for all surgeons when he stated: "In all times, even to the present day, the surgeon's chief concern during an operation has been the management of the blood vessels. The fear of death on the table from haemorrhage has deterred many a charlatan and incompetent surgeon from performing otherwise perilous operations." He was a strong advocate of surgical training and is credited with introducing the surgical residency program, one that gave increasing responsibility to neophyte surgeons.[11]

Not only were new techniques devised for dealing with traditional problems, but entire new areas began opening in surgery. George W. Crile (1864–1943) of Western Reserve perfected a method for dealing with traumatic shock during surgery and pioneered in blood transfusion and thyroid surgery. Harvey W. Cushing (1869–1939), the outstanding leader in cranial surgery during the early years of the twentieth century, helped lay the basis for neurosurgery and was largely responsible for making brain surgery a recognized specialty. His pupil Walter E. Dandy (1886–1946) contributed two major advances to brain surgery. In 1918 he introduced ventriculography, the injection of air or gas as a contrast medium into the ventricles of the brain in order to make the tissue visible. Building on this technique, he also devised pneumoencephalography, a comparable method for X-raying the subarachnoid space. A French surgeon who came to America in 1904, Alexis Carrel, is considered the founder of modern surgery of the aorta and heart. He performed basic work in physiology and physiological surgery and inaugurated the era of organ transplants. His accomplishments included a technique for uniting blood vessels, organ transplants in animals, and the culturing of cells from warm-blooded animals. His multifaceted work won him the 1912 Nobel Prize in medicine and physiology.[12]

The first American pioneer in abdominal surgery was J. Marion

Sims, whose contributions to gynecology and obstetrics were noted in chapter 8. He was one of the first to attempt gallbladder surgery and very early recognized the problems involved in opening the abdomen. The initial experiments in gastric surgery were performed by Theodor Billroth (1829–94) in Vienna, but American surgeons quickly capitalized on his work and helped begin an era of abdominal and thoracic surgery. The contributions of Matas and others in developing catgut and other types of rings for enteroanastomosis has been noted. In a further development, John B. Murphy (1857–1916) of Northwestern University in 1892 devised the Murphy button for uniting the hollow sections of the intestinal tract. One area of abdominal surgery in which American surgeons shone was in the diagnosis and treatment of appendicitis. During the nineteenth century the condition was called typhlitis, based on the assumption that the problem lay in the cecum, the blind pouch in which the large intestine begins. Although as early as 1837 individual physicians had diagnosed perforation of the appendix in cases of so-called typhlitis, it remained for Reginald Heber Fitz (1843–1913) of Boston to pinpoint the source of the problem. In 1886 he read a paper analyzing 466 cases of typhlitis and showed that the vast majority of them involved inflammation of the appendix. So convincing was his study that by the 1890s the term "typhlitis" was replaced by "appendicitis." The next step was taken by Charles McBurney (1845–1913), a New York physician-surgeon who greatly facilitated the diagnosis of appendicitis. In 1889 he identified what became known as McBurney's point, an area of tenderness localized in the right lower quadrant of the abdomen. Subsequently, in 1894, he described an operative method for removing the appendix, one still called McBurney's incision. Interestingly, as McBurney himself admitted, the method was first used by Dr. L. L. McArthur of Chicago. McBurney was also an early advocate of operating before the inflamed appendix ruptured.[13]

The American aptitude for mechanics proved of value in several medical areas, but it was particularly useful in the case of thoracic surgery. The problem of maintaining respiration and continuous anesthesia during chest surgery was solved by a series of developments. In the early 1880s Dr. Joseph O'Dwyer of New York developed a tube for passing air through the larynx and trachea in cases of acute diphtheria. When George H. Fell of Buffalo devised an apparatus for giving artificial respiration, O'Dwyer simplified and improved Fell's device by combining it with a modified version of his own tube, and it became known as the Fell-O'Dwyer apparatus. Rudolph Matas of New Orleans was the first to recognize the potential value of the Fell-O'Dwyer appliance for chest operations, and in 1900 he redesigned it to provide both respiration and continuous anesthesia during thoracic surgery.[14]

Anesthesia was another field in which Americans made notable contributions, although it should be remembered that some of the new forms of anesthesia were discovered by Europeans. In 1884 Carl Koller of Vienna publicized his pioneering work on the value of cocaine as a local anesthetic. Dr. William S. Halsted, who was then in New York, began experimenting on himself and his associates by injecting the nerve trunks with a cocaine solution. These dangerous experiments led to Halsted's addiction to cocaine, one that plagued him for the rest of his life. Yet they opened the entire field of conduction anesthesia, and other men such as George W. Crile and Harvey W. Cushing gradually began refining the technique.[15] While Halsted was conducting his studies, Dr. James L. Corning (1855–1923) of New York began experimenting with spinal anesthesia, and in 1899 Dr. Rudolph Matas first employed it for surgical purposes. Matas also developed an improved method for massive infiltration anesthesia and was a pioneer in regional anesthesia.

Dentistry

American medical practitioners in smaller towns and rural areas, at least until the end of the nineteenth century, included pulling teeth among their medical services. The professional basis for dentistry dates back to the eighteenth century when French and English surgeons, most notably Pierre Fauchard and John Hunter, removed dentistry from a state of crude empiricism and placed it on firmer foundations. In the nineteenth and twentieth centuries the development of dentistry was largely an American accomplishment. American practicality and mechanical ingenuity are part of the explanation, but a better one may lie in the lack of discrimination toward surgeons and the higher American standard of living. Surgeons still had the aura of tradesmen in Europe, and dentists ranked below surgeons. In America physicians and surgeons were one and the same, and the better dentists usually acquired medical degrees—not a hard task in the nineteenth century. The close relationship between medicine and dentistry can be seen in the 1847 decision of the Baltimore College of Dental Surgery to appoint a joint committee of five physicians and three dentists to examine candidates for the degree of Doctor of Dental Surgery.[16] Since dentistry is concerned with comfort and appearance and seldom confronts the patient with a life-or-death situation, it flourishes best among prosperous people — and Americans were relatively prosperous.

The French introduced the use of porcelain for teeth and gold for fillings in the eighteenth century, and by the early nineteenth century American dentists were familiar with both. For one reason or another, Americans concentrated on saving teeth instead of merely extracting them, and they made rapid progress in their gold filling technique. At the same time dental manufacturing companies began making porcelain teeth on a large scale, and a new industry was born.

The individual generally credited with establishing American dentistry as a profession was Horace H. Hayden (1768–1844). Hayden became interested in dentistry when he encountered John Greenwood (George Washington's dentist) in New York. In 1800 he moved to Baltimore, where he continued his studies in medicine and dentistry. The Baltimore Medical and Chirurgical Society voted in 1805 to grant licenses to dentists, and Hayden was licensed to practice in 1810. Anxious to remove the stigma of traveling quacks that still hovered over dentists, in the 1820s he began lecturing on dental physiology and pathology to medical students in the University of Maryland. His efforts to improve dentistry were finally rewarded when in 1840 he helped found the first national dental organization and the first dental college.[17]

Without detracting from Hayden's contribution, a great deal of the credit for establishing dentistry as a profession belongs to the notable work of a second pioneer dentist, Dr. Chapin A. Harris (1809–60). Harris studied and practiced medicine in Greenfield, Ohio, before turning to dentistry. Subsequently he centered his activities in Baltimore, where in 1833 he was granted a medical license by the local medical society. In 1839 he published *The Dental Art*, which he later expanded and published under the title *Principles and Practice of Dental Surgery*. This first dental textbook, periodically revised, remained a standard work for fifty years.[18]

Both Harris and Hayden were anxious to raise the level of dental education, and they first centered their efforts on establishing a dental department in the University of Maryland School of Medicine. When they were unsuccessful, in part as a result of internal problems within the medical school, they turned to the state legislature and in 1840 obtained a charter for the Baltimore College of Dental Surgery, the first school of its kind. Although the University of Maryland medical faculty had voted against establishing a dental department, the dental school received strong support from the local medical profession. In fact, two-thirds of the membership on the school's first advisory board were physicians. In the following years the school experienced a slow but steady increase in enrollment, and by the Civil War it was drawing students from all sections of the United States and even from the British Isles and France. Within the next few decades dental schools proliferated. By 1880 some thirteen schools were in operation. Despite the high standard set by the Baltimore school, none of the dental colleges had a university connection until 1867 when Harvard opened a dental department, thereby giving academic respectability to dental education.[19]

Two other significant developments aided the cause of dentistry. In 1839 the *American Journal of Dental Science* began publication under the auspices of a group of New York dentists. The following year Horace Hayden and Chapin Harris founded the first national dental association, the American Society of Dental Surgeons. Thus, with a formal system of education, a national organization, and its own publications, the American dental profession was well established by the time of the Civil War.

At the same time, several technical innovations greatly improved dental treatment. In 1838 the hand mallet was introduced, and in 1855 Charles Goodyear made the first application of vulcanized rubber as a base for false teeth. The next decade saw the development of scientific dental prostheses (artificial dentures) and the rubber dam to keep teeth dry during dental work. American dentistry continued its world leadership during the following years. In connection with the bacteriological revolution in the latter part of the century, men such as Willoughby Dayton Miller introduced antiseptic and aseptic dentistry. World War I turned dental attention to facial injuries and helped the development of maxillofacial surgery. A dental innovation that also benefited surgery was the invention of the automatic electric suction pump by Dr. C. Edmund Kells of New Orleans. Originally designed to deal with saliva in dental practice, the device was modified by Kells, Joseph Hume, and Samuel Logan in 1916 to make it suitable for general surgery.[20]

In the postwar years state and local dental societies, working through school and health centers, promoted oral hygiene and created a public awareness of the role of the mouth in relation to general health. In this connection it was dentists who first urged their patients to have regular checkups. In the past, individual dentists and dental associations have outshone the medical profession in their willingness to cooperate with school and public health authorities in promoting preventive dentistry and providing dental care. Their motives were not all pure, however, since support for school dental programs was based on a reluctance to treat children in private practice and a desire to improve their status.[21] Now that children have become an integral part of private dental practice and the profession has become more affluent, it will be interesting to see the effect on the profession's social conscience.

Radiology

As with anesthesia, the discovery of the X-ray was immediately seized upon by the American medical and dental professions. Wilhelm Conrad Roentgen first announced his discovery of the X-ray on December 28, 1895, and in January 1896 Professor M. I. Pupin of the Columbia University physics department made the first diagnostic radiograph in the United States. Within the next few years physiologists such as Walter B. Cannon of Harvard, who used X-rays to study the movements of the stomach and intestines, and dentists such as C. Edmund Kells of New Orleans began making broad-range applications of X-rays. Another American deserving mention is William Herbert Rollins, a New England physician and dentist who was among the first to recognize the danger involved in the use of X-rays. In 1901 he announced that his laboratory work with guinea pigs showed that X-rays were capable of causing death. These experiments led him to warn of the danger of overexposure and made him one of the leading advocates of X-ray housing devices.[22] The development of the X-ray and its technology was essentially an international accomplishment, but it was one in which Americans played a significant role. For example, the introduction of the Coolidge tube in 1913 opened a new era in X-ray work. Invented by William D. Coolidge while working for General Electric, the new tube eliminated the need for the hot filament required in the old gas tubes.

While physiologists such as Cannon were among the pioneers in the use of radiology, surgical services were the chief beneficiaries in the early years of radiation. In consequence, the first radiology departments were usually outgrowths of surgical units. Radiodiagnosis grew rapidly, but the development of radiotherapy was a slow and rather costly process. Many of the pioneer radiologists suffered severely from the effects of radiation. Kells, for example, developed cancer in the fingers of both hands and endured some thirty-five operations before taking his own life.[23] Radiotherapy led to many malignancies in radiologists, surgeons, and patients before improved X-ray machines, techniques, and sophisticated dosimetry made it a relatively safe and effective form of therapy.

The Early Twentieth Century

In 1884 E. M. Moore, president of the American Surgical Association, spoke of the way in which surgeons were "plunging into every cavity and recess of the body" and declared that the "current medical literature is loaded with the wonders of abdominal surgery." While commending these developments, he qualified his remarks by adding "though rashness seems often to outstrip judgment." Along with many of his colleagues in surgery and medicine, he also warned against the rise of specialism.[24] His warning proved of little avail, for, as in medicine, the ever-widening field of medical knowledge made specialization inevitable. Ophthalmology had long been a specialty. The work of Sims and others had laid the foundations for obstetrics and gynecology. The introduction of the electrically lighted cystoscope by Max Nitze vastly improved surgery of the bladder, and paved the way for urology. Orthopedics, an outgrowth of pediatrics, made remarkable progress in America, and by the early 1900s, in reverse of the usual practice, German physicians were coming to the United States to learn the latest developments. Neurosurgery and other specialties, too, were coming into their own.[25]

Among the major factors stimulating surgery in these years was the development of radiology, already touched upon. Another was the increasing use of intravenous replenishment, the injection of sterile fluids, salts, nutriments, and blood. Experiments with transfusions of blood and other liquids date far back in history, and in America such procedures were tried as early as the 1832 Asiatic cholera epidemic. Their successful use, however, awaited advances in the basic sciences. The first of these advances came at the turn of the century when Karl Landsteiner of Vienna identified blood types. The next one resulted from early studies in what was to become the field of hematology. Led by W. H. Howell and Jay McLean, a number of Americans began studying the blood in an effort to identify the substance responsible for clotting, and by 1918 they succeeded. Within a few years, a purified version, the first of the coagulants, became available for medical purposes.[26]

The history of surgery in the foregoing pages necessarily emphasizes successes, and thus gives a distorted picture to readers accustomed to the relatively low surgical mortality rates of the present. While outstanding operators were introducing new techniques and saving many lives, mortality rates for appendectomies, cesarean sections, and many other procedures considered routine today remained quite high throughout the first quarter of the twentieth century. An analysis of twenty-five cases of appendicitis presented before the Michigan State Medical Society in 1895 showed that the death rate for the twelve patients treated surgically was 33.3 percent and that the overall mortality was 40 percent. Despite great progress in aseptic procedures and surgical techniques, a study of hospital statistics in 1920 found the average mortality rate for appendectomies in the hospitals records examined to be 10 percent.[27] The cesarean section was even more dangerous, and its use was generally considered a last resort. In 1895 Dr. Thomas E. Schumpert, house surgeon of Charity Hospital in Shreveport, Louisiana, reported that in a difficult case of parturition he had first considered a craniotomy but hesitated because the child was still living. Of the 1,718 women admitted to the obstetrical wards in Charity Hospital of New Orleans between January 1, 1916, and June 30, 1918, only twenty-three were delivered by cesarean. Of these twenty-three, seven resulted in maternal death.[28]

The opening of new areas of surgery frequently encourages poorly trained or incompetent enthusiasts to move into the area, leading to abuses and, in some cases, temporarily causing more harm than good. In 1885 a distinguished New York physician declared that "the race would be better off had gynecology never been invented," and one of his colleagues agreed with him that "the injury which bunglers, enthusiasts, and charlatans have done in this connection greatly outweighs the good which others have accomplished."[29] In 1909 the president of the American Surgical Association held that "too many operations were undertaken for malignant disease, without any certainty that the patients' lives were ultimately made more comfortable or substantially prolonged," a warning that still rings true today.[30]

While the Mayo Clinic, established in the first decade of the century, and the better medical schools enabled individuals to practice surgery on a full-time basis, most surgery was still a part-time practice. Indicative of the general attitude of physicians toward surgery, in December 1909 the Boston Medical Society complained in a circular letter sent to the city's hospitals about the "rising feeling" that surgery could be performed only in institutions, "thus depriving all ordinary private physicians and surgeons of a class of cases." [31] At this time surgical training was still stressing knowledge of anatomy and surgical technique rather than surgical judgment, and dexterity and rapidity in operating were, as in the nineteenth century, the hallmarks of greatness. The American Surgical Association, founded in 1880, might have taken the initiative to improve the general caliber of surgery, but it was primarily an honor society of outstanding surgeons with little concern for the average practitioner. Recognizing the need to improve the quality of surgery and to establish a means for accrediting surgeons, Franklin H. Martin, John B. Murphy, George Crile, Charles Mayo, and others joined in 1913 to organize the American College of Surgeons. Despite the obviously sound motives of its founders, the college encountered a barrage of abusive attacks from state medical journals representing general practitioners. Nonetheless, the college steadily increased in membership. Out of necessity, since it appealed to the many physicians who practiced some form of surgery, the original standards were low, but by World War I, surgery was on its way to becoming a respectable specialty. [32]

The enormous casualties endured by the great powers in World War I led to considerable advances in the management of wound infections and abdominal, head, and eye wounds. The open management of contaminated wounds became standard, and Dakin's solution (hypochlorite), introduced by Alexis Carrel and Henry D. Dakin, provided a relatively good antiseptic. As the war progressed, surgeons rediscovered what a few observant surgeons in the eighteenth and nineteenth centuries had found—that closing an open chest wound permitted the patient to breathe. Effective means for preventing tetanus were developed, saving thousands of lives. Toward the end of the war blood transfusions were introduced, and, although used only sparingly, they stimulated the technology required for transfusions. Trench warfare, with all its horrors, led to an increasing number of facial and head injuries and gave an impetus to plastic surgery. Although not a concern of surgeons, the so-called "shell shock" created an increasing awareness of mental illness.

By the end of World War I surgery was far removed from what it had been at the close of the Civil War. Asepsis, radiology, a greater knowledge of physiology, improvements in surgical technique, and a host of other developments had literally remade surgery. While surgical intervention was rapidly increasing, advances in medical sciences and public health were beginning to eliminate certain surgical procedures. The introduction of diphtheria antitoxin drastically reduced the need for tracheotomies; surgical treatment for intestinal problems induced by typhoid were falling as a result of safe water and food supplies and vaccines; and the decline in tuberculosis was reducing the need for some surgical procedures. Yet these were relatively minor compared to the increase in the number and types of operations performed. The public image of the surgeon also had undergone a metamorphosis; the picture of the callous blood-and-pus-splattered surgeon had given way to one of the white-coated scientific practitioner. The age of the surgeon was at hand.

CHAPTER 13

Medical Education

THE PRACTICING PHYSICIAN in the second half of the nineteenth century continued to gain training from a variety of sources. The old apprenticeship system still functioned, although the ease of obtaining diplomas guaranteed that most doctors had some type of medical degree. Aside from the relatively large number of practitioners who bought their degrees from diploma mills, the quality of medical training varied widely. The better physician obtained a bachelor's degree from a reputable school, took an M.D. in an equally good institution, and then spent one to three years studying abroad. The average physician, however, had no more than a high school education—and frequently less—and had acquired a medical degree by attending the same four- or five-month course of medical lectures for two years in a row. A physician who attended the University of Michigan Medical School in 1866 later recalled that at that time there "were no clinics of instructive value, and no laboratories except the dissecting rooms." Although a few schools offered voluntary laboratory courses in chemistry, Michigan, he wrote, "was practically the only school where any laboratory instruction was required," since a six-weeks' course in chemistry was a requirement for graduation.[1]

Medical schools were still proprietary institutions in which the need to recruit students took precedence over any entrance requirements. As late as 1887 an officer of the Maine State Board of Health had an eight-year-old girl apply in her own handwriting for admission to a number of medical schools. Although she stated that she had none of the requirements for admission, over half the schools accepted her application, several of them assuring her that the examinations for a degree were not

difficult. Even in the best schools there were few obstacles to graduation. As of 1870, examinations at Harvard Medical School consisted of
nine professors spending five minutes each questioning the candidate.
To pass the examination, it was only necessary to satisfy five out of
the nine professors; thus a candidate could fail four out of nine medical subjects and still obtain his degree. In 1877 Dr. William Pepper
pointed out that it took four or five years of apprenticeship to become
a craftsman, but that one could acquire a medical degree in less than
one third of the time.[2] Dr. Simon Flexner, who acquired a medical degree from a two-year school in 1890, wrote: "I did not learn to practice
medicine . . . indeed I cannot say that I was particularly helped by the
school. What it did for me was to give me the M.D. degree."[3]

The early nineteenth-century view of medical students as a crude
and unruly group carried down to the end of the century. Dr. Edward
H. Dixon, a well-known New York physician, described the lecture
room of the Medical Department of New York University as "an ill-
constructed, dirty room, drenched with tobacco, and perfumed with
vile odors." The audience, he wrote, was "utterly indescribable." At
the end of the class hour a "most excruciating noise splits your ears"
as "the students rush forth like mad buffaloes."[4] The *Medical Record*
in 1882 carried an article entitled "The Percentage of College-Bred
Men in the Medical Profession," in which the author noted that the
percentage was declining as the century advanced. He gloomily concluded that medicine held little attraction for college graduates, adding
that it was a mistake to classify "the *medical business* among the learned
professions."[5]

A growing awareness of the inadequacy of medical training led to
the establishment of many state licensing boards during the latter part
of the century. Since these boards tended to accept almost any medical
degree, the net effect was to stimulate the rise of inferior schools. For
example, the number of medical colleges increased from 90 in 1880 to
151 by 1900. Aside from the fact that medical knowledge was in a state
of flux, the basic problem was that medical schools were all proprietary
institutions. Even in the case of those associated with a university the
connection was purely nominal. Medical departments remained under
control of their own faculties, which determined the budget, collected
student fees, and established academic standards. The only school in
which the medical faculty was willing to suffer a reduced income in
order to maintain higher standards was the Chicago Medical College.

Organized in 1863 under the leadership of Nathan Smith Davis, an outstanding reformer of medical education, the college lengthened the school year and subsequently required a third year for graduation.[6]

Despite this discouraging picture, American medical schools could not help but react to the explosion of knowledge that was drastically altering all aspects of Western society. Moreover, the general level of education in America was on the rise, and it is more than a coincidence that university presidents should have taken the initiative to reform medical education. The first of these was Charles Eliot, who became president of Harvard in 1869. Representing the new generation of men trained in science, Eliot quickly recognized the woeful inadequacy of the medical department. He surprised the medical faculty by presiding over their meetings, and then outraged the majority of senior members by recommending major changes. The faculty divided, with the younger ones supporting Eliot and the conservative majority in opposition. In the course of the debate Eliot was informed by Professor Henry Bigelow that written examinations were futile since half of the students could barely write. He was also warned, correctly as it turned out, that any reforms would lead to a reduction in the size of the student body. The arguments served only to convince Eliot of the need for change, and he finally declared that further debate was useless and that the reforms would be made.

As a result, the school year was lengthened from four to nine months, a three-year graded curriculum was introduced, and both written and oral examinations were required in all departments. As predicted, Eliot's reforms reduced the medical school's enrollment by 43 percent between 1870 and 1872. Nonetheless, Eliot persisted, and when the universities of Pennsylvania, Syracuse, and Michigan followed suit, the three-year graded curriculum was established in the leading schools. More significant, financial control of the school was placed in the hands of the Harvard administrators. This step was followed by Yale in 1880, and other universities, too, slowly began integrating their medical schools into the university administration.[7]

While medical schools were striving to raise their standards, the appearance of Johns Hopkins University profoundly affected all American education. Established in 1876 under the inspired leadership of Daniel Coit Gilman, it quickly set new standards for graduate education and brought a radical change to medical training. Gilman, with the help of John Shaw Billings, the founder of the Army Medical Library (later the National Library of Medicine), began searching for a medical faculty in the early 1880s, and his first choice was Dr. William H. Welch, a bright young man who had gone to Europe to complete his medical education and had studied with two great scientific leaders, the pathologist Julius Cohenheim, and the physiologist Willy Kuhne. Both men highly recommended Welch, and in 1884 he was appointed professor of pathology. With the help of Welch and further assistance from Billings, Gilman gradually recruited a faculty representing the best physician-scientists and clinicians available. In short order he brought in William S. Halsted to head surgery, William Osler as professor of medicine, Howard A. Kelly as associate professor of gynecology and obstetrics, Franklin P. Mall as professor of anatomy, and Henry M. Hurd as superintendent of the University Hospital.

While helping to recruit a staff for the hospital and school and engaging in his own laboratory studies, Welch was in close contact with the regular academic faculty and learned to appreciate the role of research in connection with teaching. This conditioning accorded with his own bent, and Welch shares the credit along with Eliot, Gilman, and others for making American medical schools centers for research as well as teaching.[8] Johns Hopkins was not the first school to build a teaching hospital; this honor goes to the universities of Michigan and Pennsylvania. Michigan opened a university hospital in 1869, but Pennsylvania, which established its hospital in 1874, is credited with having the first university-controlled hospital.[9] What Johns Hopkins did, however, was to make the hospital an integral part of a research-oriented medical institution. It also provided a permanent clinical staff for the hospital and established a nurses' training school in close conjunction with it.

The opening of Johns Hopkins School of Medicine in 1893 marked the first time in America that a bachelor's degree and a knowledge of French and German were required for admission to a medical school. The emphasis on laboratory and clinical research that characterized the school and hospital soon won for Hopkins a reputation for preeminence in medical education. Within a few years the school's graduates and younger faculty members were spreading the Hopkins system throughout the United States.

Well before the opening of Johns Hopkins the basic sciences were beginning to assume a greater role in medical education. In the 1870s and 1880s physiology and pathology evolved from anatomy, and the widening use of microscopes led to the development of histology and bacteriology. Medical chemistry courses, too, benefited from the introduction of laboratory work, although too much emphasis was still placed on inorganic chemistry. Efforts were made to require basic chemistry as a prerequisite for medical school, but success was not achieved until the twentieth century. In these same years more and more schools required laboratory work for all basic science courses, and these laboratories in turn made experimental work possible. The integration of medical schools into universities further strengthened the basic sciences by bringing them into closer contact with the work of academic scientists.

The few colleges who attempted to raise standards invariably suffered a reduction in student enrollment, making it evident that some type of joint action was necessary for effective reform. In 1876 the initial meeting of what was to become the American Medical College Association was held in Philadelphia. Delegates came from nearly all geographic areas, although New England was represented solely by the University of Vermont. The association attempted to standardize fees and institute a graded curriculum, and, in 1880, it voted for three years of training. The requirement of three years' work for graduation led a number of schools to resign from the association, and this fact, coupled with a split between the large schools from the East and those from the West and South, ended the association in 1882.[10]

Reform, however, was in the wind, and in 1890 a new medical college group, the National Association of Medical Colleges (later the Association of American Medical Colleges) was organized. This time some fifty-five of the ninety orthodox medical colleges sent representatives. The first decision was to create a permanent organization with relatively strict requisites for membership. All schools belonging to the association were to require entrance examinations and to offer a three-year course of instruction, a six-month academic year, written and oral examinations, and laboratory work in chemistry, histology, and pathology. Overriding the argument that mental effort involved a heavy strain on young people and that the six-month school year was "in violation of all laws of health, physical and mental," the association's members voted in favor of all requirements, an action that indicates that most of the better medical schools had already met the requirements or were in the process of so doing.[11] In 1894 the associated medical colleges voted to increase the course of study to four years beginning with the first-year class of 1895. As had been anticipated, between 1895 and 1897 twelve of the sixty-six members of the association felt they could not meet this standard and resigned, but, unlike its predecessor, the association survived. The reform movement also received help from the National Confederation of State Medical Examining and Licensing Boards, which in 1891 voted to require candidates for a license to have a minimum of three years' medical training.[12]

Meanwhile the American Medical Association was belatedly reentering the picture. Throughout the first fifty years of its existence it had been preoccupied with fighting the irregulars, most notably the homeopaths, but early in the twentieth century it turned its attention once more to the training of physicians. At the AMA's annual meeting in 1900 the delegates voted that the association's constituent societies could not admit anyone whose M.D. degree had been acquired with less than four years of training. In 1902 a committee on education was appointed, and two years later this committee was made a permanent body. Working in cooperation with the Association of American Medical Colleges and the Southern Medical College Association, in 1905 the AMA established a Council on Medical Education. The latter body began meeting regularly, and initially its annual reports presented a discouraging picture. In 1906 the council named five states with notoriously poor medical schools, and the following year it reported that only 50 percent of the 160 medical schools were equipped to "teach modern medicine," that 30 percent were doing a poor job, and that the other 20 percent were "unworthy of recognition."[13]

In 1907 the council asked the Carnegie Foundation to investigate medical education. The foundation acceded and turned the job over to Abraham Flexner, a layman who had already published one study on American colleges. Flexner was a graduate of Johns Hopkins and a great admirer of William Welch. In consequence, he began by examining the medical school at Johns Hopkins and decided to use it as a model. Flexner's study was completed in 1909 and published in 1910.[14] It came at a time when the AMA's Council on Medical Education had made the medical profession acutely aware of the inadequacies of medical training, and the *Report*, which was widely read by laypeople and physicians, marked a turning point in medical education.

Flexner made a complete and detailed analysis of each school and passed judgment on it in firm and decisive prose. Speaking of the Atlantic Medical College and the Maryland Medical College, Flexner declared: "That such unconscionable concerns should at this day continue to flourish is a blot upon the state of Maryland and the city of Baltimore." Of the South he wrote that it "is generally overcrowded with schools with which nothing can be done; for they are conducted by old-time practitioners, who could not use improved teaching facilities if they were provided." [15] While the Flexner report would undoubtedly have created a stir, it might well have aroused a brief flurry of attention and then faded away had it not been that Flexner was able to persuade the Rockefeller Foundation to make grants that eventually totaled almost fifty million dollars to those schools that Flexner considered worthwhile. Rockefeller's contributions in turn stimulated other philanthropists to support medical education, with most of the money going to those institutions designated by Flexner as worthy of support. The result was to widen the gap between the better and poorer schools, causing the latter gradually to fall by the wayside. By 1930 the number of medical schools in America had dropped from 148 to 66. [16]

While developments in the basic sciences were forcing major changes in medical education, clinical training made only limited gains until the first two decades of the twentieth century. In the nineteenth century, clinical medicine was taught in large amphitheaters or by professors parading groups of students through hospital wards for a quick glimpse at patients. The growth of municipal hospitals in a few cases offered opportunities for better students to acquire some clinical training. For example, by the early 1880s fourteen senior Tulane medical students were selected by examination for student residencies, a form of house staff training, in Charity Hospital. They were provided with free room and board and given an excellent opportunity to learn hands-on medicine. In 1890 Charity Hospital made two more positions in the outpatient clinics available to medical students. The following year the Tulane faculty appointed a committee to search for "educational facilities" in the other New Orleans hospitals and clinics. By 1893 internships were available for thirty-one of the approximately one hundred senior medical students. [17] It should be noted that Tulane was well in advance of most medical schools in this respect.

William Welch was familiar with a form of teaching akin to the present clinical clerkship, which he had learned from Palmer Howard of McGill University, and he introduced it into Johns Hopkins in the 1890s. Almost at the same time Harvard University introduced a similar program whereby senior medical students were assigned to observe and care for several hospitalized patients.[18] The problem with clinical teaching was that few medical schools had hospital connections, and for those few, it was rare for the medical school to have any control over the hospital. Fortunately the rapid increase in the size and number of hospitals solved the problem. Hospital administrators soon realized that interns, along with nurses, represented a cheap form of labor. By 1920 the internship, a year of postgraduate clinical training, had become a standard part of medical education.

Since so little clinical training was provided at the undergraduate level, in the 1880s several "polyclinics" emerged. Organized by reputable practitioners, they offered postgraduate clinical instruction in medicine. The first to open was probably the New York Polyclinic, founded in 1882. The New Orleans Polyclinic, chartered by the state to offer graduate work in medicine in 1888, was the third such clinic to offer graduate instruction. Its faculty included prominent New Orleans practitioners and most of the junior members of Tulane Medical School. The polyclinic maintained a close relationship with the medical school and with Charity Hospital. The Tulane University administration, after it had taken control of the medical school in 1904, was anxious to promote graduate training, and the growing size and reputation of the polyclinic made it a logical addition to the university. Consequently, in 1906 the polyclinic became the postgraduate department of the medical school.[19] While the residency program had forerunners in the nineteenth century, the formal residency program of today—postgraduate hospital training in a specialized area—did not develop until the 1920s.

In 1924 Flexner evaluated the changes that had taken place in medical education and rejoiced that almost half the schools in existence in 1910 had closed their doors, including nearly all of the weakest ones in the South and West. Virtually all schools, he added, were now equipped with laboratory and clinical facilities and the basic courses were being taught by qualified faculty members on a full-time basis. By this date, too, the four-year graded curriculum had become standard.[20] While Flexner could take pride in these changes, much of the credit belongs to the AMA's Council on Medical Education, which, through its annual rating system, exerted continuous pressure to raise educational standards. The work of the Association of American Medical Colleges (1890) and the rising standards required by state licensing boards also contributed to the general advance in medical education.

By 1920, aided by the spread of Hopkins graduates who held positions in so many medical schools, the Hopkins system was well established in American medical education. An undergraduate degree was becoming a prerequisite to medical training, and a three- or four-year graded curriculum was standard. Nearly all schools provided hospital facilities and clinical instruction and required their graduates to take a year's internship. The curriculum consisted of two years of basic sciences, including laboratory work, and two years of clinical training in hospitals and outpatient clinics. The constant pressure exerted by medical reformers not only weeded out the weaker schools but helped to strengthen the better ones, with the result that the average medical graduate by 1920 was far better trained than those who had graduated thirty years earlier.

Without disparaging the excellent work of Johns Hopkins, Abraham Flexner, and the AMA's Council on Medical Education, we should note that by the beginning of the twentieth century, social and scientific changes clearly were undermining the proprietary medical schools. Expensive laboratories and medical equipment were becoming essential to medical training, and the limited income of proprietary schools meant that they could neither build nor maintain these facilities. Medical education was moving into a new era, and even without Flexner, Welch, and others the change was in the making.

In recent years medical historians have tried to assess the work of Flexner upon the pattern of twentieth-century medical education. As early as 1972 Robert P. Hudson pointed out that "Flexner's contribution was not so much revolutionary as catalytic to an already evolving process." Kenneth M. Ludmerer went further in 1985 by arguing that changes in general university education and the impact of academic sciences on medical schools determined their shape long before the Flexner report. He maintained that the rise of academic medicine, the development of American research, and the integration of medical schools into universities went hand-in-hand, and he asserted that Flexner and the AMA only influenced but did not participate in shaping medical schools.[21]

There is considerable validity in Ludmerer's argument, but Abraham Flexner deserves more credit than Ludmerer gives him. E. Richard Brown makes an excellent case for showing that Flexner and the wealthy philanthropists he mobilized played a significant role in giving medical schools their research orientation. Flexner's experience at Johns

Hopkins unquestionably convinced him that the scientific model of the Johns Hopkins medical school represented the ultimate in medical education.[22] Daniel M. Fox has pointed out in his study of Flexner's writings that the latter was an educational elitist with little interest in medical practice or public health.[23] Without doubt the Flexner report generated widespread interest in medical education and served to educate the public to accept scientific medicine and to convince philanthropists to support medical research. At the time the Flexner report was made the issue was whether to have a standard form of medical education or two categories of schools, one research-oriented and the other designed to provide practical training. Flexner was largely responsible for channeling both private and state funds into supporting research-oriented scientific medical schools, thus standardizing medical education.

On the face of it, the movement to improve medical education was an intelligent and progressive step; better-trained physicians clearly meant better medicine. Yet it is evident from any perusal of medical journals in the late nineteenth and early twentieth centuries that economic and class motives provided a considerable impetus for reform. The ineffectiveness of the licensing laws before 1900 and the ease with which one could acquire a nominal medical degree guaranteed a plethora of doctors. It also insured a relatively low financial status for those in the profession. Obviously, raising entrance standards into medical schools was a prime means for reducing the number of physicians and an effective way to increase the social and economic status of the profession. This argument was set forth frequently in medical journals and may well have had more influence than the more idealistic appeals for education reform. The question of social status was almost as important as the economic one in the drive to raise standards. The better-trained physicians with college and university backgrounds were almost exclusively products of the middle and upper class, while the proprietary schools tended to recruit more from the lower economic groups. With some justice, university-trained physicians could complain about their poorly educated colleagues, but a class bias shows through many of the diatribes against doctors from the lower classes.

Whether or not physicians intended to keep members of the lower economic groups out of medicine, this was one result of reforming medical schools. The prerequisite of a bachelor's degree even as late as 1920 automatically excluded over 90 percent of the population from medical education, and, as medical training became longer and more costly, the net effect was to make medicine more and more exclusive. The selection of strongest schools by Rockefeller and other foundations added still further to the exclusiveness of medicine. The well-established eastern schools, along with a handful of leading schools in the South, Midwest, and West, were the chief recipients of foundation largesse. Since medical schools for women and blacks were generally among the weaker institutions, they were virtually swept away.

In the case of women, token acceptance of female students by a number of leading medical schools seemingly eliminated the need for separate women's medical colleges. Unfortunately, biased entrance requirements and a deliberate policy by most faculty members to discourage women students resulted in a steady drop in the number of women M.D.'s during the early years of the twentieth century. One last point worth noting in this connection is that, as the medical profession increasingly drew its membership from the upper classes, it became more and more conservative. The leadership that medicine had shown in the public health movement and other progressive reforms of the late nineteenth century was no longer in evidence by the 1920s.[24]

CHAPTER 14

The Medical Profession Organizes

T HE IMMEDIATE POST–CIVIL WAR YEARS, as indicated earlier, brought little if any improvement in the economic position or social status of the average physician. While a few outstanding individuals were able to acquire considerable wealth — usually as a result of a combination of skill and social position — the average practitioner continued to earn a minimum living from his practice. And, as they had done since the founding of America, many doctors continued to supplement their incomes by operating small businesses and farms. The growing number of medical schools actively competing for students in the late nineteenth century and the lax licensure laws gave even the lowest income groups access to the profession, thus swelling its ranks. Nonetheless, sharp social and financial barriers separated the elite physicians from the average practitioner whose academic background before entering medical school often did not include even a high school diploma.

As might be expected, medical fees were highest in urban areas, but this advantage was offset by keener competition among doctors. Charles Rosenberg estimated that physicians starting their careers in New York City in the 1860s probably earned about $400 per year.[1] Despite a general rise in living standards, the relative income of physicians improved little by the end of the century. In 1898 a Dr. Sexton, addressing the local medical society in New Orleans, asserted that seven-eighths of the city's 358 physicians made less than $1,000 per year. The situation was even worse in rural areas. A physician practicing in New

Paltz, New York, a village of about 500 or 600 inhabitants, claimed that his patients were indignant if he charged more than 50 cents for a housecall and 35 cents for an office visit. For this munificent sum, the doctor was also expected to supply them with medicine. For an out-of-town call involving a distance of up to six miles, the fee was $1. To add to Dr. Sexton's woes, patients often took from one to five years to pay their bills. He mentioned in passing that this small village had two practitioners, a fact that in itself helps to explain the relatively impoverished status of the profession.[2]

Doctors' inability to collect fees is a problem that is as old as medicine itself. In the colonial period it was not unusual for a medical bill to be carried for many years, occasionally remaining unpaid until the settlement of the patient's estate. Ancient medical authors often warned physicians to collect bills before their patients were fully recovered. In the modern period economic depressions always aggravated this problem, and the late nineteenth century was no exception. During the depressed years of the 1870s, about seventy New Orleans doctors formed a Medical Protective Association to assist them in collecting their fees. The same physicians also denounced the contract practice of medicine as demoralizing to "the profession of medicine, and ruinous to the financial welfare of us all."[3]

Contract medicine — an agreement by which physicians provided complete medical care for an annual fee — had long been traditional in the South. With the growth of unions, large-scale industries, and social organizations throughout the country, the contract method gradually spread. The sharp competition among physicians not only insured their availability for such contracts, but it also kept contract fees to a minimum. As state and local medical societies gained strength, they began prohibiting their members from engaging in contract medicine. In the twentieth century the AMA, too, threw its weight into the balance, and by 1920 this form of practice was reduced to negligible proportions. Even so, fear of the contract system continued to condition the attitude of organized medicine for many years, and it was used as a major argument against much of the proposed federal health legislation later in the century.

Another financial complaint of the medical profession arose from the appearance of free dispensaries and clinics. The impetus for these institutions came from two sources: one was simple philanthropy; the second was the specialists' need for clinical subjects. Specialists seeking to improve their skills and train their students needed access to relatively large numbers of patients. General practitioners in the late nineteenth century, however, were resentful of competition from colleagues who set themselves up as specialists, considering them a threat to an already limited practice; thus specialists sought to avoid conflict by establishing dispensaries for the poor. Since many workers lived at a poverty level, it was not easy to determine where the line should be drawn between those who could afford to pay and those who could not. This same situation held true for the general dispensaries and public hospitals. Understandably, physicians whose own incomes placed them in the category of genteel poverty argued that the dispensaries were depriving them of paying patients.

In addition to its financial troubles, the medical profession worried about its lack of prestige. Although its social status, along with that of law and theology, had never been high, physician orators in deploring the condition of their profession constantly harked back to a mythical golden past. As the new world of science and industry emerged in the second half of the nineteenth century, many physicians happily laid claim to scientific authority. A few, however, were more realistic. For example, Dr. A. N. Bell, the respected editor of *The Sanitarian*, in 1876 reprinted an article asking "Is Medicine a Science?" and answered that it was not. "It is a nice question," the article stated, "which has done the more hurt, the disease or the remedy: whether, for instance, the child's health suffers more from the intestinal parasites which vex him, or from the destructive purgatives employed as anthelmintics; whether the cancer or the knife produces death more speedily; whether calomel or quinine" are more dangerous than the illnesses they seek to cure. Dr. Bell concluded that the doctors might best serve humanity by teaching the fallacy of physic.[4] While Dr. Bell's characterization of the medicine of his day had much validity, major discoveries in nearly all areas of the biological sciences were foreshadowing fundamental changes in medical practice and the status of physicians.

In the meantime, recognizing the limitations on the prevailing medical knowledge, physicians sought to emphasize their role as moral leaders and family counselors. Dr. Clarence J. Blake told the graduating medical students of Yale in 1898: "You are going out, as each one of you realizes, to a ministry, . . . a priesthood."[5] In medical schools and at medical gatherings physicians were enjoined to heal both body and soul. They were informed that their role was similar to that of teachers and counselors, to advise on such matters as sexual problems, diet, and recreation. Dr. Andrew H. Smith, in giving the Anniversary Discourse before the New York Academy of Medicine in 1890, declared that unsanitary working conditions, excessive drinking, and other maladies of society would grow unless their "natural protectors," the members of the medical profession, assumed leadership.[6] It is ironic that precisely at a time when the profession was stressing its social role, science and technology were beginning to transform the whole field of medicine.

Although beset by problems in the nineteenth century, the medical profession made major gains during the first two decades of the twentieth. One factor was that broad advances in medical knowledge had reached a point where they could be applied to medical practice. At the same time, the profession greatly improved its economic and social position by developing strong medical organizations, first at the local level and then on a state and nationwide basis. Until late in the nineteenth century, medical societies proved relatively ineffective. The early ones attracted only a few physicians and most associations were short-lived. All too often they were torn apart by internal quarrels that not infrequently led to the founding of a competing society. It was not until the post–Civil War period that state and local medical societies began appearing on a fairly wide scale. In general, medical societies could be found only in the larger towns and cities, and, even when state societies emerged, they tended to be dominated by physicians from the state's largest city. For example, Blanton states that the "Medical Society of Virginia for the first thirty years of its existence was in reality Richmond's local association."[7] Certainly this was true in Louisiana, where New Orleans was the focal point for most of the early medical organizations. The rise of medical sects further increased the number of societies, for homeopaths, eclectics, osteopaths, and other irregulars found it necessary to organize in self-defense. By 1878, when Louisiana established a state society, every state in the Union possessed some type of state organization.[8] The strength of these groups varied widely, but the general trend was toward larger and more effective state societies. Yet nothing bespeaks their weakness better than the failure of these societies to establish official journals. Not until 1899 did the first state medical society journal appear.

While local and state societies were increasing their membership rolls and becoming better spokesmen for their profession, several regional associations came into existence, and at the national level some fifteen specialty groups were established between 1864 and 1902. During these years the AMA, organized in 1846, was struggling for survival and having little success in meeting its original objectives of improving medical education and raising professional standards. The sheer size of America and transportation difficulties tended to restrict membership to the Middle Atlantic and Midwestern states, and the AMA's attempt to become an effective national organization was further hindered by a cumbersome and ineffectual structure. The association's lack of success in promoting higher educational standards was discouraging. Some of its members fought valiantly for this reform, but the gains that had come by 1900 can scarcely be credited to the AMA. It had consistently supported public health measures at the national level, but the American Public Health Association, established in 1872, quickly became the chief spokesman for this field. The AMA, however, did continue to fight for a national health department, and many of its members were active in promoting state and municipal health laws. Nonetheless, Charles A. L. Reed, the president of the AMA, admitted in an address to the association in 1901 that the organization had "exerted relatively little influence on legislation, either state or national."[9]

The one area in which medical societies in the late nineteenth century achieved a measure of success was in the promotion of licensure laws. In glancing back over the history of American medical licensure, it is clear that from the colonial period to 1830 there were few limitations on the practice of medicine. Even these few restrictions were swept away in the era of Jacksonian democracy. For most of the century the possession of a medical degree or a certificate stating that the owner had served an apprenticeship was an automatic qualification to practice. In reality, anyone who wanted could set himself up as a physician. Moreover, as colleges vied with each other for medical students, medical degrees became successively easier to acquire. Beginning in the 1870s stronger state medical societies began emerging, and the first issue they tackled was the elimination of quacks and unqualified physicians. Enacting sound licensure laws and establishing qualified medical licensure boards, however, was a long and complicated process.

In North Carolina a State Board of Medical Examiners had been created in 1859, but to all intents and purposes it was powerless, for one clause in the enabling act specified that no one practicing in violation of the law should be guilty of a misdemeanor. In 1885 this provision was eliminated, but the new measure included a "grandfather clause" — one that declared that the law would not apply to anyone who had acquired a diploma from any medical college before 1880. Four years later all physicians were required to register with the clerk of the superior court in the county in which they practiced. The term "physician" encompassed almost every practitioner in the state, since the law described three classes of doctors: those licensed by the Board of Medical Examiners, those with medical degrees dated before March 7, 1885, and those taking an oath that they had practiced medicine in the state prior to March 7, 1885. No further change was made in the law until 1899 when an amendment prohibited anyone from applying to the examining board who was not a medical graduate. In the succeeding years the licensing law was gradually strengthened, although it was not until 1921 that the grandfather clause was eliminated.[10]

In South Carolina the first licensing law in the postwar era was passed in 1869. As with all early laws, it was a weak measure with enough loopholes to include all who wished to practice. In 1881 a new act enabled county boards of health to license physicians. Seven years later prospective doctors were given the choice of obtaining their licenses from the state examining board, the state's medical college faculty, or the local county board of health. Other modifications followed, but it was not until 1897 that a reasonably effective law was enacted.[11]

Louisiana, which had had one of the best licensing systems in the early nineteenth century, passed a law in 1862 requiring physicians to make an affidavit stating that they possessed a medical degree from a reputable school. Ten years later the penalties for making a false affidavit were increased—a futile gesture, since few physicians bothered to file one in the first place. In 1882 responsibility for licensing was transferred to the state board of health. As might be expected, a grandfather clause was included. Although subsequently a few minor changes were made, when the state medical society pushed for a stronger law in 1890 its efforts were defeated in the legislature, in part due to the objections of the homeopaths. After several unsuccessful tries, in 1894 the medical society joined with the homeopaths and secured the establishment of two state boards, one appointed from the ranks of the regular state medical society and another from the homeopathic society. The usual grandfather clause blanketed in all physicians in practice as of 1894, but the law guaranteed that henceforth newcomers to the profession must have at least minimal qualifications.[12]

The divisions within the medical profession that delayed the passage of Louisiana's first sound licensing law are even more evident in the case of New York. This state's first postwar law, passed in 1874, was a compromise between the factions within the regular medical profession and the many irregular physicians. So many compromises were made that the law was meaningless. The main issue dividing the State Medical Association was a provision in the AMA's code of ethics that prohibited its members from consulting with homeopaths and other irregulars.

As was true in some other states, the orthodox physicians in New York finally succeeded in passing a good licensure law in 1891 by collaborating with the homeopaths and eclectics. Under the terms of the 1891 act each of the three groups was given its own board. This development led the osteopaths and Christian Scientists to make a similar demand. In the face of this challenge, the allopaths (regulars), homeopaths, and eclectics united in support of a single board. The result was a new law in 1907 creating a single board with the three groups equally represented. By this date the osteopaths had raised their educational standards and were permitted to take the same examination as the regulars.[13]

The process by which the foregoing states achieved some degree of medical regulation illustrates the difficulties encountered in all of the states. Of the four, Louisiana's progress toward medical licensure best typifies the path followed by most states: first, a weak law requiring registration with local officials, a medical society, or some type of examining board; second, a new law authorizing either the state board of health or local health boards to issue licenses; and finally, the creation of a relatively effective state licensing system. Frequently this final step was made possible only when the state medical society joined with the homeopaths or eclectic practitioners. The irony of this is that the AMA and state medical societies had devoted their major efforts during the second half of the nineteenth century to fighting irregular practitioners, in particular, the homeopaths and eclectics. The regulars acceptance of the old adage "if you can't beat them, join them" was made easier, however, by the willingness of these two irregular medical sects to modify their theories and accept the new developments in medicine.

By 1900 every state had some type of medical registration law, although six of them still granted a license to anyone holding a medical diploma. More significant, about half the states required both a medical degree and an examination before granting a license. In North Carolina, Louisiana, and some eighteen other states midwives were partially or totally exempted from the licensure laws, and few if any states closely regulated them. The 1894 Louisiana law, which included a provision stating that the act was not "to apply to the so-called midwife of the rural districts and plantation practice," clearly shows a class bias.[14] Midwives practiced largely among the blacks and poor whites, and neither the medical profession nor the legislature was concerned with unprofitable patients and nonvoters.

As part of the general effort to raise professional standards, in 1891 a few members of medical examining boards organized the National Confederation of State Medical Examining and Licensing Boards. The aim of this body was to help to standardize testing programs and to encourage medical schools in their efforts to improve education. Despite this step toward standardizing licensing procedures, the qualifications required by state boards varied widely, and the problem of reciprocity soon came to the fore. A Confederation on Reciprocity was established in Chicago in 1902 to promote interboard acceptance of state medical licenses. The confederation achieved only limited success, and in 1912 it merged with the National Confederation of State Boards to form the present Federation of State Medical Boards.[15]

While the quality of medical practice was rapidly improving in the first two decades of the twentieth century, grandfather clauses in the various state licensing acts guaranteed that thousands of poorly trained and semiliterate physicians would continue to treat patients. Moreover, the enforcement of the licensing acts required public support, and many—if not most—Americans were still doubtful of laws that seemingly gave a monopoly to physicians or lawyers. A "Dr. Allen" who began practicing in rural Louisiana sometime before 1894 is a good case in point. He had no medical degree and never bothered to register as a physician. He apparently was well liked, for when a grand jury brought charges against him for practicing without a license, he announced he would give up his practice. Faced with this prospect, the grand jury withdrew the indictment, and he continued to practice until his death in 1920.[16]

While state and local medical societies were pushing for licensure laws, they also closed ranks to meet the increasing threat of malpractice suits. The legal profession, which for most of American history had commanded even less respect than medicine, was beginning to achieve a measure of respectability, and one result was an increase in the number of malpractice suits. Physicians, who are constantly making value judgments, have always been reluctant to censor their fellow practitioners, but, as lawyers increasingly began employing physicians as professional witnesses, the medical profession began viewing malpractice suits in a more serious light. In 1885 Dr. E. J. Doering, writing in the *Journal of the American Medical Association*, urged physicians to organize for their legal defense. "Let it be known that the individual physician is backed by such an organization, and he will be let alone."[17] In 1887 the Michigan state society voted that a member could not volunteer testimony against another member, and subsequently it decided to provide legal help for all members accused of malpractice. In response to what was seen as an increasing threat, in 1893 a group of Detroit doctors formed a Physicians Protective Association. County societies in New York and Philadelphia soon followed suit, and by 1910 some thirteen state medical societies were providing legal defense for their members. Reflecting a not uncommon attitude, Dr. J. E. Stubbs, in addressing the Physicians Club of Chicago in 1899, asserted that it was in the best interests of the profession to conceal medical errors from the public.[18]

For over fifty years the AMA had been struggling to become the major representative of the medical profession. Aside from the sheer size of the United States, which made it difficult to organize on a nationwide basis, another obstacle was the AMA's fight against the irregulars, which harmed its public image and caused divisions within its own ranks. The American public, fearful of monopoly, was highly suspicious of licensing laws and resentful of any attempt to place restrictions on homeopaths and other irregulars. As mentioned above, the AMA's code of ethics, which was made compulsory for membership in 1855, prohibited its members from consulting with irregulars. Over the years contacts with unorthodox physicians were restricted even further, and constituent societies were forbidden to admit them to membership. The effect was to create divisions within the AMA's own ranks. In the first place the distinction between orthodox physicians and irregulars was not clear. For example, Dr. Morton Robinson of Newark, New Jersey, began practicing as a botanic physician in the early 1850s. He was listed in the city directory among the botanics from 1851 to 1871. In 1872 he was classified under the heading "allopath" (or regular). In 1877 he was head of the Eclectic Medical Society of the State of New Jersey, and from 1883 he was simply described and "physician and surgeon."[19]

In many areas, homeopaths, eclectics, and orthodox physicians were often on friendly terms and relied on each other for consultations. In smaller communities regulars often had no choice but to consult with a homeopath or an eclectic.

The reaction of local medical societies to the AMA decree was mixed. In 1870 the AMA formally censured the Massachusetts Medical Society for admitting homeopaths. The society conceded its error and responded by resolving to expel them. The homeopaths, with help from some of the regulars, made the society's action a public issue. After considerable soul-searching and an extensive public debate, the society confirmed its original decision and voted to dismiss the homeopaths. Most state societies accepted the AMA's code and refused all contacts with irregulars. In New York, however, the homeopathic issue split the state society wide open. In 1882 the Medical Society of the State of New York voted in favor of a modified code of ethics that permitted its members to consult with any "legally qualified practitioners of medicine." A bitter quarrel ensued within the society, leading the minority group, which favored the AMA code of ethics, to establish a new association, the New York State Medical Society. Over twenty years elapsed before the two groups finally merged.[20]

The year 1901 marked the second of two developments that placed the AMA in the forefront of the medical profession. The first had been the appearance of the *Journal of the American Medical Association* in 1883. This publication gave the association an effective voice and generally enhanced its status within the profession. The second was the constitutional reorganization in 1901, which made the association both more representative and at the same time more effective as a national body.[21] As of 1900 only about 25 percent of the over 100,000 orthodox physicians belonged to local or state societies and less than 9 percent were members of the AMA. Moreover, the western and southern states were scarcely represented in the organization, and specialists were rapidly establishing their own associations. Under the leadership of President Charles Reed, who recognized the need for drastic reform, the AMA began a restructuring of its organization. The first aim of the reformers was to bring the specialists back into the fold. Their second objective was to strengthen local and state societies by increasing their membership, coordinating their activities with each other and bringing them into close association with the national organization.[22]

In 1901 a reorganization committee presented its recommendations to the AMA convention. The committee's report first stated that county medical associations should be the basic unit of the profession. Up to this date medical societies had tended to be exclusive and elitist. The committee, however, declared that membership, instead of being a privilege, was to be the right of any reputable licensed physician. Furthermore, membership in a county medical society automatically gave membership in the state society. Whereas the AMA had formerly admitted representatives of all state and local societies, henceforth the state societies were to be the only constituent members. The AMA's House of Delegates was made the legislative body of the association, and each state society was allowed a certain number of delegates with voting rights. The delegates to the convention accepted all of the committee's main recommendations. This structural overhaul was not without risk, since the specialists had already organized, and the right to limit membership in state and local organizations had a long tradition behind it. In fact, the immediate result was a decline in AMA membership, largely due to the loss of many specialists, but the specialists were too dependent upon the general practitioners to remain apart for long. Objections were raised by a number of state and local societies, but the advantages of a united profession were all too obvious, and the opposition quickly dissipated.[23]

The next important step in strengthening the AMA was taken in 1903 when the association's detailed code of ethics was replaced by a statement of principles. Physicians were now given discretion in the matter of consulting with other practitioners, the effect of which was to include licensed homeopaths and eclectics among the ranks of the regulars. As indicated earlier, acceptance of medical sectarians was made easier by the advent of scientific medicine, which tended to standardize medical education and practice. Once medicine became based on a better understanding of physiology, pathology, and the other biomedical sciences, the theories that had divided physicians were no longer tenable. The sectarian medical schools that survived in the twentieth century were those recognizing the need for training in the basic sciences.

While the reorganization of the AMA was a major event in its history, of equal importance was the appointment of Dr. Joseph N. McCormack, the dynamic secretary of the Kentucky Board of Health, as official organizer for the association. An individual with a strong social conscience, McCormack had been appointed to the Kentucky State Board of Health in 1880. Within the next twenty years he was largely responsible for all of Kentucky's early public health laws, pushed a medical practice law through the legislature, and strengthened the state medical association. As secretary of the Kentucky State Board of Health, McCormack, along with other AMA reformers, had seen how Dr. Jerome Cochran had created a powerful medical association in Alabama, one that was able to elect a majority of physicians to the state legislature in 1873 and rewrite Alabama's medical and public health laws. McCormack was determined to build equally strong state and local societies throughout the country.

McCormack, a man of boundless energy, was all too aware that personal enmities and bitter rivalries among physicians were a prime cause for the weakness of the profession, and in his travels he constantly appealed for professional unity, urging physicians never to speak disparagingly of each other. Conscious of the serious economic problems besetting the profession, he encouraged the establishment of modest fee schedules to limit ruinous competition among physicians, and he inveighed against abuses such as fee splitting, unethical advertising, and quackery. He was also a major advocate of strengthening medical licensure laws, medical education, and other means for reducing the number of incompetent practitioners.

Along with strengthening local medical societies and unifying the profession, McCormack recognized the need to improve the profession's image. He was a charismatic speaker, and he followed an exhaustive schedule addressing physicians and laypeople. To the latter, he spoke of medical ethics and of the public services performed by the profession, preaching the need for sound health, preventive medicine, and public health. Following the path laid out by McCormack, the AMA in 1910 created a Council on Health and Public Instruction, which included separate bureaus for medical legislation, public relations, and organization. In summarizing his work, James G. Burrow, the authority on the AMA, states that McCormack "projected the image of the new physician, one trained by advancing scientific standards, sensitive to social issues, and culturally mature."[24]

The reformed AMA, as noted early, immediately threw its weight into the fight for better medical education through the work of its Council on Medical Education. At the same time it launched an attack on quacks and irregulars. Although the long fight against the homeopaths and eclectics was on its way to resolution, new medical sects had arisen to challenge the orthodox profession. Osteopaths, chiropractors,

Christian Scientists, and optometrists presented a major challenge in the early years of the twentieth century, and they had strong support from the National League for Medical Freedom, an organization supported primarily by the patent medicine manufacturers. To meet the threat, the AMA sought to strengthen the medical licensure laws, and in the process became involved in bitter political battles at all levels of government. The public still had reservations about medical licensure, and the irregulars and the patent medicine manufacturers proved effective lobbyists in state legislatures. Consequently the AMA and its societies did not win all of the battles against the irregulars, but it gained considerable experience in the art of lobbying and mobilizing public opinion.

The medical profession was fortunate in that many of its own best interests coincided with those of the public. The need to regulate the vast patent medicine industry and to control the sale of potentially dangerous medicines was of public concern. At the same time, requiring prescriptions for many drugs was to the advantage of the physicians. In fighting for pure food laws, physicians were both demonstrating their civic consciousness and asserting their authority on matters pertaining to health. Local and state medical societies began agitating for pure food and drugs in the latter part of the nineteenth century, and in the early years of the twentieth the AMA joined the struggle and became an important element in the coalition that secured the Pure Food and Drugs Act of 1906.[25]

Although individual physicians supplied much of the leadership in promoting public health during the nineteenth century, medical organizations played only a minor role. The revived AMA and its associated societies, not without some dissension within the ranks, now became a major force in battling for public health measures. Medical societies supported the gathering of vital statistics, local health units, stronger state health boards, pure water and sewer systems, and school health. In fact, motivated in part by altruism and in part by the milieu of the Progressive Movement, the AMA and many of its member societies were involved in the fight for almost every public health reform in the period up to World War I.

One of the earliest public health crusades was against the sale of impure and adulterated milk, a major cause of the enormous infant mortality rate in the nineteenth century. The milk crusade began with a drive against swill milk shortly before the Civil War. Swill milk was derived from cows kept in incredibly filthy conditions and fed solely on the waste from distilleries and breweries. In this same period it was becoming evident, too, that milk from all sources was often adulterated with water and other substances. The discovery of bacteria in the 1870s and 1880s provided additional incentive to regulate the sale of milk, and beginning in New Jersey in 1892 medical societies unilaterally began taking it upon themselves to inspect milk supplies; milk given a medical society's seal of approval was then sold as "certified milk." [26]

The late nineteenth century also saw the beginning of school health inspection. Originally designed to identify contagious diseases among schoolchildren, the program was broadened in the early 1900s, and medical societies were in the forefront of those advocating the appointment of school nurses, health inspectors, and school hygiene programs. They also backed the movement for child health and actively lobbied for the establishment of child health bureaus at the state and national levels. The AMA, along with the American Public Health Association, was equally active in the legislative battles for a national health department and until 1917 strongly supported the principle of national health insurance.

It is to the credit of the AMA that it promoted public health and preventive medicine despite the fact that these programs decreased the demand for medical services. The wider use of vaccines, improved sanitation, and better and safer supplies of food and water were sharply reducing the incidence of typhoid, scarlet fever, diphtheria, and the other debilitating and fatal disorders of earlier years. Many physicians, viewing the relative poverty of their profession, had serious qualms about the AMA's policy, but a genuine sense of social concern motivated most of the association's leaders. Whatever may have been their qualms, the majority of physicians recognized that by asserting leadership on public health matters the profession was strengthening its authority and gaining greater public respect. While supporting many aspects of public health, the medical profession managed to place sharp limits on the medical care rendered by public health departments. By the end of World War I the AMA emerged as an effective political lobby and the powerful voice of a strong and unified medical profession. It had greatly improved the profession's image and effectively preserved the fee-for-service system.

The successful effort to maintain the fee-for-service system at all costs was a major factor in the decline of the public dispensaries (outpatient clinics). As noted in chapter 11, medical developments contributed to changing the structure of hospitals and enabling physicians to assume control. These same changes also helped to undermine the public dispensaries, which, by providing medical care for the poor and lower paid working class, were considered a serious threat to private medical practice. By World War I it was no longer feasible for a physician in an office with a handful of medicines to provide adequate care for a wide range of disorders. The medical profession seized upon this argument to justify closing the dispensaries, and, in the process, eliminated a threat to the fee-for-service system.

In his perceptive study *The Transformation of American Medicine*, Paul Starr points out that the medical profession benefited from the rise of professionalism and the advances in science and technology, which underlay what he terms its cultural authority. Yet science, he adds, did not guarantee the rise of medical authority for "the growth of science might have reduced professional autonomy by making doctors dependent upon organizations." While the medical profession capitalized on the new medical knowledge, he asserts that it achieved its present status by gaining control of both the market for its services and virtually all health agencies. The profession regained occupational control through reforming medical education; won authority over medication by fighting against proprietary drugs (ethical drugs can be advertised only to physicians); gained control of hospitals, technology, and technologists; resolutely fought against all efforts by middlemen to come between the doctor and patient; and placed limitations on public health.[27]

While Starr tends to dismiss the desperate need for reforming medical education and the conscientious efforts of many physicians to promote licensing and drug control for the benefit of patients, there can be little doubt that a reorganized and greatly strengthened AMA was a major factor in creating a strong and politically powerful medical profession.

CHAPTER 15

The Advancing Front
of Medicine

THE CLOSE INTERRELATIONSHIP between the biological
sciences and the ways in which each of them has contributed to major advances in medicine and surgery make it difficult to
present an organized account of the drastic changes that medicine has
undergone during this century. The first forty years saw the refinement
of the bacteriological revolution and the broad-scale application of the
new science of bacteriology to the great epidemic diseases that for centuries had been the major concern of medicine. Probably of more importance in these years were discoveries that broadened the traditional
fields of anatomy, physiology, pathology, chemistry, and pharmacy. As
the rate of discovery accelerated, it was no longer possible to encompass
all the knowledge gained in any one particular area, and a host of new
fields emerged: biochemistry, immunology, biophysics, pharmacology,
virology, genetics, and neurobiology.

In conjunction with these developments, the past fifty years have
witnessed major advances in clinical testing. Well designed and managed clinical trials are now available for all types of illnesses, ranging
from cancer to behavioral problems. This type of testing has been
possible through the use of major clinical establishments such as the
National Institutes of Health (NIH), Food and Drug Administration
(FDA), Army Medical Department, various foundations, and the cooperation of physicians, hospitals, and patients. For the first time therapeutic efficacy and safety can now be determined in a more rational,
scientific manner, rather than by relying on anecdotal therapy as in
the past.

The structure of medical education in which students start with the basic sciences and then move into clinical medicine would appear to be a logical sequence for a chapter on twentieth-century medicine. The line between clinical and basic research, however, is no longer sharply delineated and discoveries in the biomedical sciences quickly move into the clinical area. In consequence this chapter will follow both a topical and chronological approach, summarizing developments in certain basic fields and citing examples to show the application of these discoveries in the area of therapeutic and preventive medicine. Any overview of the leading edges of medicine necessarily is predictive, since it shows the major areas in which current research is concentrated.

Early research in physiology, which may well have been the foundation of modern scientific medicine, centered primarily on normal physiology. Pathophysiology did not come into its own until the present century and at times almost obscured the fact that to understand abnormal physiology, one must first understand normal physiology. Experimental physiology started in nineteenth-century France with François Magendie and Claude Bernard and quickly spread to England and Germany. Late in the century American students returning from Europe, most notably Germany, helped to professionalize physiology in the United States, founding the American Physiological Society in 1887 and the *American Journal of Physiology* in 1898. In the twentieth century, general physiology spawned a host of specialized areas of study: biophysics; cellular biology; comparative physiology and nutrition; digestion; and renal, endocrine, reproductive, muscular, and nervous physiology.[1]

In the nineteenth century, clinical departments concentrated their efforts on teaching medicine and used laboratories solely as diagnostic aids. Due to the efforts of men such as Llewellys F. Barker of Hopkins and his disciple Rufus Cole, director of the Rockefeller Hospital, these departments in the early 1900s became centers for both teaching and research. This research led to a proliferation of distinct areas of study. One of the more interesting aspects of the ever-widening horizon of biomedical knowledge is that intensive specialization, particularly as it involves molecular structures, has led to blurring the distinctions between the traditional basic sciences. Moreover, in the past forty years medicine has come to draw upon the knowledge gained in areas such as physics, metallurgy, and engineering. The net effect of this increasing knowledge has been to make it possible to gain some understanding of many of the constitutional, degenerative, and debilitating disorders plaguing the human organism.

One of the newer fields of medicine that has developed through the collaboration of clinicians and basic scientists is endocrinology. Endocrine disorders form a special category of diseases, although they overlap with other categories. They can contribute to psychosis, immune system regulation, and susceptibility to infectious disorders. They may also be hereditary. Endocrinology also illustrates the interaction between the many areas of medicine. Some neoplastic diseases, both benign and malignant, are characterized by the overproduction of certain hormones, and certain cancers stimulate the production of ectopic hormones. In the process of studying tumors and cancer, much has been learned about normal endocrinology and insights have been gained into immunology. Research on myeloma, cancer of the plasma cells, led directly to an understanding of the molecular biology of antibodies and to the work of César Milstein, Geörges J. F. Koehler, and Niels K. Jerne, who received the Nobel Prize in 1984 for their monoclonal antibody discovery, the fusion and cloning of cells.

Endocrinology also relates to immunology in other ways. Powerful inflammatory hormonelike substances called cytokins are released from immune cells following stimulation by many environmental agents, bacteria, and viruses. These immune cytokins can attach to receptors in the brain and influence nervous-system function. Another example is provided by juvenile diabetes and other autoimmune disorders, which, under experimental and clinical conditions, can be mitigated if treated early with immunosuppressive drugs.

Endocrine disorders, those caused by an excess or inadequate flow of hormones, had been recognized at least as early as the nineteenth century, although their exact cause was unknown. Harvey W. Cushing was one of the first American clinicians to realize that the ductless glands played a major role in the physiological processes. He made a number of fundamental discoveries concerning the pituitary gland and recognized that it had a measure of control over the other endocrine glands. Meanwhile early biochemists were attempting to determine the nature and effect of the substances released by the glands. Despite Cushing's studies of the pituitary gland, it was not until the 1920s that researchers began identifying the various pituitary hormones, and it was not until after World War II that improved technology made it possible to produce them in pure forms.

Although the term "hormone" was not introduced until 1905, efforts to identify hormonal substances had been going on for ten years. The first breakthrough was made by two British scientists in 1895 when they discovered that an extract of the adrenal glands caused a rise in blood pressure. Two years later, John J. Abel and Albert Crawford of Johns Hopkins reported that they had isolated the active principle, which they called epinephrine. The adrenal glands produce a number of different hormones, and many researchers from several countries contributed to identifying them. By World War II over twenty-five hormones had been isolated in their pure crystalline forms, but their precise role was not clear. During the war, Merck and Company began a major effort to produce adrenal steroids and succeeded in creating a substance that was subsequently named cortisone. In 1948 E. C. Kendall of the Mayo Clinic, who had isolated thyroxin, administered cortisone to a patient with severe rheumatoid arthritis. The treatment brought rapid relief and demonstrated that cortisone was an effective anti-inflammatory.[2]

The high incidence of goiter in certain geographic areas, with its gross swelling of the throat, had early drawn attention to the thyroid gland. First attempts to treat the disease surgically had proved disastrous when surgeons had removed the entire gland. The first breakthrough in medical treatment came in 1909 when D. Marine and C. H. Lenhart were able to prevent goiter in experimental animals by administering iodine. Subsequently Edward C. Kendall, an American biochemist, in 1914–15 chemically identified the thyroid hormone and showed that it contained a high percentage of iodine. Two years later, Marine and O. P. Kimball successfully used iodine to treat a human patient. This discovery not only made it possible to relieve patients suffering from hypothyroidism, but also led to the introduction of iodized salt in the 1920s. This great prophylactic virtually eliminated goiter in the Great Lakes area and other sections of the country where the disease was endemic.[3]

The role of the parathyroids in disease was first uncovered by William G. McCallum and C. Voegtlin of Johns Hopkins in 1909, and the hormone produced by this gland was identified and named parathormone in 1925 by a Canadian, James B. Collip. Subsequently it was learned that parathormone regulated calcium and phosphorous metabolism, thus helping to explain the clinical symptoms of hyper- and hypoparathyroidism. McCallum, building on the work of the Germans, Joseph von Mering and Oscar Minkowski, and of his colleague

Eugene L. Opie, confirmed in 1909 that a substance produced by the islets of Langerhans was responsible for preventing diabetes. Subsequently, two Canadians, Frederick G. Banting and Charles H. Best, in 1921 were able to extract what became known as insulin from animal pancreatic tissue. By injecting this substance into dogs with induced diabetes, they were able to lower the animals' blood sugar. With help from J. R. Mcleod and J. B. Collip, in 1922 a refined form of insulin was produced and injected in a young boy dying of diabetes. His miraculous recovery demonstrated that regulated doses of the hormone insulin could preserve the health of diabetics. Whereas diabetic children had rarely survived beyond the age of fifteen, once the problems of mass-producing insulin were solved, it became possible to give diabetics a relatively normal life.[4]

The growing knowledge about physiology and metabolism, the sum total of all processes by which the body maintains itself, inevitably led biochemists and others to investigate the role of food, and this in turn created the field of nutrition. German scientists in the nineteenth century were the first to make significant progress in this area, and Americans who studied under them introduced the new methods of research on metabolism into America—although, as with science in general, medical research continued to be a multinational endeavor. One of the first of these Americans was Wilbur O. Atwater, a chemistry professor at Wesleyan University in Connecticut. He improved the calorimeter, a device originally designed to measure heat produced during metabolism, and along with Francis G. Benedict was able to demonstrate that fats and carbohydrates were the source of energy during exercise.[5]

For a good part of the twentieth century the basal metabolic rate was determined by a relatively crude and expensive clinical laboratory test to assess thyroid function. In the second half of the century it was replaced by simpler and more effective methods. First a measurement of radioactive iodine was used to determine the metabolic rate, but the ubiquitous presence of iodine in hospitals eventually led to more sophisticated tests for measuring the non-iodine part of the thyroid hormone.

The study of the digestive process led directly to biochemistry. Its emergence in the twentieth century was largely an American development, and not until the 1930s did the field gain a place in British and European universities. Russell Chittenden of Yale established the first laboratory of physiological chemistry and made significant contributions to the study of protein requirements in humans. In 1906 he became president of the newly formed American Society of Biological Chemists. Biochemistry remained under the aegis of medical schools because academic chemistry departments regarded biochemistry as an aspect of medical chemistry and hence did not seek to annex it. Biochemistry may also have had a symbolic value in America, since it exemplified the ideals of the movement toward scientific medicine.[6]

Beginning in the sixteenth century, it was discovered and rediscovered time and time again that scurvy, a deficiency disease, could be cured by fresh fruits and vegetables, most notably citrus fruits. In the nineteenth century two new dietetic disorders, although they were not immediately recognized as such, were identified in the United States, beriberi and pellagra. As noted in chapter 11, in 1911 Casimir Funk derived a substance from rice hulls that cured beriberi. His discovery, which ultimately proved to be thiamin or vitamin B_6, pointed the way to eliminate the disorder.[7] Similar biochemical research also discovered the precise food element essential to prevent scurvy. Although improved diet had almost eliminated the disease from advanced Western nations, it was not until 1928 that ascorbic acid (vitamin C) was isolated and not until 1932 that it was positively identified as the causative agent for scurvy.

Epidemiological studies in the early 1900s showed that pellagra was a much more serious threat to the health of poor southerners than beriberi. Assuming that pellagra was contagious, the United States Public Health Service in 1914 assigned Joseph Goldberger to investigate its cause. As mentioned earlier, by perceptive detective work he soon demonstrated that pellagra was a dietetic disorder of the poor and could be prevented by the addition of milk and meat to the diet. Southerners generally rejected his findings, considering them a reflection on the South. At first Goldberger believed the essential element was one or more of the amino acids until he discovered in 1923 that the disease could be cured by the addition of yeast to the diet. The specific antipellagra factor was not found until 1937, eight years after Goldberger's death. In that year Conrad A. Elvehjem of the University of Wisconsin identified nicotinic acid, part of the B-complex, as the essential factor. Subsequently it was discovered that a lack of the amino acid tryptophan as well as nicotinic acid could cause pellagra.[8]

Research on diet led two groups of scientists, Elmer V. McCollum and Marguerite Davis of the University of Wisconsin and Thomas B.

Osborne and Lafayette B. Mendel of Yale, independently to discover a fat soluble substance in dairy products that was essential to growth. Subsequently McCollum and his group found two essential food factors, the fat-soluble substance known as vitamin A and a water-soluble one known as vitamin B. In the succeeding years it was shown that vitamin B consists of a number of water-soluble vitamins. One of the more significant vitamins of the B complex was folic acid. Recognizing that animal livers contained a growth-producing substance, between 1941 and 1943 scientists at Lederle Laboratories isolated a small amount of pure folic acid and by 1945 were able to synthesize it. In the meantime, clinical trials demonstrated that folic acid was an effective treatment for nutritional anemias and sprue.[9]

Rickets is a deficiency disease with a long history and one that was clearly identified clinically in the seventeenth century. As with some other disorders, it became a more serious problem during the industrial revolution. Early in this century scientists began searching for its cause, and their work led to the discovery of vitamin D. Building on the work of two English scientists and of his colleagues in the departments of pediatrics and biochemistry at Hopkins, in 1922 McCollum and his associates were able to isolate this vitamin. About the same time observers noted that sunshine could cure rickets, raising questions about the validity of the vitamin D thesis until it was discovered that ultraviolet light causes the body to produce vitamin D. As with vitamin B, in later years vitamin D was broken down into several forms.[10]

Vitamin K, essential to the production of prothrombin, a constituent of blood that enables it to clot, was first recognized by a Danish biochemist in 1934, but Americans played the key role in its identification and application. In 1939 Dr. Edward A. Doisey, a biochemist at St. Louis University, completed the work of fellow researchers in Rochester, New York; Marquette, Wisconsin; and the Mayo Clinic by isolating vitamin K, determining its chemical structure, and synthesizing it in his laboratory. Since a small percentage of newborns lack vitamin K, the synthesizing of this vitamin made it possible to save many infant lives and facilitate infant surgery.[11]

The discovery of vital food elements led to enriching certain basic foods. The first step in this direction resulted from the finding by Harry Steenbock of the University of Wisconsin in 1924 that vitamin D could be added to food by exposing it to ultraviolet radiation. By the late 1920s bakeries began using irradiated yeast in bread, and food processors began irradiating their products. By the mid-1930s, for example, the use of irradiated milk was general in the United States. World War II greatly stimulated an interest in nutrition, and wartime measures resulted in enriching bread and flour with the essential B vitamins. An unintended result of the discovery of vitamins has been their wholesale ingestion by the American public, probably the major food fad of the twentieth century.

Banting and Best's discovery of insulin came just in time to save the life of George R. Minot, who had developed diabetes in 1921, and by so doing it hastened the development of a cure for pernicious anemia. Minot, a member of the Harvard medical faculty, was familiar with the work of George H. Whipple, at that time director of the Hooper Foundation for Medical Research in San Francisco, whose studies showed that anemia in dogs could be cured by adding liver to their diet. Beginning in 1924 Minot and his colleague William P. Murphy began experimenting with diets high in liver on patients with pernicious anemia. By 1926 it was clear that the experiments were successful, although it was necessary for the patients to remain on the diet. Shortly thereafter William B. Castle demonstrated that two factors were involved in pernicious anemia, one substance supplied by the stomach (gastric juice) and the second by diet. In 1950 the essential factor supplied by a diet of liver was identified as vitamin B_{12}.[12]

A basic field of medicine that has contributed notably to many other disciplines is hematology, a specialty that has emerged in recent years. Until the 1920s it was essentially a descriptive field, but in that decade improved methods of blood examinations were introduced, including the hematocrit devised by M. M. Wintrobe. It now became possible to establish standards for normal blood, opening the way to studying blood disorders. Studies on the inhibitory effect of mustard gas upon the growth of blood cells and subsequent observations on the destructive effects of mustard gases on lymphoid tumors during World War II laid the basis for modern chemotherapy and the development of oncology. Hematology provided the first example of a "molecular disease" when Linus Pauling and his associates in 1949 were able to demonstrate that an abnormal hemoglobin protein was responsible for sickle cell anemia. Their work opened the way to recognizing hundreds of other abnormal hemoglobins, some of which were potentially harmful. Molecular biology made it possible to peer into the lymphocyte and find that it was a highly specialized family of cells. This knowledge gave rise to the field of immunology and helped explain how one of the ribonucleic acid (RNA) viruses alters the functioning of lymphocytes in acquired immune deficiency disease or AIDS.[13]

As James Bordley III and A. McGehee Harvey have pointed out, many of the dramatic developments in medicine have been made possible by advances in technology and technique. Credit for the first successful tissue culture belongs to Ross G. Harrison of Johns Hopkins, who in 1907 was able to culture frog embryos. On learning of Harrison's technique, Alexis Carrel of the Rockefeller Foundation improved on it and laid the basis for modern tissue culture. This development made possible a wide range of medical advances and has been invaluable in virology. The 1920s and 1930s saw the introduction of instruments for micromanipulation that, in conjunction with advanced microscopes, made possible the dissection of individual cells. These and other developments in micropuncture and microchemistry helped pave the way for a new era of biomedical research.[14]

Of equal importance to biomedical advances was the invention of the electron microscope. Developed largely in Germany in the 1920s and 1930s, the first commercial instrument was produced in the United States by the Radio Corporation of America in 1941. In the 1940s two new scientific tools were introduced, chromatography for segregating minute amounts of organic matter and the spectrophotometer for determining the identity of matter in a solution by measuring the amount of light absorbed. These two inventions, along with the electron microscope, contributed notably to the emergence of molecular medicine.

Although Americans made only limited contributions to the explosion in medical knowledge in the latter part of the nineteenth century, they were in the forefront of the discovery of insect vectors. Theobald Smith of the federal Bureau of Industries and his associate F. L. Kilbourne, after a series of careful experiments, were able to prove conclusively that Texas cattle fever was conveyed by ticks infected with the disease. Their report in 1892 undoubtedly added to the growing suspicion that insect vectors were also responsible for human diseases.[15] During these years British and Italian scientists were beginning to unravel the connection between mosquitoes and malaria, and, as mentioned in chapter 12, the Walter Reed Commission in 1900 identified the *Aedes aegypti* mosquito as the yellow fever vector.

While bacteriology was gradually bringing the great epidemic dis-

eases of the nineteenth century under control, those caused by rick-
ettsiae and viruses awaited the development of new techniques and
improved technology. By 1900 the name "viruses," a term used for
centuries as a synonym for poison or venom, was applied to minute
pathogenic organisms small enough to pass through a porcelain filter.
Smallpox and the infectious agents for several plant and animal diseases
already had been placed in this category, and in the course of its investigation of yellow fever, the Reed Commission had added this fever
to the list of viral diseases. The first significant American contribution
to virology was made by George M. Sternberg in 1892 when he discovered that the amount of smallpox antibodies in the blood could be
determined by how much vaccine matter it took to neutralize it. This
neutralization technique has since had a wide range of applications. In
the years from 1900 to 1915 research was concentrated on proving the
filterability of disease agents and in searching for a medium to culture
these "invisible" viruses.[16]

Most of this early work was undertaken by Europeans, although the
Rockefeller Institute began working on polio and other viruses beginning in 1907. In 1922 Thomas M. Rivers joined the staff of the hospital
of the Rockefeller Institute, and under his leadership the institute became a leading center for virus research. His textbook *Filterable Viruses*
(1928) summarized virtually all existing knowledge on the subject and
in effect established virology as a separate field.[17] In 1931 Ernest W.
Goodpasture of Vanderbilt University Medical School along with Alice
Woodruff showed that fowl pox virus could be cultivated in chicken
embryos and then demonstrated that eggs were also suitable for growing human viruses. This major advance simplified all viral research and
opened the way for the production of vaccines.[18] Using the chicken
embryo technique, in 1936 Max Theiler at the Rockefeller Institute developed a vaccine for yellow fever, and during this same year Albert
Sabin and Peter Olitsky succeeded in growing poliovirus in neural tissue. The 1930s also saw some progress in understanding the nature of
influenza.

The establishment of the National Foundation for Infantile Paralysis
in 1938 concentrated large funds on studying poliomyelitis and in the
process benefited all viral research. In 1949 John F. Enders, Thomas H.
Weller, and Frederick C. Robbins of Harvard developed a technique
for keeping tissue alive in test tubes and growing poliovirus on it. By
1951 the three major strains of polio had been typed. More important,

the ability to culture viruses in test tubes was a major step forward for virology. With the help of the new scientific instruments, it was possible within the next few years to pinpoint the essential differences between viruses and bacteria. In these same years evidence was accumulating indicating the role of viruses in certain forms of cancer.[19]

Rickettsial diseases such as typhus and Rocky Mountain spotted fever, as with viruses, grow only within cells, and it was not until 1938 that the first rickettsias were cultivated in chick embryos, a step that helped both to study rickettsias and to produce vaccines. The 1930s also witnessed the beginning of research into coccidioidomycoses, one of the few fungal diseases in which American research has played a leading role.

Among the new fields coming to the fore in the twentieth century is pharmacology, the study of the properties and reactions of drugs, as differentiated from pharmacy, the dispensing and preparation of them. Although its origins can be traced further back, pharmacology began in nineteenth-century Europe and arrived in America largely in the person of John J. Abel (1857–1938). Abel, one of many Americans to complete his medical education abroad, returned to America in 1891 to accept an appointment to the first American chair in pharmacology at the University of Michigan Medical School. Two years later he was lured away by Dr. William H. Welch to become professor of pharmacology in the newly established Johns Hopkins Medical School. The work of Abel, along with that of his associates and students, laid the basis for present-day American pharmacology. Among his many contributions, he and E. M. K. Geiling first succeeded in obtaining insulin in a crystalline form. Abel also helped found the *Journal of Experimental Medicine*, was cofounder and editor of the *Journal of Biological Chemistry*, and founded and edited the *Journal of Pharmacology and Experimental Therapeutics*. Other outstanding American pharmacologists include Otto Loewi, who received the Nobel Prize in 1936 for his research on the vagus nerve; Julius Axelrod, winner of the Nobel Prize in 1970 for his work on catecholamines; and Earl W. Sutherland, who inaugurated the era of modern endocrine pharmacology and was awarded the Nobel Prize in 1971 for his work on hormone action at the molecular level. Included within this group should be Selman A. Waksman, a soil microbiologist, biochemist, and incidental pharmacologist, who won the Nobel Prize in 1952 for his discovery of streptomycin and other antibiotics.[20] Waksman and his work will be discussed below.

In the area of therapeutics some progress had been made in the nineteenth century. A number of important drugs, such as aspirin, atropine, cocaine, morphine, quinine, and digitalis, were in use by 1900, but few significant additions were made during the next thirty-five years. Paul Ehrlich in Germany was the first to concentrate on finding what he termed "magic bullets," drugs that would act directly on pathogenic organisms. His compound 606, or salversan, which was first tested on syphilitic patients in 1909, was hailed as a major breakthrough. Unfortunately a high toxicity and other disadvantages limited its effectiveness, but Ehrlich's approach opened a new vista in the search for better drugs. Nonetheless, other than the discovery of insulin and a treatment for pernicious anemia, no major addition was made to the armamentaria of physicians for the next thirty or so years.

The first significant breakthrough in the fight against infections was the discovery in 1935 of the sulfa drugs. A young German, Gerhardt Domagk, was examining certain coloring agents, looking for one that would affect bacteria in living tissue, and in the process discovered the first of the sulfonamides. French, British, and American scientists quickly followed up his work, and a host of new sulfa drugs were created. Although the sulfa drugs were a marvelous discovery, they had definite limitations, and a search was already under way for even better therapeutics. The discovery by Alexander Fleming of the antibacterial qualities of a substance produced by a mold in 1928 is well known. It proved exceedingly difficult to extract the substance, which he named penicillin, from the mold, and his discovery languished for ten years. While Fleming continued to work on penicillin, in 1931 Rene Dubos and Oswald Avery of the Rockefeller Institute reported finding that an extract from a soil bacillus was capable of breaking down the capsule of one type of pneumonococcus. The extract, unfortunately, proved too toxic for use in humans, but its discovery encouraged further research on antibiotics.

In 1938 two researchers at Oxford University, Howard W. Florey, an Australian, and Ernst B. Chain, a German refugee, stimulated by the findings of Fleming and others, began a search for antibacterial substances produced by microorganisms. The following year they decided to concentrate their efforts on penicillin, and in 1940 were able to produce enough of it to make a successful test on streptococci-infected mice. Early in 1941 they gave penicillin to their first human patient, a policemen riddled with a staphylococcus infection. The patient rallied almost miraculously, but not enough penicillin was available to save him. Spurred on by the wartime need for more effective means to deal with wound infections and unable to interest British pharmaceutical firms in penicillin, Florey and Norman Heatley, a biochemist who was working with the group, came to the United States. Here support from the Department of Agriculture led to a joint undertaking to mass-produce penicillin by the Committee on Medical Research of the Office of Scientific Research and Development and three pharmaceutical companies. Many problems had to be solved, but by the time of the Allied invasion of France in 1944 enough penicillin was available to treat all severe casualties among the Allied troops. By 1950 penicillin was being produced by the ton, and, as the new miracle drug, regrettably was being prescribed widely and needlessly for common colds and a host of other minor infections.[21]

While research on the sulfa drugs and penicillin was underway, Selman A. Waksman, a Russian emigré and professor of biochemistry at Rutgers University with an interest in soil microbiology, began a search for products of soil bacteria capable of destroying pathogenic organisms in man. In 1943 he and his associates obtained a substance from a strain of actinomycetes, microorganisms about halfway between bacteria and fungi, which he named streptomycin. Testing in 1944 demonstrated that it was effective against human tuberculosis, and by 1948, streptomycin was being produced by eight pharmaceutical companies. The drug, however, was expensive to produce and not always effective. About the same time as the discovery of streptomycin, a Swedish scientist found that a modified form of salicylic acid could inhibit the growth of tubercle bacilli. Subsequent clinical tests showed that the new drug, called PASA, in combination with streptomycin was often more effective than either one separately. In 1951 three pharmaceutical companies, two American and one German, almost simultaneously discovered still another antitubercular drug, isoniazid. As the search for new drugs intensified, by 1973 five more antibiotics and two more chemical remedies for tuberculosis became available, making it possible to cure nearly all cases.

The postwar years opened what has been termed the era of antibiotics. American pharmaceutical companies, cut off from Germany and the Continent, were forced to step up their research, and their success with penicillin gave them further encouragement. In 1947 Parke, Davis, and Company announced the discovery of the first broad-spectrum antibiotic, chloromycetin, a drug effective against many rickettsial disorders as well as bacterial diseases such as typhoid fever. In short order other broad-spectrum antibiotics appeared on the scene, aureomycin, terramycin, and tetracycline. As the screening for new antibiotics became less productive, the next step, made possible by the emergence of molecular biology, was to modify the penicillin molecule. In the early 1940s it was discovered that resistant strains of bacteria produced an enzyme called penicillinase, which inactivated penicillin. By modifying the nucleus of various penicillins it was possible by 1960 to produce a number of synthetics resistant to penicillinase. Subsequently the discovery of the cephalosporins, broad-spectrum therapeutics, have proved effective in enabling severely immune-suppressed patients to survive.[22]

In addition to the sulfa drugs and antibiotics, the succeeding years saw the appearance of a host of new families of drugs. Anticoagulants, diuretics, beta and calcium blockers, amphetamines, steroids, tranquilizers, and other chemotherapeutics were either discovered by chance or designed to treat specific disorders. Whereas formerly physicians had but one or two drugs to treat a particular condition, they were now given a wide choice—and many of the drugs can be taken in combination. The choice may have become almost too great; the 1966 *Physicians Desk Reference* listed over twenty-five hundred prescription drugs.[23] By the 1980s developments in genetics and molecular biology were opening up even wider vistas in the area of therapeutics.

The remarkable achievements of antibiotics in the fight against infections were not an unmitigated good. Drug companies, anxious to cash in on medical discoveries, actively promoted their products via newspapers, television, and lay and professional journals, and as each successive wonder drug was announced in the news media, physicians, often pressured by their patients, tended to overprescribe it. Aside from possible side-effects, which were serious enough in themselves, the result was to increase the speed with which resistant infections have developed. Tranquilizers and the other powerful therapeutics, too, have been and are still being abused, despite efforts by medical leaders and public health officials to educate physicians and patients. The task is no easy one, with almost weekly media reports of new miracle drugs. An even worse result is that every medical breakthrough opens the way for new forms of quackery, a problem intensified in recent years by the deemphasis on federal regulation.[24]

Americans have made significant contributions to the neurosciences, but in doing so they have drawn on the findings of many other nationals. One of the chief founders of American neurology was S. Weir Mitchell (1829–1914), noted for his studies relating to the peripheral nerves and the central nervous system. The early neurology departments, particularly on the East Coast, tended to have a strong clinical orientation. The University of Chicago, which opened in 1892, included a professorship of neurology in the biology department. When the university affiliated with Rush Medical College, the neurology professor, H. H. Donaldson, was able to create a neurology department centering its research on microscopic anatomy of the nervous system. His successor, Charles Judson Herrick, who was given charge of a merged neurology and anatomy departments, initiated a new research program of evolution-based comparative neurology, thus continuing the department's strong basic-science tradition.

Indicative of the merging of scientific fields, the first two Americans to receive the Nobel Prize for their work in neurology were Joseph Erlanger, a physiologist, and Herbert Gasser, a pharmacologist, who received the award in 1944 for "their discoveries regarding the highly differentiated functions of single nerve fibers." In 1967 H. K. Hartline, a physiologist, and George Wald, a biologist, shared the Nobel Prize for their work on the chemical and physiological visual processes. Julius Axelrod, a biochemist with the National Institutes of Health, shared the Nobel Prize in 1970 with an English and a Swedish scientist for their work on neurotransmitters. An American endocrinologist, Andrew V. Schalley, along with two other Americans, Rosalyn S. Yarrow and Roger C. L. Guillemin, won the Nobel Prize in 1977 for their work in isolating and characterizing neurohypophyseal hypothalamic "releasing" hormones. In so doing, they showed how substances released from the brain (hypothalamus) controlled the master endocrine glands (pituitary) which in turn controlled the peripheral glands.[25]

The discovery of neurotransmitters, the substances that transmit nerve impulses across the synapses, and their gradual explication helped to explain the precise way in which certain drugs affected the brain, paving the way for new drugs to treat nervous disorders. L-Dopa for Parkinson's disease and a number of antipsychotic drugs were among the first of these. By 1960 enough was known about the brain to permit neuroendocrine control of ovulation, making possible the development of the birth control pill.[26]

Advances in the neurosciences profoundly altered psychiatry in the 1950s, but other developments, reinforced by the experiences in World War II, had an equally significant impact upon it. At the end of the nineteenth century, psychiatry generally accepted a somatic view of mental disease. The demonstration by Hideo Noguchi and J. W. Moore in 1913 that paresis resulted from a chronic progressive infection of the meninges and brain by the syphilis spirochete lent further credence to this belief.[27] The introduction from Europe of shock therapy for schizophrenia and the prefrontal lobotomy in the 1930s were in accordance with the somatic approach. The first form of shock therapy was that induced by intramuscular injections of insulin. In America electroshock therapy, first used by the Italians in 1938, was the preferred method of treatment, and a modified form of this strenuous procedure still has adherents today. The heroic surgical procedure, prefrontal lobotomy, an operation that certainly calmed patients but at a rather large cost to them, has not stood the test of time, although microsurgery may open the way for a greatly modified form of this operation.[28]

As a result of social and cultural changes and alterations in financing care for the aged, mental hospitals for the first sixty or more years of the twentieth century tended to be filled with aged and chronically ill patients. The majority of psychiatrists in the pre–World War II years were associated with mental institutions and relied on somatic therapies to treat mental diseases. Since mental ills were assumed to have a physical basis, psychiatrists accepted the traditional concept of a sharp dividing line between health and disease. A few of them, such as Sigmund Freud in Vienna and Adolph Meyer and William A. White in America, began suggesting that a continuum existed between normal and abnormal behavior. If such were the case, then early outpatient psychiatric help in community facilities might well prevent the onset of serious illness and thus reduce the need for institutionalization.[29]

Among public health and social workers there was also a growing recognition that social conditions affected the incidence of mental illness. In 1920 Harry A. Moore suggested that unemployment, congested populations, and child labor were factors in nervous disorders, and Dr. Haven Emerson in discussing mental health problems in 1929 declared that "public effort has not yet reached the stage where recognition is given to social problems as a whole."[30] By this date a number of private and government social agencies were concentrating their attention on delinquent and disturbed children, using the services of psychiatrists, psychologists, and psychiatric social workers. In the 1930s the national government, through the Social Security Act, began subsidizing mental hygiene programs, most of which were aimed at children, in the belief that early intervention was the most effective way to deal with mental ills.

As had been true to a lesser extent of the First World War, World War II, during which some 1,750,000 men were rejected for neuropsychiatric reasons, created an awareness of the high incidence of mental illness and stimulated research in all areas of psychiatry. The psychodynamic and psychoanalytical concepts were already gaining ground when the many cases of combat stress in World War II clearly demonstrated that the environment was a significant cause of mental maladjustment. Wartime experience also showed that early intervention in noninstitutional settings was the most effective way to treat combat stress. Equally important in drawing attention to the mentally ill was the influence of some 3,000 conscientious objectors to the draft who had been assigned to work in mental hospitals. Here they found patients living in atrocious conditions and often victimized by brutal staff members. Their reports horrified the public and helped make Congress receptive to supporting mental health programs.[31]

In the postwar years a new generation of psychiatrists influenced by psychodynamic and psychoanalytic concepts began emphasizing the role of social factors and the community in mental health. They sought the early identification of nervous disorders and their treatment in the community setting. As Nolan D. C. Lewis stated in 1948: "We as civilians should insist (not merely request) on the establishment of more child guidance centers and treatment clinics in cities and towns over the country." Public mental hospitals for years had been suffering from underfunding, staff shortages, and overcrowding. Under these conditions care was largely custodial. Social activists joined with psychiatrists in their efforts to replace traditional mental hospitals with new forms of community care and treatment. The first successes in the fight for better health came with the passage of the National Mental Health Act of 1946 and the formal creation of the National Institute of Mental Health in 1949. Stimulated by federal grants, many states began developing community health programs in the 1950s, and psychiatric and psychological services grew rapidly.[32]

Precisely at the time when the federal government was promoting community health programs, medical scientists were laying the basis for the emergence of antipsychotic drugs. Modern drug therapy dates back to 1951 when a French scientist synthesized chlorpromazine, the first of the tranquilizers. Soon after, reserpine, a member of the rauwolfia group, was added to the list of antipsychotic therapeutics. The 1960s saw the introduction of benzodiazepine (Librium) and varialion (Valium). With the number of these drugs rapidly increasing, chemotherapy became the preferred method of treatment for schizophrenic, manic-depressive, and certain other types of severely ill mental patients. The effect was to reduce drastically the use of prefrontal lobotomy and to minimize electroshock therapy.[33] The success of chemotherapy in relieving symptoms and enabling patients to function more or less normally was also a major factor in reducing the length of time patients spent in hospitals. At the same time, as mental illness came to be less stigmatized, admissions to all mental hospitals rose and more individuals were willing to accept community mental health services.

As the movement for community health programs gathered strength, the Joint Commission on Mental Illness, a group of interested professionals and laypeople, issued a report in 1961 urging a national system of community mental health centers. Congress responded in 1963 by providing matching funds on a limited basis for the development of these centers. Between 1967 and 1980 some $2.7 billion was appropriated, making it possible to open 789 mental health centers. The failure of the federal authorities to oversee these programs has negated much of the intended benefits. Many of the federally supported community health centers largely treat alcoholism and substance abuse and what are essentially counseling problems. Probably no more than 15 percent of their clients suffer from severe mental illness. It has been estimated that by 1990 only about 5 percent of these federally funded mental health centers were functioning as originally intended.[34]

In their enthusiasm for the new program, which emphasized prevention and cure within the community, psychiatrists and social activists overlooked the fact that thousands of chronically mental ill were incapable of functioning on their own. To make matters worse, the writings of men such as Erving Goffman and Thomas Szasz helped convince the public that mental hospitals were not only useless but positively harmful. As the public became convinced that mental hospitals were bad, a movement for patient rights emerged. Idealistic lawyers, aided by a number of court decisions, contributed notably to deinstitutionalizing the mentally ill. The result was a mass exodus of patients who were discharged into communities that were ill-prepared to receive them. The extent of this exodus is shown by the drastic reduction in the state mental hospital population, which dropped from 559,000 to 138,000 in the years between 1955 and 1980.[35]

Ideally these discharged patients should have received counseling and help from psychiatric social workers and nurses and other trained professionals, and they should have had access to halfway houses and community mental health centers. Unfortunately no provision was made for coordinating the various federal, state, and community mental facilities. Often patients were discharged from state institutions without any notification to local authorities. In a few areas these patients received some help, but the majority of them were shown how to get on welfare and then left to sink or swim.

Unfortunately, the establishment of community health centers depended on the willingness of local authorities to support the programs. Often poorer areas where the centers were most needed showed little interest, and those states that have cooperated have had to pay an increasing share of the costs due to the Reagan administration's reluctance to support social programs. The result is that many individuals incapable of functioning in society have simply been tossed onto the streets. A 1985 study of 132 individuals discharged from an Ohio state medical hospital showed that within six months 47, or 36 percent of them, had become homeless.[36]

Despite community mental health programs and advances in chemotherapy, admissions to mental facilities increased by almost one-third between 1969 and 1987. Originally Blue Cross–Blue Shield and private health insurance companies provided only minimal payments for mental illness, but gradually they have been forced to increase their coverage. The rising availability of insurance money combined with the increase in substance abuse has led to the multiplication of for-profit psychiatric centers. One critic has suggested that these "mental units market themselves in response to voguish social and personal problems (eating disorders, sexual abuse, 'co-dependency') and have become dumping grounds for adolescents whose parents want nothing more to do with them." Others have charged that far too many poorly disciplined, rebellious, or troubled children are diagnosed as mentally ill and placed on drugs or hospitalized. As early as 1974 E. Fuller Torrey asserted that many of the problems classified as mental illness have nothing to do with medicine or brain diseases, but were simply unwanted behavior, such as alcoholism, anxiety, hypochondria, drug addiction, and antisocial activity. These problems, he believes, can be handled by psychologists, trained social workers and nurses, and other nonmedical personnel.[37]

A major criticism of the psychiatric profession is that the majority of psychiatrists have found treating the middle and upper classes for what used to be called "neuroses" (a term that has now joined "neurasthenia" on the ash heap of psychiatry) a much more pleasant and profitable business than dealing with the severely mentally ill. Government support has increased the number of psychiatrists in the past forty years by a factor of ten, and billions of dollars of government funds has been spent, and yet it is doubtful that the severely mentally ill have received much benefit.

Estimates vary, but possibly as much as one-third of the homeless are severely mentally ill. The more fortunate ones periodically are arrested and sent to mental hospitals, only to be returned to the streets until their conduct again becomes too outrageous. Other mentally ill patients are periodically jailed, where they at least receive a measure of custodial care. Fortunately two national organizations, the National Alliance for the Mentally Ill and the National Mental Health Consumers Association, both representing mental patients and their families, are now lobbying to improve mental health services. Their success will depend upon their ability to create an informed public. Despite considerable progress, care of the mentally ill still has a long way to go.[38]

Of the new sciences in the twentieth century, biochemistry provided the basis for most medical advances in the pre–World War II years. In this period biochemistry dealt largely with small molecules such as amino acids, vitamins, and hormones, which flow in and out of cells. In the postwar years molecular biology, which deals with the macromolecules made and retained within the cells, has affected all of the life sciences. Molecular biology can be said to have started from Oswald Avery's study of the pneumococcus. In 1944 he reported his discovery that the material that transmits traits from one generation to another is DNA (deoxyribonucleic acid) and could be transferred between the pneumococcus cells. This finding opened the way for the fields of molecular genetics and bacterial genetics. In the meantime extensive research on the *Escherichia coli* bacteria had shown that bacteria were subject to viruses (bacteriophages). By 1950 several American researchers had demonstrated that these phages consisted largely of DNA. In consequence, bacteria became a model for studying the principles of molecular genetics. They were relatively simple and multiplied rapidly, and the billions of cells provided ample numbers of rare mutants.[39]

In 1953 an American, James D. Watson, and a Britisher, Francis H. C. Crick, building on the work of crystallographers and other scientists, were able to describe the structure of DNA, thereby setting the stage for a revolution in molecular genetics. They discovered that four base pairs of nucleic acids, linked together in a double helix, formed a code, analogous to the dots and dashes in the Morse code, that spelled out the order of amino acids in proteins. Subsequent research has provided an enormous amount of detailed information on the chemical and biological properties of DNA. Nonetheless, only a fraction of the code has been deciphered. Moreover, scientists are only beginning to understand the interaction between cell membrane receptors and the DNA system in the nucleus. If this interaction can be fully understood, it may lead to methods for preventing the malignant changes that distinguish the cancer cell from the normal one. The effect of the Watson-Crick discovery on genetics was enormous. Writing in 1976 James V. Neel estimated that 90 percent of solid information on human genetics had been discovered in the preceding thirty years. He noted also that only two American medical schools offered a sequence of lectures on medical genetics before World War II, whereas by 1976 over 80 percent of them were teaching the subject.[40]

In 1974 the development of recombinant DNA techniques almost overnight made possible the practical application of the vast amount of fundamental knowledge acquired in the preceding years. Bioengineering has made it possible to modify bacteria and use them for a wide variety of purposes. In medicine it has created a wide range of possibilities, including the development of monoclonal antibodies to attack cancer cells and those infectious bacteria resistant to antibiotics. The widening knowledge of human genetics has resulted in identifying about two thousand hereditary diseases caused by defective genes. It is currently possible to predict the probability of several hundred of these disorders based upon prenatal diagnosis of fetal cells cultured from the amniotic fluid. More important, bioengineering is now being used therapeutically to provide healthy replacement genes. The patients' cells are engineered to manufacture certain missing growth factors such as those responsible for producing insulin or causing haemophilia. Thus the engineered cells serve as a sophisticated drug-delivery system.

Gene therapy holds enormous promise, too, for treating many other disorders such as Parkinson's disease, malignant melanoma, and certain severe immune deficiency diseases. In addition to the medical area, the new knowledge of genetics is also being applied widely in industry and agriculture. For example, plants are now being tailored to make them resistant to frost or to certain diseases, and genetically altered bacteria have been designed to clean oil spills and remove fats from plumbing lines.[41]

Another major area to benefit from the major developments in cell biology in this century has been immunology. Although immunization against smallpox by inoculating healthy individuals with smallpox pus dates back to antiquity, relatively safe vaccination began with Edward Jenner's announcement in 1798 of the use of cowpox (vaccinia) to prevent smallpox. No further progress was made until 1880 when Louis Pasteur found that an attenuated chicken pox virus could ward off the disease in fowls. The crudeness of laboratory techniques in those days made the process risky. Fortunately, as mentioned earlier, six years later Daniel E. Salmon and Theobald Smith of the federal Bureau of Animal Industries discovered that a heat-killed vaccine was equally effective in protecting against disease. By World War II the collaboration of scientists from various countries led to the development of effective vaccines against typhoid, tetanus, and diphtheria, and useful ones against certain other bacterial diseases.

Even before the development of vaccines, European researchers discovered that toxins produced by certain bacteria caused animals infected with the disease to produce antitoxins, and that these antitoxins could be used to neutralize the toxins in other animals and humans. The first successful therapeutic use of antitoxins was in the treatment of diphtheria and tetanus patients, and, until the advent of antibiotics, these serums proved useful in treating pneumonia and meningococcal meningitis. Fortunately the growing use of vaccines and the appearance of newer and more effective drugs sharply reduced the need for serums. Nonetheless, the research associated with their development contributed notably to improving medical knowledge.

Rickettsial diseases, the most fearful of which was typhus, proved more difficult to prevent. The basic research of Howard T. Ricketts on Rocky Mountain fever, described in chapter 12, led to the development of a vaccine from infected ticks, but it was difficult to produce. The first breakthrough on the vaccine front was made by Harold R. Cox in 1938. Cox, who identified the rickettsial disease Q fever, was able to cultivate the organisms in chicken embryos by injecting the rickettsias into fertile hens' eggs. His technique opened the way to large-scale production of vaccines for typhus, Rocky Mountain spotted fever, and most rickettsial diseases.[42] The vaccine for typhus came just in time to be of major benefit. Typhus had been a major killer in World War I, but the wide use of vaccine in World War II almost eliminated the disease among American troops.

Efforts to achieve vaccines against viral diseases in the period before World War II were not quite so productive. Much was learned about influenzas and polio, but the only success, other than smallpox, was Max Theiler's attenuated vaccine against yellow fever mentioned earlier. Using the chicken embryo technique, enough of this yellow fever vaccine was produced to protect the troops in tropical areas during World War II. The war provided a great stimulus to research on viral and rickettsial diseases, and notable successes were achieved by the Army Medical Department Research and Graduate School at Walter Reed Army Medical Center and at the NIH's Bureau of Biologics. The vaccines they produced against the various forms of typhus, encephalitis, and other disorders saved thousands of military and civilian lives.

The early research in virology, which led to the culturing of virus in eggs and test tubes, paved the way for effective vaccines against poliomyelitis. That polio was singled out for intensive study was undoubtedly due to the crippling of President Franklin D. Roosevelt and the creation of the National Foundation for Infantile Paralysis. Simon Flexner of the Rockefeller Institute, the leading center for viral research, was convinced that the disease entered the body through the respiratory tract, and the result was to send researchers off in the wrong direction for many years. By the 1930s it was becoming evident that the virus attacked the digestive tract. The technique of cultivating poliovirus in nonneural tissues developed in 1949 made possible the typing of the three major polio strains and led teams of scientists into a race to produce a vaccine. One group, headed by Jonas Salk and supported by the National Foundation, aimed to produce an inactivated vaccine, while the other, under the leadership of Albert B. Sabin, sought to make a vaccine from attenuated virus. By 1953 the Salk vaccine was ready for large-scale clinical trials. Despite a temporary setback due to one faulty lot of vaccine, the tests demonstrated the success of the vaccine. In the meantime Lederle Laboratories was pushing ahead with the development of an oral vaccine made from an attenuated virus. After extensive testing overseas, in 1961 the Sabin vaccine was licensed by the Public Health Service, and, because it was so easy to administer, became the vaccine of choice.[43]

The many strains of influenza have made it a difficult disease to control, since the organism mutates so easily. Nonetheless, three major types of the virus were identified by World War II, and the 1940s and 1950s saw the development of a number of vaccines, largely by Joseph E. Smadel and his group at the NIH. Aided by the vaccine developers and the international surveillance network now housed in the World Health Organization, which provides early warning of new strains of influenza, the vaccines have been quite successful in limiting the ravages of influenza epidemics, especially among the young and the elderly. The accumulated knowledge gained from polio research and other areas of virology have also been applied successfully to other viral disorders.

Building on the early work of John F. Enders and Thomas C. Peebles, in 1963 an attenuated measles vaccine was made available in the United States. The same techniques produced a comparable vaccine for rubella by 1968, and shortly thereafter for mumps.[44] The common cold, caused by the rhinoviruses, as with influenza, consists of many different antigenic forms, and so far has thwarted attempts to create an effective vaccine. Pneumonia too has presented serious problems with respect to vaccines, although some success has been made in immunizing older people with capsular carbohydrates (antigenic fractions) derived from types I, II, and III pneumococci.[45] This development indicates the possibility that similar vaccines for other disorders may be developed in the near future.

In the past forty years immunochemistry has been slowly unraveling the mysteries of the immune system. The process has been facilitated by the technique of immunofluorescence developed by Albert H. Coons in 1941.[46] This technique has contributed significantly to explaining the interaction between antigens and antibodies, and has facilitated organ transplants, led to the development of immunosuppressive drugs, and provided an insight into the autoimmune diseases.

The one disease that, because of its multicausation, has become a focal point for nearly all fields of biomedical research is cancer. Cancer received only limited attention during the early years of this century since tuberculosis or consumption was still the most feared disease. Although cancer aroused dread, the public assumed it was hopeless and tended to be apathetic. Little was known about its cause or cure, and surgery appeared the only hope for its victims. A number of theories about cancer emerged, but the first specific evidence about its cause was Peyton Rous's discovery in the years 1910–12 that a certain tumor in chickens was caused by a virus. Little attention was paid to this discovery until Richard E. Shope, a virologist at the Rockefeller Institute, in the early 1930s found that infectious papillomatosis in cottontail rabbits was a viral disease. Rous, a leading figure in American oncology for over fifty years, then gave further support to the virus theory by showing that the Shope papilloma virus could cause malignancies in domestic rabbits. These findings were not fully appreciated until the field of virology was stimulated by polio research in the 1940s and 1950s.[47]

Cancer research took on a new direction when in 1932 a French scientist working with mice demonstrated the relationship between hormones and cancer. Aware of this development, Charles B. Huggins began experimenting with dogs and gave further proof to the hormone theory by showing that castration resulted in reducing the size of the prostate gland. His findings opened the way to treating a number of forms of cancer by "physiological surgery," i.e., the removal of a particular gland to remedy a disorder, or by hormonal therapy.[48]

By 1933 cancer had become the second leading cause of death and had replaced tuberculosis as the most dreaded disease. As public concern increased, the national government responded by passing the 1937 Cancer Act creating the National Institute for Cancer. In the post–World War II years money, both private and public, began pouring into cancer research. By this time dissension had emerged among advocates of cancer research. One group was convinced that environmental factors and personal habits were responsible for cancer, and that the emphasis should be on prevention. On the other side were the majority of medical scientists who believed that research funds should be devoted primarily to finding a cure. As early as 1932 Dr. William McNally of Rush Medical College suggested that smoking was a factor in the increase incidence of cancer of the lungs. Six years later Drs. Raymond Pearl, Alton Ochsner, and Michael DeBakey made the same point. It was not until the 1960s and 1970s, however, that advocates of cancer prevention through modifying the physical and social environment were able to gain a hearing.[49]

By this time cancer researchers were bringing to bear the entire knowledge of the new biological sciences. Molecular virologists in the

1970s were able to explain the precise way in which the genes in the RNA of a virus were incorporated into the DNA of a cell. Immunologists learned more about the immune systems' ability to resist neoplastic cells and began investigating methods to enhance the systems. Geneticists were studying the role of heredity, and, in addition, it became clear that the environment was responsible for many cancers. As early as the 1940s testing began to survey compounds for carcinogenic activity. As this search broadened, it became evident that pollution of the air and water by chemicals, ultraviolet light from sunshine, and ionizing radiation were all contributory factors to the rising incidence of cancer.

Until about 1940 the only treatment for cancer was surgery and/or radiation. Since then better methods for controlling shock, improved blood replacement techniques, and antibiotics have permitted more radical and safer surgery. In these same years radiation technology has become more sophisticated, and it too has assumed a larger role in cancer treatment. A major development in the past thirty years has been the emergence of chemotherapy, which has added a new weapon in the fight against cancer. At the same time, new rehabilitation methods, such as restoring the voice after removal of the larynx, have improved the quality of life after surgery. Today the cancer patient is aided by a medical team consisting of oncologists, radiologists, surgeons, pathologists, and other professionals.[50] Much still remains to be done before the threat of cancer can be reduced or removed. Despite the steady progress against cancer, the present methods of treatment are still heroic, and future generations may well view them with the same horror that reading about the bloody and painful surgery of a century and a half ago arouses in us today.

Happily the prospects for cancer patients are brightening, particularly in view of many recent advances in immunotherapy. One of these involves so-called tumor-infiltrating lymphocytes, or TILS, the lymphoid cells that actually infiltrate solid tumors. The cells can be grown in culture suspensions under the influence of certain cytokins called interleukins (IL). Given intravenously, they survive for several months in the blood or at the tumor site. Thus, one theoretically takes these TILS from the tumor of the patient, grows them in tissue culture, expands them numerically, and gives them back to the patient so that they home in on the tumor and kill it. In a recent study, TILS therapy plus one of the interleukins was used to treat fifty patients with a certain kind of malignant melanoma known to be uniformly fatal; a 38 percent survival rate, or remission rate, resulted. TILS holds even further promise because certain cytokines that are powerful toxins, such as a substance called tumor necrosis factor, can actually be genetically grafted into the TIL to make it even more powerful.[51]

Other immune cells, such as Natural Killer (NK) cells, are now believed to play a role in preventing tumor growth and resisting the metastatic spread of tumors. Monoclonal antibodies are proving to be important in tumor therapy, because they provide a degree of specificity not previously possible with conventional antibodies. They are also being used to classify tumor cells, tissue biopsies, and body fluids, as well as to isolate and characterize various tumor markers that identify the tumors or cancers.

Cancer is only one area that may benefit from the recent major developments in immunology. Researchers are beginning to understand the way in which the body defends itself from its own cells (autoimmune disease), to make the immune system tolerant to certain foreign tissues, and to turn off or regulate inflammatory responses in the body. Many of the cytokines from immune cells, such as T cells, are quite important in causing inflammation throughout various tissues of the body. For example, marked increases in one of the cytokines, interleukin-2 (IL-2), have been noted in patients with autoimmune diseases, whereas a decreased amount of the cytokine has been found in certain immune deficiency diseases. Since a sharp increase in the receptors for these interleukins, such as the IL-2 receptor, characterize many inflammatory diseases, including autoimmune conditions, certain infections, parasitic diseases, malignancies, multiple sclerosis, and related disorders, it is now possible to test for these substances for diagnostic purposes.

Another promising area is the prospect of toxin-interleukin therapy. In this procedure, the toxin is bound to the IL-2 or IL-2 receptor, and the fusion protein is taken into the cancer cell, causing it to die. These immunotoxins may offer new therapeutic perspectives for treatment of certain forms of cancer and autoimmune diseases. In general, they consist of a wide range of growth factors, antibodies, and hormones that are coupled to these toxins. The toxins themselves are usually of bacterial or plant origin and are specifically designed to target selected cancer cells, cells infected by a virus, or other abnormal cells. These and other experimental forms of therapy on the frontiers of medical research may well revolutionize medical treatment.[52]

As with cancer, most of the gains in the fight against cardiovascular diseases have come since World War II. It was not until then that the electrocardiograph, invented early in the century, came into common use as a diagnostic tool. Close cooperation between cardiologists and surgeons combined with major advances in therapy and technology have been responsible for a vastly improved treatment for heart patients. Hypertension, a significant factor in cardiovascular disease, is now amenable to diuretics, beta blockers, and a host of new drugs. The same is true for arryhthmia, for which therapeutics are also available. The discovery of the role of cholesterol in atherosclerosis has led to the creation of medicines and diets designed to prevent or slow down the process. Equally important has been the recognition of life styles as a significant factor in cardiovascular problems. Health education about dangers such as smoking, obesity, and lack of exercise is beginning to contribute to the reduction of cardiovascular disease. One other important advance that has saved many lives is the growing use of cardiopulmonary resuscitation. By 1960 both electroshock and cardiac massage were available. Surgery and technology also have been responsible for much of the improvement in cardiovascular treatment.

One of the most notable developments in the twentieth century has been the way in which the United States has forged to leadership in the biological sciences. No Americans were represented among Nobel Prize winners in fields of physiology or medicine from 1901 until Karl Landsteiner, a naturalized citizen, won the award in 1930. From 1930 to 1960 Americans either won or shared no less than seventeen of the annual prizes. During the period from 1960 to 1990, Americans were listed among the winners on twenty-four occasions. Clearly the growing wealth of the United States contributed to the explosion of medical research, but large-scale philanthropy, a uniquely American trait, deserves part of the credit. The rise of medical centers in the early twentieth century was to a considerable degree the result of funds provided by foundations and individual philanthropists. These same sources also poured money into state and private universities, and in the process encouraged state and local governments to support research institutions. The successes achieved in medicine by World War II led to massive federal grants, and in the last forty years the federal government has been the single major source of research funding.

CHAPTER 16

Surgery and Medical Technology since World War I

SURGERY UNDERWENT a rapid transformation in the years from 1870 to 1920, but the pace of change slowed in the next twenty years, awaiting further developments in the ancillary sciences. Surgical training, as it had in the past, continued to emphasize knowledge of anatomy and surgical technique, and speed and dexterity were the qualities most admired. Some justification existed for this since even in the 1920s and 1930s operating rapidly was still a necessity. Without blood banks, anticoagulants, and effective means for controlling infection, lengthy operations presented serious risks. By this date surgery was established as a specialty, but many surgeons were simply general practitioners with some manual dexterity and a flair for surgery.

The number of half-trained surgeons was increased by medical schools offering graduate courses in surgery for general practitioners, most of whom proceeded to perform surgery despite their lack of hospital residency training. Since surgery was one of the more lucrative branches of medicine, the situation encouraged general practitioners with limited surgical skills and comparable moral scruples to venture into the field. Some interesting questions arise in connection with medical schools' offering graduate work in surgery. Were they making the best of a bad situation by giving some training to physicians already engaged in surgery or were they encouraging practitioners with limited surgical training to operate? Whatever the case, many skilled surgeons with intellectual curiosity were gradually expanding surgical knowledge and techniques. Unfortunately, with a few exceptions, they viewed their field narrowly, and it was not until after World War II that surgeons became fully aware of studies in related fields and began to participate actively in medical research.[1]

Despite this discouraging picture, individual surgeons were attempting to raise standards, and some progress was made in the pre–World War I years. As noted in chapter 13, the American College of Surgeons (ACS) had been founded in 1913. It had sought to draw as many surgeons into its ranks as possible, and in consequence its qualifications for membership were relatively low. Candidates were required to have had a one-year internship, two years' experience as a surgical assistant, a minimum of seven years' experience in which they devoted more than half of their practice to surgery, and were to submit a hundred case records. The major weakness of these requirements was that they emphasized surgical technique and showed "only token concern for the basic medical knowledge supporting . . . surgical judgment."[2] The significance of the American College of Surgeons transcends its contribution to raising surgical standards, since it established the precedent that qualifications for medical specialties should be determined by the profession rather than the state.[3] The college, however, was basically a professional society, and it remained for the specialty boards that were established beginning in the 1930s to set the standards for cognitive ability and clinical competence.

Despite attacks by state medical societies and a lack of support from the AMA and the American Surgical Association, the College of Surgeons grew rapidly, reaching a membership of seven thousand by 1924. As it did so, academic surgeons and members of the older medical societies began criticizing its low admission standards. Reflecting this growing sentiment, Dr. J. M. T. Finney of the American Surgical Association in his 1924 presidential address urged that the various surgical societies cooperate in promoting better surgical training and in certifying qualified surgeons. The most outspoken critic of the profession was Dr. Evarts A. Graham of Washington University. In an address delivered before the Southern Medical Association in 1924 he decried the emphasis on operative technique, and sharply criticized fee splitting and the inclination of certain surgeons to operate for financial reasons. He also insisted that surgeons should have both a broad medical background and some research experience.

In 1932 Graham began a movement to reform the College of Surgeons and to bring academic surgeons into its fold. He also sought the help of the American Surgical Association in raising certification standards for surgeons. The task was far from easy; old enmities and the opposition of conservatives to change hindered the movement, but Graham and his associates persevered. By 1935 they were able to bring together representatives of the ASA, the ACS, and the Surgical Section of the AMA to design an independent certification board. After considerable — and often acrimonious — debate, the American Board of Surgery was created. The board was to consist of three representatives from each of the national organizations, the ASA, the ACS, and the AMA, and one member from each of the four regional surgical associations. Aside from a number of senior surgeons blanketed into membership, candidates for certification were required to have had three years of training beyond an internship and either two years of experience or two more years of additional training. Among the other requirements was a written and oral, or practical, examination. The first meeting of the board was held in January 1937. Within a short period the American Board of Surgery became a major force in shaping surgical education and in setting standards for hospital staffs.[4]

While surgical societies were seeking to raise professional standards, developments in the ancillary medical sciences were preparing the way for further advances in the field of surgery. Before longer and more complicated operative procedures could be attempted, some means had to be devised to compensate for the patient's loss of blood, and more effective ways had to be found to combat infection. Limited successes had been achieved with person-to-person blood transfusions, but the availability of a ready source of blood required finding a way to preserve it. The first step in this direction came during World War I when it was discovered that the addition of sugars extended the useful life of blood. In the 1920s refrigeration proved an effective method of preserving blood, and, as this and other preservation techniques gradually improved, in 1937 the first blood bank in the United States was established in Chicago's Cook County Hospital.[5]

An equally important step toward making blood transfusions feasible was the development of anticoagulants. The work of W. H. Howell, Jay McLean, and their associates on isolating the clotting factor in blood was noted in chapter 13. In 1922 Howell and Emmett L. Holt, a distinguished pediatrician and public health leader, succeeded in producing heparin, the first of the anticoagulants.[6] In the succeeding years more and better anticoagulants and transfusion techniques were developed, and, stimulated by the casualties during World War II, blood transfusions became a standard procedure.

Meanwhile the appearance of still another specialty area, anesthesiology, was facilitating the work of the surgeon. Most of the advances in anesthesia in the early years of the century were made by Europeans, but Americans, particularly those working in the basic sciences, shared in the research. Intravenous anesthesia had been tried earlier, but it was not until the introduction of barbiturates in 1903 that it came into more general use. The early twentieth century also saw researchers from other fields beginning to study the physiology of anesthesia and the body's reaction to the various anesthetic agents. As the number of barbiturates and other anesthetic drugs multiplied, experimental work soon demonstrated that the use of multiple agents could provide safer and more effective anesthesia. At the same time continuous improvements were made in the types of apparatus required for administering anesthetics. One of the more significant advances in anesthesia was the discovery of the value of curare as a muscular relaxant. It came to the attention of scientists at the Squibb Institute for Medical Research in the late 1930s, and after several years of research they produced a curare extract suitable for anesthetic purposes. Although curare has since been supplanted by better drugs, it served to introduce muscular relaxants to the field of anesthesia.

As the knowledge and skills required for administering anesthesia increased, a few physicians began to specialize in the area. As early as 1912 the American Association of Anesthetists was organized, and by 1914 a *Quarterly Supplement of Anesthesia and Analgesia* was added to the *American Journal of Surgery*. The first endowed chair of anesthesia was established at Harvard in 1917, although, reflecting the state of anesthesiology, it was not filled until 1936. Despite the multiplication of anesthetic agents and the ever-widening field of knowledge relating to anesthesia, it did not achieve recognition as a specialty until the post–World War II period.[7]

The 1930s witnessed three developments that were of both immediate and far-reaching significance to surgery: blood transfusions become more available; improvements were made in anesthesiology; and the appearance of the sulfa drugs sharply reduced the danger of infection in cases of trauma or during surgical procedures. These developments proved of immense benefit to America during World War II, but more than that, they helped lay the basis for a second surgical revolution in the postwar years.

The emergence of surgeons as specialists had aroused the opposition of general practitioners, and in turn the rise of specialties in surgery encountered opposition from general surgeons. The leading American neurosurgeon for the first thirty years of the twentieth century was Harvey W. Cushing of Johns Hopkins and Harvard, who is generally credited with making brain surgery a specialty and originating many of its techniques and procedures. In 1918, when Cushing and Walter E. Dandy, his former student and assistant, had already done much of the pioneering work in brain surgery, Dr. Arthur D. Bevan, speaking before the American Surgical Association, denounced specialism in general and declared: "There is no such thing in existence today as a specialty of brain surgery."[8]

Neither Bevan nor anyone else could hold back the tide of specialism, and today general surgeons are finding their field of work steadily narrowing. Cushing was both an imaginative surgeon and an outstanding teacher. His former student Walter Dandy contributed much to neurosurgery, including devising a method for localizing brain tumors by means of air contrast ventriculography, a major advance in the field. In the late 1940s George Moore of the University of Minnesota provided a more precise method for identifying and locating brain tumors by using radioactive iodine in connection with cerebral X-rays. In recent years advanced scanning techniques have facilitated the surgical treatment of brain tumors. In part arising from the many spinal injuries in World War II, neurosurgeons have since been successful in dealing with tumors, ruptured or prolapsed disks, and other problems involving the spinal column.

Ophthalmology, the oldest specialty, has made its greatest strides in the past twenty years. Couching for cataract dates at least as far back as 500 B.C., but it has been only in recent times that implants of synthetic lenses have restored vision to thousands of the elderly. An equally significant advance in ophthalmology has been the use of laser surgery to treat retinal and other eye defects. The newly developed microsurgery also holds the possibility of the surgical correction of myopia and other vision problems.

Urology became a medical specialty largely as a result of the cystoscope, a European device invented in the early 1800s and made more effective late in the century by combining it with an electric light. Prostatic surgery, however, remained in the hands of the general surgeons until American surgeons in the twentieth century developed the transurethral method for treating enlargement of the prostate. In 1913 Hugh Young reported treating an enlarged prostate by means of a punch operation using a lighted cystoscope. In the succeeding years other American urologists simplified the procedure by improving the cystoscope so that the surgeon could see the entire field of operation. By 1920 electric cautery replaced the knife, and in 1928 M. Stern further improved the cystoscope and used a wire-loop electrode to excise the tissue. Other improvements followed, and by the time of World War II transurethral prostatectomy became the standard method of treatment.[9] These technological improvements also established urology as a surgical specialty.

Probably no aspect of surgery demonstrates the drastic changes in surgery since the 1870s so well as that pertaining to the abdominal cavity. In 1886, following a long discussion in the annual meeting of the American Surgical Association, the participants agreed that an exploratory laparotomy was necessary in cases of perforating wounds of the abdomen. Twenty years later Albert Vander Veer, then president of the association, declared that before this time such an operation was "believed too hazardous, and in fact, impossible."[10] Despite considerable advances by the time of World War I, the danger from shock, blood loss, and infection continued to make abdominal surgery risky. In the early years of World War I conservative treatment for abdominal wounds, involving rest, morphine, and the withholding of food, was the standard treatment. The result was a tragically high mortality rate of 94 percent for intestinal wounds. As the war progressed, it became evident that operating as soon as possible reduced the mortality rate by more than half.

The development of the endoscope, one of the more significant advances in the medical field of gastroenterology in the twentieth century, has proved a boon to surgery. The basic principle of the endoscope originated late in the nineteenth century when Chevalier Jackson of Philadelphia solved the problem of removing foreign bodies from the lungs and air passages without surgical intervention by means of a tube known as a bronchoscope. The next step was the development of the endoscope, a lighted flexible tube, which, by permitting an examination of the gastrointestinal tract, eliminated a good part of exploratory surgery. The addition of fiberoptics to endoscopes now provides the gastroenterologist with a clear view of the insides of the GI tract and the peritoneum. In more recent years the laparoscope evolved from the endoscope, permitting abdominal surgery with a minimum of trauma. The past seventy years have seen steady improvements in the surgical handling of gallstones, ulcers, diverticulosis of the colon, cancer, and other types of abdominal problems. In addition, many new methods have been devised for diagnosing and treating gastrointestinal problems. One example of this is percutaneous catheterization of the pancreas and gallbladder ducts; another is gallstone "lithotripsy," a means by which gallstones are disrupted sonically. Fortunately, the use of greatly improved drugs for treating infections, hyperacidity, and metabolic and autoimmune disorders has reduced the need for many former surgical procedures, and the quickening pace of discoveries in all areas of medicine encourages hopes for still further reductions.[11]

At the 1909 meeting of the American Surgical Association ten papers were presented on thoracic surgery, marking the beginnings of what would become a new specialty.[12] Among the early American pioneers in these years were Rudolph Matas, whose work has already been noted, John B. Murphy of Chicago, and Charles E. Eisberg of New York, all of whom contributed to solving the problem of maintaining respiration while the chest was open. General surgeons performed most thoracic operations for the first four decades of the century, although increasingly individual surgeons began to specialize in chest surgery. Tuberculosis was the major cause for surgical intervention, although occasional operations were performed for bronchiectasis, chronic infections, and cancer. In the 1920s artificial pneumothorax, a method of collapsing a tubercular lung in order to give it rest, was used extensively. It was supplanted in the 1930s by thoracoplasty, an operation allowing the lung to rest by collapsing the chest wall. The 1940s saw the increasing use of pulmonary resection, made possible in part by the introduction of more effective drugs for controlling tuberculosis and other infections.[13]

In the past fifty years antibiotics have largely eliminated bronchiectasis, pulmonary tuberculosis, and other pneumonic infections. However, the appearance of lung cancer in the 1930s and its explosive rise in the following years, along with the emergence of cardiac surgery, have created an even greater need for thoracic surgeons. It was these developments that were largely responsible for making thoracic surgery a specialty in 1947. By that date cardiovascular surgery was well on its way to be coming a specialty of its own.

Alexis Carrel, a brilliant French scientist who came to the United States early in his career, in the years between 1902 and 1912 anticipated developments in cardiovascular surgery and organ transplantation by over fifty years. Experimenting on dogs, he and his associate, Charles C. Guthrie, performed a series of successful operations on the aorta and heart, discovered a method for successful vascular anastomosis, and then turned to the study of organ transplantation. Dr. Richard H. Meade in his excellent history of surgery states that had Carrel "not become interested in organ transplantation and philosophy, it seems likely that surgery of the heart and aorta would have reached its present state many years earlier." [14] Unfortunately, Carrel's early work received scant attention until the post–World War II era.

Before World War II, heart wounds were treated conservatively and the case mortality rate was high. During the war, Dr. Dwight E. Harkin, faced with seemingly fatally wounded soldiers, began removing fragments of bullets and shrapnel from the heart. By so doing he greatly increased the recovery rate and at the same time he and other army surgeons gained valuable experience. Shortly after the war several American surgeons began attempting to operate on the mitral valve. In 1948, using the knowledge and skills required for cardiac surgery that they and others had acquired during the war years, Charles Bailey of Philadelphia and Dwight Harkin almost simultaneously performed successful operations to open the mitral valve. In short order knowledge of the operation spread widely, making it possible for the first time to treat mitral stenosis. In the meantime, Alfred Blalock and Helen B. Taussig of Johns Hopkins in 1945 had devised a bypass operation for blue babies in which the subclavian artery was anastomosed to the pulmonary to increase the oxygenation of the blood. [15]

A medical development in the 1940s that helped clear the way for cardiac surgery was the introduction of the cardiac catheter, a major diagnostic instrument. In more recent years cardiac diagnosis has been facilitated by the use of ultrasound (echocardiography) and by various scanning methods. By the outbreak of the Korean War in 1950, which itself gave further stimulus to cardiovascular surgery, intracardiac surgery was already established. Despite this, heart surgery could make only limited progress until some type of circulatory support system was devised. A number of researchers had been working on the problem, one of whom, John H. Gibbon, Jr., of Jefferson Medical College, had spent almost twenty years on the task. His efforts were rewarded in 1953 when his heart-lung machine made it possible to inaugurate open heart surgery on humans. Within two years it had become practical to stop the patient's heart for repair purposes. In this connection the work of Bernard Lown, who solved the problem of "defibrillating the heart" with an electric jolt of a refined impulse curve, should be mentioned. Today, with Lown's machine paramedics do a closed-chest resuscitation routinely outside of the hospital. By the 1960s new, improved devices for maintaining blood circulation and better anesthetic procedures were facilitating the work of the cardiac surgeons. Today various enzymes and anticlotting compounds can dissolve blood vessels' clots and eliminate the need for surgery or else simplify the work of the surgeon.[16]

Meanwhile cardiovascular surgery was rapidly forging ahead. In the late 1950s the number of papers relating to the subject at the annual meeting of the American Surgical Association increased rapidly as Michael E. DeBakey of Houston, Denton A. Cooley, and others began reporting the results of their new techniques and procedures. Among the successes in vascular surgery were the new methods first used in the 1950s to deal with aortic aneurysms, and the introduction of dacron grafts in 1964 by Michael DeBakey and his associates in Houston. This same year saw the next major development in cardiac surgery, the coronary bypass, an operation in which sections of the patient's veins or arteries from elsewhere in the body are used to circumvent a blockage in one or more of the coronary arteries.[17] By the 1960s surgeons were successfully treating a number of genetic and valvular heart problems. The steady growth of vascular surgery, along with comparable developments in other medical areas, set the stage for two further advances in cardiac repair, organ transplants, and the reattachment of limbs and other parts of the body.

Before successful transplants could be performed, two basic problems had to be solved. First, an effective method of anastomosing or joining the blood vessels had to be devised, and second, some means for preventing the immune system from rejecting the foreign tissue had to be found. Early in the century Alexis Carrel and Charles C. Guthrie had made considerable progress in solving these problems, but, aside from Carrel's discovery in the 1930s of how to maintain organs *in vitro*, little further was done. It was not until major progress had been made in immunology and genetics that the problem of tissue rejection could be solved. Peter B. Medawar, elaborating on the work of Sir MacFarlane Burnet, in the 1940s demonstrated his theory of actively acquired immunity against grafted tissue, i.e., that the body literally strengthens its defenses against foreign tissue, resulting in a quicker rejection of a second transplant. The discovery in 1951 that cortisone suppressed the immune system and its resistance to foreign tissue marked the beginning of drug-induced immunological tolerance.[18]

Although kidney and other organ transplants had been performed on animals earlier, the first successful kidney transplant in humans was performed in 1954 by Joseph E. Murray of Boston, who first solved the problem of organ rejection. In this instance, he transplanted a kidney from one identical twin to another. The early transplants were made only between identical twins, but, as more effective immunosuppressive therapy became available and surgical technique improved, by 1962 surgical teams in Boston and other cities were turning kidney transplants into a routine procedure.[19] Shortly after Murray's kidney transplant, another Boston scientist investigating the immune system, E. Donnel Thomas, in 1956 successfully performed the first bone marrow transplant. This procedure is now the standard treatment for most forms of leukemia and certain types of cancer. It also holds promise for treating a wide range of other disorders. Murray and Thomas were awarded the Nobel Prize in medicine in 1990 for their contributions. By the early 1960s accumulated knowledge in the fields of surgery, genetics, immunology, physiology, and other areas made it possible to attempt the transplantation of other organs. In 1963, after extensive testing with animals, human transplants of both liver and lungs were performed. Although the early patients survived only briefly, in the succeeding years further improvements in surgical technique, immunosuppressive therapy, and control of infection steadily yielded better results.

The next logical step was the transplantation of human hearts. The way had been well prepared by the emergence of intracardiac surgery, and in 1964 it was planned to transplant the heart of a dying patient into another patient suffering from terminal cardiac disease. When the prospective human donor remained alive and the intended heart recipient went into shock, the heart of a chimpanzee was substituted. The cardiac patient lived only briefly, but the operation demonstrated that heart transplantation was feasible. Three years later, in 1967 the first human heart was transplanted. As was the case with other organ transplants, the survival rate of the early heart-transplant patients was low, but, as cardiac surgeons gained more experience, heart transplants changed from surgical experiments to complicated but feasible surgical procedures.[20] The introduction of cyclosporin, which has reduced the chances of both rejection and infection, has turned heart transplants into a routine operation. Today in over half the states Medicare pays for heart transplants, and the major problem, as with other organs, is a shortage of donor hearts. It should be mentioned that cyclosporin is not the perfect answer. The problem of eventual kidney failure secondary to the drug has not been solved, and there is the usual increased risk of infections with any immunosuppressive agent. Currently an anti-T cell serum (anti-"CD3," a monoclonal antibody) is used to inhibit the rejection of grafts.

The continuing progress in the treatment of coronary heart problems is shown by the appearance in recent years of less traumatic methods than the cardiac bypass for dealing with blocked arteries. Angioplasty, a method for opening arteries by means of inflating a minute balloon, is quite successful in many cases. Two experimental techniques presently undergoing evaluation are the use of a rotating, cylinder-shaped blade to shave away deposits in the arteries and the use of laser beams to literally burn away the fatty deposits. Along with these technological devices, the introduction of the heart pacemaker has added years of quality life for patients suffering from various forms of arrythmia. Gradual improvements in the design of pacemakers and their batteries now enable these implantable devices to provide many years of service.

It is clear from the foregoing that technology, which has contributed to the world's productive capacity, has also helped to shape medicine. Its first medical application was in the diagnostic area. During the nineteenth century the stethoscope, the ophthalmoscope, and the sphygmomanometer were introduced, and in 1901 the electrocardiograph came on the scene. The first laboratories to start diagnostic tests for infectious diseases were established in the 1890s. It was in this decade, too, that laboratories started producing vaccines and actively engaged in medical research. By the early twentieth century, clinical laboratories had became an integral part of hospitals, and private clinical laboratories were multiplying. As early as 1944 a physician complained of what he termed "the present-day tendency towards a five-minute history followed by a five-day barrage of special tests in the hope that the diagnostic rabbit may suddenly emerge from the laboratory hat." Starting in the midcentury, the number of laboratory tests began accelerating. For example, the Yale–New Haven Hospital performed 48,000 laboratory procedures in 1954; by 1964, despite only a slight increase in the patient census, the number of tests rose to 200,000.[21]

The 1970s saw an ever-greater increase in laboratory work. Public faith in science and technology and the introduction of automated laboratory analysis, along with a rising number of malpractice suits, encouraged physicians to order more and more tests. It was in these years that the term "defensive medicine" was coined as the medical profession sought to defend itself from unjustified malpractice suits and huge awards by jurors to whom insurance companies were vague abstractions. Standardized and speedier laboratory tests and such devices as photofluoroscopy also made possible multiphasic screening in the late 1940s, a method by which large numbers of ostensibly healthy people were given a barrage of tests.

By the 1960s the computer had added a new dimension to the mechanization of medicine. Its most obvious use was in medical research and the collection of patient and hospital records, but it soon became clear that the computer had a useful function as a diagnostic tool. As biophysics became a significant area of medicine, it became possible to devise machines to monitor continuously the physiological changes taking place in the patient. The problem of watching and evaluating the results of these continuous physiological observations was solved by combining these devices with computers that could record, evaluate, and make the results readily available. Subsequently, computers were programmed to sound an alarm in case of any significant physiological changes. In the past thirty years the computer has become omnipresent in medicine, particularly in combination with X-ray machines such as the Computer Tomography Scanner (CT scanner).

Technology has also made possible the miniaturization of surgical instruments and the emergence of microsurgery. In the past forty years microsurgery has had a profound effect on many areas of surgery. As early as the 1920s Swedish audiologists began using microscopes to help in correcting ear defects, and in the 1940s ophthalmologists, as noted earlier, began using microscopes for delicate work on the eyes. By the 1950s the need for connecting minute blood vessels led to the increasing use of microscopes in a number of fields. In addition to specially designed microscopes, microsurgery required a host of miniature instruments and new operating techniques. Aided by advances in microsurgery, in 1962 Dr. Ronald A. Malt in Massachusetts General Hospital performed the world's first successful limb attachment, one involving a boy whose arm had been ripped off while he was attempting to jump a freight train. In the succeeding years steady improvements in medical instruments and surgical techniques meant that by the 1980s a high degree of success was being achieved in reattaching various parts of the body and in transferring skin and other tissues from one section of the body to another. By this time, too, Johns Hopkins and other schools were offering courses in microsurgery.[22]

As might be expected, nephrology and neurosurgery have greatly benefited from microsurgery, since it has facilitated the difficult tasks of repairing kidneys and reconnecting nerves. Microsurgery has been particularly effective in dealing with vascular problems and tumors affecting the brain. The carotid bypass, a means for improving blood flow to the brain, owes its existence to this new method of surgery, and it has been particularly effective in dealing with cranial aneurysms and tumors. Aside from its other advantages, microsurgery, in conjunction with such devices as the laparascope, has created what has been termed "noninvasive surgery." This type of surgery is probably best known for its association with sports medicine, since the phrase "arthroscopic surgery" has become common on the sports pages. A flexible viewing instrument called an arthroscope is inserted through a small opening and in conjunction with other flexible devices can excise or cauterize tissue with a minimum of trauma. Many orthopedic procedures that formerly required a major surgical invasion and lengthy hospitalization can now be done with a minimum of trauma and a relatively short recovery time.

Noninvasive surgery has also led to major advances insofar as surgery on women is concerned. It has drastically reduced the discomfort and extent of hospitalization required for correcting blocked fallopian tubes and the excision of tubal pregnancies. Menorrhagia, which in some cases required a hysterectomy, can now be treated on an outpatient basic by cauterizing the uterus with a laser beam. In the area of obstetrics electronic fetal monitoring has enabled many women to bring a healthy child to term, and amniocentesis, along with other methods for examining the fetus in utero, provides considerable information on the health of the fetus. Thus, microsurgery has led to new surgical procedures and greatly reduced the trauma attendant to many of the more traditional ones.

Another significant technological development is the growing use of ultrasound waves for diagnostic purposes and as a substitute for invasive surgery. For centuries physicians have sought a lithotriptic, a drug or other method for pulverizing urinary calculi (bladder stones). In 1739, when the grim operation known as lithotomy was the only cure for this fairly common disorder, the English Parliament awarded five thousand pounds to Joanna Stephens for discovering a medicine for "the Cure of the Stone."[23] It scarcely need be said that the money was wasted. Fortunately, antibiotics and other forms of treatment have greatly reduced the occurrence of this once common disorder, but the problem of calculi formed in the kidneys, urinary tract, and gallbladder still remains. Using sound waves, it is possible in certain cases to pulverize these calculi to facilitate their washing away. Although still in an early stage of development, this new form of noninvasive treatment may prove a significant addition to medicine.

The laser beam, mentioned earlier, has already contributed notably to surgery and appears on the threshold of becoming a major surgical tool. It has helped microsurgery by providing the surgeon with a clear field of vision through its ability to seal extremely small blood and lymph vessels and has proved equally valuable in dealing with minute tumors and aneurysms. Not only microsurgery, but virtually all fields of surgery have been affected by laser. Aside from its well-known use in correcting a wide range of eye and ear problems, obliterating tumors, and sealing blood vessels, laser is now used in such operations as laparoscopic cholecystectomies, a procedure in which diseased gallbladders can be detached from the body by lasers and removed through a small incision. A laser method for clearing blocked blood vessels has already been tested on the legs and holds promise for opening blocked coronary arteries.

One of the more radical changes brought about by medical technology occurred with the introduction of kidney dialysis. The small number and high cost of artificial kidney machines at first limited the extent of dialysis, forcing arbitrary choices as to which patients should benefit from it. Aware of this problem, in 1973 Congress voted to extend Medicare to cover nearly all patients suffering from severe chronic kidney disease. At that time the annual cost was estimated at between $200,000,000 and $250,000,000. By 1981 the cost was well over one billion dollars, and by 1990 it was in excess of three billion. The only alternative to dialysis is kidney transplantation, an expensive procedure in itself, but the number of available donors is far below the demand.

During the past few years, a series of studies has shown that from 20 to 40 percent of dialysis patients are severely debilitated. In view of the rapidly rising cost of dialysis, the question has been raised as to whether all patients, regardless of their general health, should be placed on dialysis. Britain and other countries with national health insurance systems limit the use of dialysis, basing it upon the age and condition of the patient.[24] So far, Americans have been reluctant to face up to the realities of medical economics.

For centuries physicians have sutured open wounds, a tedious procedure. In the late 1960s an American surgical company began marketing a surgical staple gun. The stapling technique was slow to win adherents until studies in the 1980s showed that the higher cost of staple over sutures was more than compensated by the patients' reduced recovery time. In the medical area the development of miniature implantable pumps placed under the skin is another promising development. They can be used to allow cancer victims to control their painkillers or to administer drugs directly to the cancer site. These pumps also hold promise as an effective method for delivering insulin to diabetics, and conceivably may be useful for other medical problems.[25]

Medical technology usually conveys the impression of X-rays, radiation, computers, and electronics, yet many technical fields, such as engineering, metallurgy, and plastics, have made significant direct contributions to orthopedics and other surgical areas. Metallic rods and plates to support or replace damaged bones, artificial hip joints, and a wide variety of prosthetic devices illustrate the benefits derived from cooperation between clinicians and researchers in nonmedical fields. Computers, sensing devices, lightweight metals and plastics, and other technological developments have made possible the creation of prosthetic devices that provide a large measure of mobility and freedom of action for the disabled.

Among the newer and more esoteric technologies are nuclear magnetic resonance (NMR), which presents a more detailed and refined picture than the CT scan, and a somewhat experimental procedure, position emission tomography (PET). The latter is a method of quantitative imaging of regional function and chemical reactions in various organs of the body. It has great potential, since it is the only technique capable of giving quantitative information about biochemical and physiologic processes. A machine of enormous importance, the fluorescence activated cell sorter (FACS), has revolutionized the counting of blood and other cells when they are first labeled with a monoclonal antibody. As a diagnostic tool it has a wide range of use against disorders such as cancer, leukemias, and immune deficiency diseases. The treatment of localized tumors such as melanomas has benefited from newer "perfusion" and "filtration" techniques, for which some of the pioneering work was done by Dr. Edward Krementz of Tulane University.

The heart-lung machine itself is a tribute to technology, but in the invention of the artificial heart, technology may have overreached itself. Large amounts of money and research time have been poured into a project of benefit for relatively few patients. At present the mechanical heart's chief value is to enable a severely ill heart patient to survive while awaiting a donor heart. The small number of patients helped by a permanently installed artificial heart and the quality of life of patients who received them have led the Food and Drug Administration to remove artificial hearts from its list of approved devices.[26] It is likely that eventually an artificial heart small enough to permit the recipient to live a relatively normal life may be available. This possibility leads one to speculate whether or not some limitations should be placed on replacement parts for the human body.

Innovations of any kind invariably find detractors, and it is not surprising that a considerable literature has appeared on medical technology in recent years, much of which expresses serious reservations. Critics have charged that certain diagnostic machines are extremely costly and provide insufficient additional diagnostic information to justify their high cost. Moreover, these elaborate machines often become prestige items, leading to excessive duplication as hospitals acquire them whether or not the patient census justifies the outlay. Having bought them, medical institutions are inclined to encourage needless use of the machines and to charge high fees in order to amortize their cost.

The Computer Tomography Scanners developed by the British in the 1970s, which require a special operating staff, illustrate one of the economic objections to new technological devices. Since the CT scanners were a prestige item, many hospitals rushed to buy them. By 1978 Great Britain had 52 scanners while the United States had 1,254. In the preceding year a health research group sponsored by Blue Cross argued that the approximately 1,000 CT scanners installed or on order in the United States far exceeded the need for such sophisticated machinery, and that in consequence thousands of unnecessary expensive scans would be performed.[27] The report was probably correct, although the CT scanners have since proved to be a valuable addition to medicine.

A valid criticism of the rapid growth of medical technology is that the very flood of new technologies and the refinement of existing ones makes it almost impossible to evaluate them medically or to test them by cost analysis. In consequence the use of a particular medical technology is too frequently determined not by a rational health policy but by "the aggregate decisions made by individual doctors about single patients day by day." Since technology can be quite profitable, corporate hospitals have been accused of promoting its use. And since physicians are often investors in medical technology and laboratories, they too are inclined to emphasize the profitability of a technological procedure rather than its medical value. The same factor enters into the use of the computers. While computer software is invaluable for medical purposes, it can be and is being used to maximize hospital and physician income. In these days of third-party payment, a slight variation in, or an alteration in the sequence of, diagnosis can bring in thousands of extra dollars.[28]

Another justifiable criticism of an excessive reliance on technology is that it can lead to an impersonalization of medicine by encouraging too great a dependence on tests, and a deemphasis of the patient's medical history. Moreover, medical devices are only as effective as the technicians and professionals who operate them and evaluate the results. The machines, too, are far from infallible, and it takes only a slight variation in calibration to provide inaccurate results. While the Food and Drug Administration was given authority in 1976 to determine the safety and efficacy of medical devices before their release, periodic inspection of them is performed largely by state and local health offices, and the quality of inspection varies widely. Somewhat belatedly, in 1988 Congress instructed the Department of Health and Human Services to establish quality standards and personnel requirements for the operation of the approximately 200,000 medical laboratories. But it was not until 1992 that the department issued final regulations requiring biannual federal inspection of laboratories performing moderate to highly complex medical tests.[29] Whether the department, in these days of financial stringency, has adequate funds and the staff to enforce the regulations remains to be seen. Finally, no machine can take into account the wide range of intangible human factors that the physician becomes aware of by thoroughly questioning and observing the patient.

Some thirty-five years ago Jurgen Thorwald published a history covering the period from 1846 to 1956 entitled *The Century of the Surgeon*. Two factors provided a measure of justification for Thorwald's title. First, from the patients' standpoint surgery did and can achieve immediate and dramatic successes, and second the one hundred years following the introduction of anesthesia did witness many remarkable surgical advances. In the past forty years, however, the biological sciences have surged ahead and profoundly affected all areas of clinical medicine, and surgery must share the limelight with medicine. While antibiotics and other drugs have drastically reduced the number of many former common operations such as those for tonsillitis and mastoiditis, and thoracic surgery for pulmonary tuberculosis is rare, surgeons have opened a wide range of new procedures and simplified traditional operations. Microsurgery and noninvasive techniques have already made great strides, and, along with other advances, hold great promise for the future.

A review of the surgery conducted during the past 150 years reveals that the first major advance resulted from the introduction of anesthesia followed by antiseptic and then aseptic procedures. With quiescent patients and the possibility of infection greatly reduced, it was possible by the end of the nineteenth century for surgeons to invade all areas of the body. In the first half of the twentieth century, the increasing use of blood transfusions and significant improvements in anesthesia, largely due to a better understanding of hematology and respiratory physiology, led to even more complicated surgical procedures. The introduction of sulfa drugs and antibiotics in the World War II era further reduced the danger of postoperative infections. The midcentury saw the introduction of the heart-lung machine, which opened the way for heart surgery, and the emergence of immunology, which paved the way for transplants. The last major advance in surgery owes much to technology, the use of fiber-optic devices to view all parts of the body, and minute surgical tools and laser beams to correct defects. Along with the latter have come a variety of imaging devices that have eliminated the need for many exploratory procedures. In the late nineteenth century, surgeons were reluctant to open the abdomen and considered the thoracic cavity sacrosanct. One hundred years later medical technology is enabling us to perform many surgical procedures within these areas with only minimum trauma.

Medical Education since the Flexner Report

BY THE EARLY 1920S the basic pattern of medical education was firmly established. Medical schools, if not integrated with, at least were affiliated with hospitals and universities, and minimal entrance standards had been established. Medical students were expected to have taken at least two years of premedical work at the undergraduate level, and their studies in medical school included two years of basic sciences and two years of clinical work, followed by a year of internship. In the succeeding years few major changes occurred in medical education except for those gradually brought about by the multiplication of specialty courses and the growing emphasis on medical research. With the increase in specialty courses came a corresponding increase in the number of required course hours. One unfortunate result was that as departments offered more and more courses and fought to obtain additional class time, the late nineteenth-century movement to create a profession well rounded in the humanities steadily lost ground. A few individual professors sought to keep the flame alight, but the advancing front of scientific medicine left neither classroom time nor funds for subjects such as history or ethics.

As indicated earlier, the internship was well established by the 1920s and became a standard part of medical education by the 1930s. At the same time, residency programs expanded and multiplied. Specialty training, however, took two main directions: one under the auspices of schools and universities and another in connection with hospitals having no medical school connections. This apparent divergence of training raised the question of regulating specialty training, but the issue was resolved by the emergence of specialty boards.[1] The snowballing of medical research raised yet another problem that had not beset earlier physicians—the need to keep abreast of new developments. In response medical schools began offering postgraduate education: short courses, clinics, and seminars designed to keep practicing physicians aware of the latest findings in their particular areas.

Among the improvements by the 1920s were the general acceptance of the clinical clerkship and an effort to introduce a preceptorial system. At Harvard, Stanford, Michigan, Wisconsin, and Vermont, third- and fourth-year students were required to work with clinical professors or general practitioners. Beginning in these years, however, the general practitioners who served as part-time faculty members were slowly replaced by specialized full-time medical researchers. In consequence, some of the benefits from preceptorial work were lost as the medical researcher, rather than the practitioner, became the role model for the students.[2]

A few sporadic attempts were also made to integrate preclinical and clinical work. Unfortunately the well-meaning attempt by state licensing boards and medical schools to standardize medical education by specifying detailed course requirements inhibited any significant reforms. Nonetheless, a number of modifications were made in the curriculum. In the basic sciences the general tendency was to move away from a clinical orientation toward a more purely scientific one, with instruction handled by Ph.D.'s. Medical chemistry was gradually taken over by biochemistry, and basic physiology was taught as a biological science with little reference to its clinical application. As teaching hours in basic physiology were reduced, new elective programs in physiology were introduced along with a number of interdisciplinary courses integrating physiology with the other basic sciences. Another area losing ground was gross anatomy. A study of 41 medical colleges in 1903 showed that on average, 549 hours were devoted to gross anatomy; by 1955 the number of teaching hours had declined to 330.[3]

Obstetrics and gynecology received scant attention in medical schools until the post–World War I years. Flexner's pronouncement that "the very worst showing is made in the matter of obstetrics," ensured that change would come. The leader in reforming the teaching of obstetrics and gynecology was John W. Williams of Johns Hopkins. Following the lead of the Flexner report, he surveyed departments of obstetrics in American medical schools and estimated that the average medical student witnessed only one live birth before graduation. He also discovered that over one-third of all professors of obstetrics had no specialty training. Williams advocated combining obstetrics and gynecology, and although he was not immediately successful in this, in 1919 he was instrumental in organizing America's first full-time obstetrics department at Johns Hopkins. He and his disciples were largely responsible for establishing obstetrics and gynecology as specialties and for raising the standards of teaching. As the field of obstetrics and gynecology broadened and subspecialties emerged, the question was raised as to precisely what aspects of the field should be taught to medical students and how much time should be devoted to it, an issue that is not unique to OB-GYN.[4]

Traditionally surgical training was provided by practicing on cadavers and by witnessing occasional operations from a distance in large surgical amphitheaters. Additional experience was gained by what was essentially an apprenticeship. The first major breakthrough in surgical training was initiated by William Halsted and Harvey Cushing at Johns Hopkins. Shortly after the turn of the century, Cushing introduced the use of dogs instead of cadavers in his surgery courses. Dog surgery, which required the use of anesthetics, surgical cleanliness, the prevention of hemorrhage, and all the other considerations incident to human surgery, quickly became the standard method for basic surgical training. As the nature of surgical work changed over the years and surgical subspecialties emerged, surgical training was acquired more and more at the postgraduate residency level. Here again the question has arisen as to the amount and nature of the surgical training required of undergraduate medical students. Since nearly all physicians have occasion to perform at least minor surgery and the licensure laws place no limitations upon the right to operate, a minimum of surgery must be taught at the undergraduate level. Moreover, it has been argued that basic surgical training helps to give students a fundamental understanding of the entire field of medicine.[5]

With a few exceptions, such as the program at Columbia's College of Physicians and Surgeons in the late 1920s, psychiatry and neurology received little attention in American medical schools until the 1930s, and it was not until the post–World War II years that full-time departments came into existence. The high percentage of military draftees rejected for reasons of mental health resulted in large-scale federal funding for both research and training in these areas. In consequence, by the 1960s some training in psychiatry and neurology became basic to undergraduate medical education. Materia medica, one of the original subjects taught in medical schools, in the years from 1920 to 1950 was transformed into pharmacology. This transformation was brought about in part through the impact of biochemistry and a host of radically new drugs. In the process pharmacology moved closer to the basic sciences, and in so doing drew more of its professors from the ranks of the Ph.D.'s. In recent years, as pharmacology has become more specialized, its undergraduate teaching has tended to be integrated with the basic sciences.[6]

Three areas of teaching—public health and preventive medicine, medical ethics, and medical history—have traditionally been stepchildren in medical schools. Public health, or hygiene as it was called, was the first to attract attention from medical educators. In the late nineteenth century the sanitary movement and the introduction of bacteriology stimulated medical professors to offer lectures and courses on hygiene. The subject, however, never became an integral part of medical education. An increasing demand for student time as a result of the multiplication of course work combined with the emphasis upon healing left little room for teaching public health or preventive medicine. In addition, the appearance of public health schools in the World War I era helped medical schools to justify relegating the subject to an inconsequential role. In 1946 a committee of the Association of American Medical Colleges defined public health as relating to community health and preventive medicine as the promotion of individual or family health. This definition left community health to the public health schools and preventive medicine to medical schools. Most students and faculty members in medical schools consider their roles to be those of healers rather than watchmen. Moreover, the definition of what constitutes promoting individual health is somewhat amorphous. In consequence, preventive medicine has only a small place in medical education.[7]

In the nineteenth century, medical history was considered a fundamental source of knowledge, and medical professors often urged their students to return to the original truths. As late as 1846 Dr. Samuel Cartwright of Mississippi advised southern physicians to study the works of Hippocrates, the fountainhead of knowledge.[8] Toward the end

of the century many educated physicians, acutely conscious of the ignorance of so many of their colleagues, advocated that medical schools
train humanistic physicians, individuals versed in the humanities and
the history of their profession. The movement regrettably conflicted
with the rise of "scientific" medicine, whose supporters rejected all past
knowledge as erroneous. Nonetheless, the number of history courses
and lectures slowly increased in the 1920s and 1930s, but they were
generally elective and taught by retired professors or individuals with
some particular interest in the subject. The establishment of the Johns
Hopkins Institute for the History of Medicine in 1929 marked the first
time a medical school employed a medical historian, and it was also the
first step toward developing trained medical historians. Since then, a
number of schools have added medical historians to their faculties, but
the subject is still viewed askance by most faculty members.

Medical ethics is another area that came belatedly to medical schools.
Courses in medical jurisprudence in the latter part of the nineteenth
century occasionally included some mention of ethics, but as late as
1910 not a single course on the subject was offered by medical schools.
The 1930s witnessed a much greater interest in the subject, although
ethics was often taught in conjunction with medical history, jurisprudence, and economics. As medical sociologists were added to the faculty
in a few schools in the 1950s and 1960s, the teaching of ethics was assumed to be in their domain. During these years interest in humanistic
medicine revived, and one result was the introduction of formal courses
in ethics. The revolutionary developments in medicine and changes in
society during the past thirty years have raised a great many ethical
problems, and the last twenty years have seen medical ethics assuming
a more significant place in the curriculum.[9]

While the curriculum was slowly undergoing changes, there was a
comparable shift in the status of the faculty from part-time to full-time.
This movement was initiated by Abraham Flexner and the Rockefeller
General Education Board, when the Rockefeller Foundation in 1913
gave one million dollars to enable Johns Hopkins to place the clinical
faculty on a full-time basis. Few schools could afford to pay the relatively large salaries necessary to keep the clinical faculty, and in the
1920s the geographic full-time system emerged. Under this method,
clinical professors were paid a base salary and were permitted to maintain a private practice. The usual practice was to allow them to keep a

certain percentage of their fees, the rest going to their respective departments. In some cases, to allay the dissatisfaction of the basic science faculty, these extra earnings reverted to the school.[10]

When the issue of full-time faculty came to the fore, the University of Michigan in 1920 sought to raise the necessary funds by establishing a university clinic in which the fees collected were assigned to the professors' departments. The preclinical faculty, however, objected to the relatively large salaries paid to the clinical faculty, and local practitioners were equally resentful of competition from the clinic. Consequently, the university was soon forced to revert to the geographic full-time system. Michigan's fault lay in attempting something ahead of its time. In the late 1960s and the 1970s, as federal money for medical schools began a relative decline in a time of soaring expenses, the concept of the university clinic was revived. These clinics today not only help to employ the majority of clinical faculty on a full-time basis but are contributing to easing general budgetary problems.[11]

By 1950, despite limited progress in curriculum reform, student complaints about the overcrowded curriculum, few electives, and little free time began to reverberate through faculty meetings. The first school to respond to these complaints was Western Reserve. In 1950 it received a five-year grant from the Commonwealth Fund to undertake a major revision of its curriculum. The chief objectives were to reduce the core courses, to integrate basic courses not only with each other but with clinical work, to allow more time for electives, and to give students a greater role in developing their programs.[12] In these years medical schools generally were engaged in a massive soul-searching, characterized by the use of outside consultants, study groups, faculty workshops, and curriculum committees. The nature of instructional problems does not permit permanent solutions, but some progress was made toward the major objectives.

Although World War II had little direct impact on medical education other than to speed up medical training, it brought a renewed interest in medical research, a development that was to have a profound effect on medical schools in the succeeding years. The wartime gains made by the National Research Defense Council and its successor, the Office of Scientific Research and Development, convinced Congress and the public that money spent for research was a sound investment. The development of atomic energy was the most striking success of government-sponsored research, but the appearance of a host of miracle drugs, led by the sulfa compounds, antibiotics, and synthetic antimalarials, encouraged the belief that with sufficient funds American medical scientists could create a brave new healthy world.

Enthusiasm for medical research in the postwar years led to a massive increase in government funding. Spending for medical research increased more than twentyfold between 1947 and 1966 with the federal government providing over two-thirds of the funds. While the National Institutes of Health and other agencies conducted a good part of the research, the tradition of research-oriented medical schools started by Johns Hopkins meant that university medical centers played a major role in the expanding research. They not only supplied most of the manpower, but with federal help they greatly enlarged their own facilities. The effect was to strengthen medical school faculties and to make possible a sharp increase in the number of medical graduates. In the fifteen years from 1951 to 1966 the annual number of medical degrees awarded rose by 25 per cent.[13]

Even though medical education was receiving indirect benefits from the funds voted for medical research, Congress, while willing to provide money for cancer or heart research, was reluctant to provide appropriations for the more prosaic task of medical education. Hence medical deans and administrators were compelled to shuffle research funds in order to pay their teaching faculties. It was not until 1963 when the Health Professions Educational Assistance Act was passed that any significant money was appropriated for medical education per se. Even today medical administrators are compelled to give a broad definition as to what constitutes research in an effort to balance teaching and research responsibilities. A side effect of the availability of federal and state funding has been a proliferation of medical schools. The 87 medical schools operating in 1967 have now increased to 127.

The flood of government funds for research was far from an unalloyed good. The appeal of research money made medical schools even more research-oriented and tended to turn them away from the equally fundamental task of teaching. Moreover, grant money was given to institutions on the basis of the research abilities of individual faculty members. Understandably medical schools recruited new professors and evaluated existing ones on their ability to attract research grants. A side effect of this was to increase the disparity between the better and poorer schools, since wealthier schools with more nationally recognized faculty members attracted a greater portion of government funds.[14]

One other significant development in the past thirty years has been an administrative one. The rising cost of technology combined with inflation has placed severe budgetary strains on the various health schools. These institutions tend to be located in major urban centers where expansion is difficult. When, for example, the University of Pittsburgh and Tulane University considered moving to the suburbs, civic and business leaders, all too aware of the economic loss to the city, promptly took action. They helped to raise funds, offered tax and other advantages, and provided administrative assistance. Thus, rising costs provided a further stimulus to the growth of health centers. These centers, which place all health schools and their hospitals and clinics under one administration, minimize budgetary problems through greater efficiency and at the same time help to integrate health care services and teaching.

The rapidly advancing front of medicine necessitates comparable changes in medical education. Within medical schools, as within universities, tradition, empire building, personality clashes, and disagreements as to the role of the physicians and the form medical care should take all complicate the task of educational reform. The job is a difficult one, but during the past few years an encouraging sign of progress has been the increasing awareness of the need to make constant adjustments in the curriculum.

In glancing back over medical education for the past ninety years, one cannot help being impressed with the vast improvement in the training provided young physicians. A good share of the credit can be ascribed to fundamental changes in medicine itself. The bacteriological revolution was only one of a series of advances that drastically altered the practice of medicine. The image of the physician at the bedside of the patient has been replaced by that of the white-coated surgeon in the operating room or the research scientist in the laboratory. Encouraged by television and by the medical profession itself, the public considers medicine a science and expects precise diagnoses and quick cures. In the first flush of enthusiasm arising from the discovery of bacteria and the development of antitoxins, many medical school professors forgot that patients were complex human beings and concentrated on pathogenic organisms. As laboratories and technology began playing a greater part in medicine, it was inevitable that medical training tended more and more toward science and technology; and, as the curriculum became overcrowded with laboratory and technique courses, it was perhaps inevitable that humanistic training would be pushed into the background.

One of the sharpest critics of medical education today, William G. Rothstein, argues that medical schools have decentralized their administrations to such an extent that it is impossible to achieve a coherent set of objectives, policies, and priorities. While federal research funding has been invaluable, at the same time it has led to an emphasis on training researchers rather than medical practitioners. Clinical professors, who should be preparing students for medical practice, have isolated themselves from the local medical community, and instead of treating ordinary patients, they deal with the extremely poor or those requiring highly specialized care. Rothstein maintains that in attempting to model themselves on liberal arts colleges, medical schools have forgotten that their role also includes teaching a body of knowledge suitable for practical application. Finally, Rothstein decries the emphasis on sciences and mathematics required by medical-school admissions committees.[15]

While there is much truth in Rothstein's assertions, it was an awareness of the need for curriculum revision that led to the reform movement of the 1950s and 1960s. As a result of this movement more time is now assigned to such topics as community medicine, social medicine, medical ethics, and medical history. The number of hours allotted to these courses varies widely, as does the form of these courses. Medicine, by its nature, is conservative, and many institutions are still content to pay lip service to the humanities and the rubric of social medicine. Yet the omens are promising, and medical education may be returning again to the Hippocratic concept of dealing with the whole patient.

CHAPTER 18

Women in Medicine

THE UNITED STATES has the distinction of granting the first medical degree to a woman, yet, far more than most countries, it has a history of discriminating against females in medicine. The awarding of the first medical degree came in 1849, during a period of great social ferment—the 1830s and 1840s—in which zealous advocates of many reforms were attracting followers. The dominant reform movement was the abolition of slavery, but reformers were fighting against tobacco and alcohol, urging women's rights, and seeking reforms in clothing, diet, and many other aspects of American life. The health crusade of the 1840s advocated fresh air, exercise, comfortable clothing, and moderate diet, and sought to give some understanding of physiology. Of particular concern to intelligent women reformers was the effort to give females some understanding of their anatomy and physiology, subjects that were taboo in polite society.

One development in British and American medicine in the late eighteenth and early nineteenth centuries was the substitution of the physician for the midwife in obstetrical care. How this came about in a society that rated modesty as the prime womanly virtue and in which a respectable female carefully covered herself from head to toe is difficult to explain. It is even harder to understand when one realizes that physicians in the early nineteenth century were not allowed to examine females with gynecological problems visually, and were compelled to assist in deliveries with their hands under a sheet or some other cover. As this form of prudery gained wider acceptance, many "modest" women with serious female ailments were reluctant to call in a physician. The obvious solution to the problem of female modesty would have been to train women physicians to deal with obstetrics and gynecology, but the idea was not considered seriously until women began forcing their way into the medical profession.

The best explanation for the movement of male physicians into midwifery is implicit in Lamar R. Murphy's study, which maintains there was a transformation in the relations between doctors and laypeople beginning in the late eighteenth century. She argues that in the colonial period the boundaries between professional and domestic medicine were not sharply defined. When, in the post-Revolutionary years, elite physicians sought to assume authority over medical treatment, their views clashed with the more common assumption that medical care should be vested in individuals demonstrating practical skills reinforced by folklore. The early health writers, largely physicians, were not opposed to domestic medical practice. Rather they sought to improve it, but at the same time to restrict it to definite areas. They emphasized the role of women in preventing disease and maintaining family health, yet at the same time claimed healing authority over matters traditionally exercised by women. Even the irregular medical practitioners, including the Thomsonians, supported the concept of two medical spheres, a professional one and a domestic one. Murphy states that an unanticipated result was to provide justification for excluding women from formal medical training.[1]

Not only were women excluded from formal medical training, but the medical profession made little effort to provide training for midwives, the one female group still providing a form of medical care considered within the physicians' sphere. This was true despite the fact that midwives continued to deliver the majority of babies throughout the nineteenth century and were delivering approximately 50 percent as late as 1910. In the early twentieth century, municipal public health departments, concerned over the high infant mortality among the lower income groups, advocated training and licensing of midwives. Two problems troubling health officials in New York City were the inadequate reporting of births by midwives and physicians and the failure of midwives and some physicians to use a mild solution of silver nitrate to prevent eye infections in newborns. In 1907 the New York Health Department was given licensing authority and subsequently established the Bellevue School for Midwives.[2]

Other city health departments, too, sought to give some training to midwives. A controversy then developed between public health administrators, who recognized that the poor could not afford specialists and hospital care, and the medical profession, led by the obstetricians, which insisted that birthing should be in the hands of professionals. Changing social conditions, brought about by the decline in immigration, a trend to smaller families, and a demand by women for better medical care, eventually enabled physicians to gain the upper hand. The process, however, was a gradual one. In New York City the elimination of the traditional midwives took over fifty years. In 1923 midwives still delivered over 21 percent of babies, and it was not until 1962 that the Board of Health ruled against licensing untrained midwives. A special exception was made for the last two midwives in this category, which allowed them to deliver only their own grandchildren.[3]

The chief impetus leading women to fight their way into the medical profession was the movement for women's rights. The majority of women who pioneered in medicine were active in the reform movements of the 1830s and 1840s, and their interest in medicine reflected their liberal outlook. The widespread belief that women were sickly and frail, incapacitated by a "periodic sickness," and subject to "female complaints" led to the rise of "Ladies Physiological Institutes," which in turn brought a demand for women teachers versed in anatomy and physiology.[4]

The state of medicine in America at the midcentury both facilitated the entrance of women into it and at the same time aroused opposition to the idea of lady doctors. The emergence of irregular medical schools, such as the eclectic and homeopathic, was an advantage, since these institutions were more inclined to accept women in an effort to gain support for their particular school of medical thought. Moreover, the excessive number of proprietary medical schools anxiously trying to build their enrollments facilitated the acceptance of women, and the minimal academic work required of all students guaranteed them a degree. In the majority of states, possession of a medical degree was an automatic license to practice. Against these advantages, the ease with which an individual could enter the profession meant an excess of practitioners, and the fear of additional competition in an already overcrowded profession undoubtedly contributed to the opposition encountered by women.

The first woman to obtain a medical degree was Elizabeth Blackwell. The product of a liberal English background, she came with her family to America at the age of eleven. She began her career as a teacher, but, motivated at least in part by her zeal for women's rights, decided to study medicine. She found a friend and guide in Dr. Samuel H. Dickson of the Charleston Medical School who helped her to "read" medicine. She tried unsuccessfully to gain entrance to various medical schools and was delighted when in 1847 Geneva Medical School of Western New York accepted her application. Medical schools were a male preserve, and nineteenth-century medical students were notorious for being coarse and rowdy. In this male-dominated atmosphere, only an attractive and strong personality enabled Elizabeth Blackwell to overcome the suspicion, resentment, and ridicule of her professors and fellow students. A correspondent to one of the medical journals reported in December that Miss Blackwell "comes into class with great composure, takes off her bonnet and puts it under the seat (exposing a fine phrenology), takes notes constantly, and maintains, throughout, an unchanged countenance. The effect on the class has been good, and great decorum is preserved when she is present." [5] Upon graduation in 1849 Blackwell was unable to find a hospital that would admit her for clinical training, so she set off for England and the Continent to continue her studies. On her return in 1850 she began practicing in New York City, where she met with considerable opposition from local physicians. Excluded from hospitals, she opened a private dispensary for women and children.

A second major hurdle preventing women from obtaining medical training was the refusal of hospitals to accept them. To remedy this situation, Dr. Blackwell, along with her sister Emily and Marie Zakrzewska, both of whom had earned medical degrees from the Cleveland Medical College (Western Reserve), founded the New York Infirmary for Women and Children. Despite initial difficulties, the infirmary flourished, and in 1868 the three women opened the Woman's Medical College of the New York Infirmary. Shortly thereafter, Dr. Blackwell, who had been commuting between England and America, returned to England to carry on the fight for the health of women and children.

Once Dr. Blackwell had broken the barrier, women began making rapid progress in medicine. The woman's rights movement was gaining strength, and Geneva Medical College gained a historical first by sheer chance. The year Dr. Blackwell graduated, 1849, three women were admitted to Central Medical College in Rochester, New York, a school established by eclectics. One of the early women graduates of the college, Dr. Myra King Merrick, returned to her home in 1852 to become the first female practitioner in Cleveland. The eclectics opened all their schools to women in 1855 and fifteen years later admitted women to membership in their national association.[6]

Reflecting the general ferment of the 1840s, a group of liberal physicians, lawyers, and businessmen, several of whom were Quakers, began planning a women's medical school in Philadelphia. After some preliminary steps, the Female Medical College of Pennsylvania was chartered in 1850. The majority of students during the first year were females interested in learning something about their own anatomy and physiology, but eight of them sought medical degrees. Opposition from conservative male practitioners and a suspicion that the school was tinged with eclecticism made the first few years difficult. The outbreak of war in 1861 forced it to close, but at the end of hostilities, the institution reopened as the Woman's Medical College of Pennsylvania under the able leadership of one of its first graduates, Dr. Ann Preston. It survives today as the last of the female medical schools.

Meanwhile, in 1848 a group of enlightened Boston physicians interested primarily in teaching midwifery opened the Boston Female Medical College. The chief founder, Dr. Samuel Gregory of Boston, two years later secured a charter for the Female Medical Education Society to promote the cause of women's medical education. In 1856 the original school was rechartered as the New England Female Medical College. It struggled along for a few years and finally merged in 1874 with the Medical Department of Boston University, at that time a homeopathic institution.[7]

By the Civil War at least three medical schools for women were granting degrees (the third one was Penn Medical University, an offshoot of the Woman's Medical College of Pennsylvania), and a number of schools, largely irregular ones, had gone coeducational. Even Harvard, affected by the general reform movement, in 1850 accepted a female and three black students. When their fellow students rioted in protest, the four individuals withdrew their applications. In consequence, Harvard Medical School waited until 1945, almost one hundred years later, before admitting women.[8]

While the majority of physicians opposed the entrance of women into their profession, a highly articulate minority actively supported the women's cause. An Atlanta physician in 1854 argued that female physicians were essential to "the safety and happiness" of a large portion "of the most refined and lovely women." Every practitioner, he wrote, almost daily saw cases that had "become incurable on account of the reluctance of females to submit" to examination. Most female diseases, he asserted, could not be cured because of "the almost insuperable objections of the fair sufferers, to the inevitable exposure of their sexual secrets to a male physician."[9] The *Boston Medical and Surgical Journal* took a moderately favorable stance at first. It published letters and articles on both sides of the issue, including one from Mrs. Paulina Wright Davis, a leading exponent of women's rights. A subsequent change in the editorship altered the journal's viewpoint, for the new editor strongly opposed the participation of women in any area of medicine—even midwifery.[10]

Unfortunately, the voices raised in opposition to women were far more numerous and strident. They repeated and embellished all the traditional arguments. Women were too frail, too sensitive, too emotional, and too lacking in rational ability. Physicians asked what would happen to female modesty and chastity if women medical students were exposed to the details of their own anatomy and—inconceivable as it seemed—to male anatomy. Even as the diehards fought for morality and decency, some opponents of women's rights manfully faced reality, for, as the editor of the *Medical and Surgical Reporter* conceded, "in some degenerate age of the world women may be received into favor as practitioners of medicine."[11]

While women were gaining acceptance into medical schools, they were not so successful with respect to hospitals and medical societies. As part of their fight to raise professional standards, the AMA and local medical societies tried to prevent their members from consulting with irregular practitioners. They also used this weapon against women physicians. In 1859 the Philadelphia County Medical Society forbade its members to consult with professors and graduates of female medical schools, and the state society concurred in the action. All was not harmony, however, for the Montgomery County society protested the decision. When the issue was raised again in 1866–67, the Montgomery County society resolved that females were as well fitted for medicine as males and instructed its delegates to vote in favor of consultations with females.[12]

Although the tide was gradually turning in favor of women, the conservatives gave ground grudgingly. When the council of the Massachusetts Medical Society voted to admit women in 1870, the editor of the *Boston Medical and Surgical Journal* commented in sorrow: "The Society [has taken] a long step downward from the dignified attitude which it has hitherto assumed, and its moral tone will have been perceptibly lowered." He need not have worried, for the conservative members delayed action, largely on constitutional grounds, for fourteen years. In 1882 Dr. James R. Chadwick recapitulated the actions of the society with respect to the admission of women and reported that he had sent a questionnaire to the secretaries of all state medical societies asking for information on their society's position with regard to women physicians. Of the 29 state societies responding, 11, largely in the South, reported that no woman had applied for membership. The other 17 state societies reported a total of 115 women members. Chadwick, who favored the admission of women, also quoted a paper on women physicians read before the American Social Science Association in 1881 stating that 390 of the 430 female graduates of medical colleges were in active practice, and that only 11 had never practiced medicine. Nonetheless, in 1883 the Massachusetts society rejected the admission of women by a vote of 62 to 58. The following year, however, the supporters of women physicians mobilized their forces, and by a vote of 209 to 123 the society admitted female physicians.[13]

At the national level, the AMA first considered the issue of female membership in 1868 and 1870, but the resolutions favoring women were tabled. In the latter year another motion was also introduced that would have permitted consultation with female physicians. According to the correspondent for the *Boston Medical and Surgical Journal*, the resulting discussion "assumed an uproarious character, and an incessant din took the place of legitimate debate." At the next annual meeting the president reflected a common attitude when, in citing the issues facing the association, he declared: "Another disease has become epidemic, 'The Woman Question.'" This "question" continued to be raised in the succeeding sessions of the AMA and always a substantial minority could be counted on to support the admission of women. In 1876 the Illinois Medical Society sent a female delegate, Dr. Sarah Hackett Stevenson, who was received with considerable misgivings. Despite consistent minority support for female physicians within the AMA and slow but steady gains at the local and state levels, the national society did not admit women until 1915.[14]

Notwithstanding conservative opposition and the reluctance of the AMA to admit women medical graduates, as Dr. Chadwick's survey demonstrated, women physicians were generally accepted by the public and by most members of the profession. In 1881 Dean Rachel Bodley of the Woman's Medical College of Pennsylvania sent questionnaires to 244 of the school's graduates and received answers from 189. Of the 189, 166 were actively engaged in medical practice, most of whom concentrated largely or in part on gynecology and obstetrics. A total of 150 of the 189 considered that they received "cordial social recognition" and only 7 reported a negative reception. Approximately one-third, 68, were members of a state, county, or local medical society. The average income for the entire group was around $3,000, with four of them reporting annual earnings of between $15,000 and $20,000.[15] In terms of income and membership in medical societies, female medical graduates would appear to have been doing better than their male counterparts. This success probably speaks more for the strength of character needed for women to enter medicine and their middle- or upper-class background than any other factor. The many semi-illiterate, lower-class males who had access to the medical profession at that time were not too likely to build a profitable middle-class practice.

In the post–Civil War years a number of women's medical schools appeared, although most of them were short-lived. Altogether nineteen schools were established between 1850 and 1895. As of 1890, eight of them were in operation. Among the better schools were the Chicago Women's Hospital College, organized in 1870; the New York Free Medical College for Women, begun in 1871; and the Woman's Medical College of Baltimore, founded in 1882. By this latter year women's position in the medical profession was steadily improving. For example, the *Journal of the American Medical Association* carried a favorable account of the 1884 graduation ceremonies at the Women's Hospital Medical College of Chicago, adding: "The institution is enjoying a fair degree of prosperity and we are informed that a new college building will be erected during the present season." The journal's correspondent from Philadelphia the following year praised the exceptionally high standards maintained by the Woman's Medical College in that city. Well before other medical schools, he wrote, the college offered a three-year graded course and an eight-month school year. Showing the ambivalence of its editors, however, *JAMA* editorialized in 1886 against higher education for women, pointing out that professional education required "an enormous outlay of physiological force; much more than a woman can afford if she is to perform her proper function as a producer of men."[16]

In the District of Columbia most women, white and black, obtained their medical degrees from Howard University, although the rise of Jim Crow drastically cut back on the number of white females. In the 1880s, as a result of a financial crisis, white women were permitted to enroll in Georgetown and George Washington universities, but once economic conditions improved, the schools returned to a strictly male policy. The homeopathic and eclectic schools actively appealed to females when it was expedient to do so but closed their doors to women when their tuition was no longer needed or male students objected. In the District of Columbia, as elsewhere, women physicians encountered constant obstacles to professional advancement. They were denied residencies and clinical appointments and were forced to open their own dispensaries and clinics. Even the black medical associations refused to admit women.[17]

Meanwhile many established institutions and newly formed schools were becoming coeducational. Medical departments were opened to women at Syracuse University in 1870, the University of Michigan in 1871, and the University of California in 1874. Except for teaching, in these years medicine offered the best prospects for women, and the number of women physicians increased dramatically. Between 1870 and 1900 the number of female doctors rose from 544 to 7,382. These felicitous numbers were no forecast for the future. By the mid-1890s a reaction was setting in against women physicians, and female enrollment in medical schools fell by one-third between 1894 and 1904.[18]

While state universities and schools west of the Appalachians in the postwar years were liberalizing their admissions, the old and well-established schools in the Northeast continued to resist. Harvard, which had shown a brief sign of weakness in 1850, was sorely tempted in 1879. The offer of a gift from the estate of Mr. George O. Hovey amounting to ten thousand dollars was made contingent upon the admission of women to the medical school. A committee appointed to look into the matter divided, with the majority favoring acceptance of the gift and the minority recommending the establishment of a separate medical school for women. Subsequently the faculty met and voted thirteen to five that it was "detrimental to the school to enter upon the experiment of admitting female students." The overseers concurred with the faculty, although they did vote sixteen to ten to admit women for medical studies "under suitable restrictions."[19] The faculty, determined to uphold the standards of decency, remained adamant, and the admission of women awaited another sixty-odd years.

The first major eastern school to make a concession was Johns Hopkins, a relatively new institution. Having made the decision to establish a medical school and having appointed a faculty, the university in 1892 was unable to raise enough money to begin operation. A group of able and wealthy women, led by M. Carey Thomas, Mary Garrett, Elizabeth King, and Mary Gwinn, the organizers of Bryn Mawr College, decided to take advantage of this financial crisis to further the cause of women's rights. They raised $100,000 and offered it to Johns Hopkins on condition that women be admitted to the medical school on an equal basis with men. The reluctant administrators and trustees agreed to accept the offer providing that the women raised a total of $500,000, expecting that this would end the matter. When a national appeal brought only about $200,000, Mary Garrett personally offered over $300,000 to complete the requisite half-million dollars, but she insisted that admission standards be raised to include a bachelor's degree or its equivalent, a knowledge of French and German, and some premedical studies. The trustees and faculty were horrified, convinced that these prerequisites for admission were far too high. Garrett and her cohorts refused to make any concessions and finally won the day. The victory gained by this determined group of women was not only an advance for women's rights, but it profoundly affected the entire course of American medical education.[20]

The decision by Johns Hopkins was a straw in the wind, and other schools soon began modifying their admission policies. Tulane University was authorized by the state legislature in 1894 to grant diplomas in law, medicine, and pharmacy to women. The medical school faculty, while willing to grant Ph.D.'s in pharmacy, could not bring themselves to admit women to medicine and delayed until 1915.[21] Cornell University, a combination private and land grant institution, opened its medical school on a coeducational basis in 1898. As more and more schools accepted female students, the raison d'être for separate women's schools ceased to exist, and they soon began closing. By 1909 only three were still in operation: the Woman's Medical College of Pennsylvania, the Woman's Medical College of Baltimore, and the New York Medical College and Hospital for Women.

Ironically, as Abraham Flexner observed, women's interest in medical education appeared to decline in direct ratio to their ability to obtain it. Between 1904 and 1909 both the number of women medical students and those graduating showed a steady decline. Whereas a total of 254 women received medical degrees in 1904, only 162 graduated in 1909. On a percentage basis, women represented 4 percent of all medical graduates in 1905, but by 1915 this figure was down to 2.6 percent. The percentage climbed to 5.4 in 1927 and then dropped below 5 until 1940. The enrollment of women in medical schools began rising again in 1945, peaked in 1948, and then declined until 1952. It held steady until 1960, when it again began a slight upward trend. In consequence, the percentage of women graduates reached a high point of 12.1 in 1949, only to decline below 5 percent in 1955. In the 1960s, the number of women enrolled in medical schools increased slowly, but in the early 1970s the relative percentage of women students moved sharply higher. In 1972–73 women represented 16.7 percent of medical students, and the following year the figure rose to 19.8 percent. This percentage almost doubled by 1989–90, when women constituted 38.2 percent of students admitted to medical schools and 36.1 percent of all medical students.[22]

Obviously many factors were at work limiting the entrance of women into medicine in the twentieth century. The tendency for medical schools to require a bachelor's degree as a prerequisite and the increasing cost of medical school education itself undoubtedly prevented many young women from entering medicine. Most parents were reluctant to spend a relatively large sum to give their daughter a professional education when they hoped and expected that she would make a "good" marriage and become a mother and housewife. Furthermore, graduate education for women was thought to reduce their chances for marriage. Regina M. Morantz-Sanchez suggests further that since occupational status is a means for measuring social class, the medical profession consciously made itself into an elite class by excluding women, the poor, and minorities.[23]

Over and above social and economic factors were deliberate efforts by medical school faculty members and administrators to discourage women students. Unofficial quotas played some role in this, but probably more important was the attitude of many professors who openly proclaimed and demonstrated their distaste for teaching women. Medicine for many of them was still considered a masculine domain, in which coarse and sometimes macabre humor was used to relieve the tension and grimness of anatomy and related fields. A not uncommon practice in medical and dental schools to awaken drowsy students, stupefied by four consecutive hours—or even as many as seven or eight—of lectures and labs during the day, was to flash pictures of nude women on the screen in the midst of serious slide presentations. Obviously "humor" of this sort was poorly suited for any classes, let alone coeducational ones. More important, it bespoke the attitude of many instructors. Happily, women students no longer feel compelled to accept slights and disparagement, and the rise of a new generation of faculty members is contributing to an improved atmosphere. If one can extrapolate the present trend, women are destined to play a larger and larger role in medicine.

One can scarcely leave a chapter on women in medicine without mentioning a few of those who have had a major impact upon medicine and public health. Dr. S. Josephine Baker of the New York City Health Department in 1908 inaugurated a program of sending nurses into tenement homes to advise mothers on how to care for the children. Out of this program came the Division of Child Hygiene, the first health unit of its type and the forerunner of the United States Children's Bureau established in 1912.[24] Her contemporary Dr. Alice Hamilton played a major role in inaugurating the field of industrial health in America. Her studies on the health of men and women working with phosphorous, lead, radium, and other dangerous substances are landmarks in occupational health. In addition, she was active in the fight for all of early twentieth-century laws for occupational safety.[25]

In the field of pediatrics Dr. Helen B. Taussig, after graduating from Johns Hopkins in 1927, became interested in congenital heart disease, particularly those defects associated with cyanosis—the so-called blue babies—and by 1940 had established herself as an authority in the field. Believing that an operation could be devised to increase the flow of blood to the lungs of blue babies, she joined forces with a surgeon, Alfred Blalock. The first operation was performed in 1944, and it opened an entire field of heart surgery. In consequence, thousands of children have been restored to health.[26] An outstanding public health figure in the midcentury was Dr. Leona Baumgartner, who served as health commissioner for New York City from 1954 to 1962. As was the case with Josephine Baker, Baumgartner had a vital interest in child health, and as director of the city health department's Bureau of Child Health for sixteen years she maintained the bureau's performance at a high level. As health commissioner she overhauled the administrative structure, fought to attract able professionals, and recognized that good public relations was essential to any successful public health policy.[27]

Nursing

Women have nursed the sick since time immemorial, but, as an organized profession, nursing is less than one hundred years old. The best nursing care for most of the Christian era was provided by religious orders, both Catholic and Protestant. The Ursulines who came to manage the Royal Hospital in New Orleans in 1727 were the first nursing group within the present United States, although Catholic religious orders have played an important role in Canadian hospitals since the establishment of Hôtel Dieu Hospital in Quebec in 1639.[28] Another important Catholic nursing order is the Sisters of Charity, whose American branch dates back to Mother Seton and the founding in 1809 of the Sisterhood of St. Joseph at Emmitsburg, Maryland. In the nineteenth century, Protestant nursing orders representing the Episcopalian, Lutheran, and Methodist churches also began work in America.

Secular nursing began in the mid-nineteenth century and owes much to the great Englishwoman Florence Nightingale. Her example helped make American women aware of the atrocious conditions that characterized most hospitals and inspired them to attempt to rectify these conditions. Hospitals in the nineteenth century, as noted earlier, were charitable institutions, designed to care for the sick poor. With the exception of those managed by religious orders, they were dirty, crowded, and underfinanced. Any nursing given was provided by convalescent patients or by ignorant and impoverished women, most of whom were of dubious character. Until better women could be attracted to the nursing field, there was little hope for improving hospital conditions.

The first effort to train nurses in America was made by a group of Quakers, who in the 1850s organized the Nurse Society of Philadelphia and appealed to young women to enter nursing. With the help of a local physician, the society also offered some practical training. A few years later, shortly before the outbreak of the Civil War, the Woman's Hospital in Philadelphia, the New England Medical College, and the New York Infirmary began giving elementary instruction in nursing.[29] The war halted further progress in nursing education, but it brought large numbers of women into hospitals, most of whom received their only training in the field. Dr. Elizabeth Blackwell, an intimate of Florence Nightingale, at once began organizing women volunteers in New York for warfare nursing, and she was the logical choice to head the Union army nursing corps. The army surgeons, however, were doubtful of a "female doctor," and the choice fell upon Dorothea Dix, a great personality and promoter whose major field of activity, care of the insane, did not intrude upon the medical profession. As superintendent of nurses in the Union army, Dix performed reasonably well despite the rigidity of many army physicians and their resentful attitude toward female nurses. While Dix was able to provide a limited training for some of her nurses, her work resulted in neither a nurses' training school nor a permanent army nursing corps. In the Confederacy thousands of women served as nurses, but they worked as individual volunteers.[30]

Following the war, the AMA appointed a Committee on the Training of Nurses headed by Dr. Samuel Gross, and in 1869 the committee advocated the establishment of a nurses' training program under the direction of the medical profession. Nothing came of the report, but it did show a developing interest in the subject.[31] In 1872 the New England Hospital for Women and Children began giving a graded course in nursing and it graduated its first class in 1873. In this same year three other hospitals established nurses' training schools, Bellevue in New York, Massachusetts General in Boston, and the New Haven Hospital in Connecticut. The Bellevue school resulted from the discovery by a group of women visitors of the atrocious conditions in the hospital. The school was modeled on the Nightingale pattern with an emphasis upon uniforms and military discipline. Unlike the English system, which maintained class distinctions, Bellevue sought, through its educational requirements, to attract middle-class students.[32]

The post–Civil War years saw a proliferation of hospitals, a growth resulting from urbanism and improvements in medicine and surgery. As the curative power of medicine increased, serious cases began moving from the home to the hospital, and private patients began to occupy more hospital beds. In 1873 the United States had 178 hospitals; by 1923 the number had grown to 6,830. Hospital administrators soon discovered that better nursing care improved a hospital's mortality rate and that student nurses provided a source of cheap labor. By 1880 the number of nurses' training schools had increased to 15, by 1900 the figure had jumped to 432, and by 1923 there were over 1,700.[33] Whereas the original concept of the training school for nurses had been one in which systematic classroom and practical instruction would be given, most hospitals provided little or no formal teaching, relying upon what was essentially an apprenticeship. By providing little more than room and board, hospitals gained the services of young women for incredibly long daily hours, six or seven days a week. In the process of producing large numbers of graduates with a limited educational background, these schools were responsible for the low social and economic status of nurses.

If nursing was to achieve a respectable position in society as the original founders of nursing schools intended, educational standards had to be raised. The first step in this direction was the establishment of a nursing school at Johns Hopkins Hospital in 1889. This school not only provided a standard for nursing education, but it gave three outstanding leaders to the nursing profession, Isabel A. Hampton (Mrs. Hunter Robb), Mary Adelaide Nutting, and Lavinia L. Dock. Despite its emphasis upon formal instruction, the Hopkins nursing school insisted on the customary rigid discipline and rigorous routine. Students had to be up for breakfast and morning prayers and be ready for duty by 7:00 A.M. to begin a twelve-hour day, with one hour off for "lunch, rest, and study." The only relief from nursing duty was provided by the twice-weekly classes held from 5:00 to 6:00 P.M. In addition, staff physicians gave lectures from 8:00 to 9:00 P.M. The first lesson students were taught was "absolute and unquestioning obedience" to their superiors and complete deference to physicians.[34] This tradition, which survives in a modified form today, has hindered the development of nursing and has not been productive of sound medical care.

Several Johns Hopkins nurses took the initiative in establishing the first national nursing association in 1894. Its purpose was to improve educational standards and to raise nursing to professional status. The next step was the establishment of a journal, a course of action advocated by Mary Adelaide Nutting as early as 1893. By valiant efforts, in 1900 the *American Journal of Nursing* began its long and successful career. As nurses started to organize, they recognized the need to distinguish between the graduates of good nursing schools and self-trained practitioners. Nursing groups within the states began pressuring legislatures, and by 1915 virtually all states had nurse registration laws.

Recognizing that professional status could not be achieved without college training, Mary Adelaide Nutting and Isabel Hampton Robb in 1899 persuaded Dean James Earl Russell of Teachers College, Columbia University, to institute a course in hospital economics. In the process of negotiating Nutting made an excellent impression upon Dean Russell, and in 1907 she was appointed to the college's newly established professorship of nursing, the first of its kind in the United States. In the ensuing years nursing schools steadily raised their academic standards. The University of Minnesota in 1909 established a nursing school, and by 1920 nearly two hundred nursing schools had some university affiliation.[35]

The struggle to raise nursing standards encountered considerable difficulties within the nursing profession itself. First of all, nurses were divided by class. The rank-and-file nurses were graduates of hospital training schools that required little in the way of an academic background. Most of these nurses were concerned primarily with pay and working conditions and had little in common with the articulate elite nurses, who envisioned nursing as a profession. Moreover, hospital training instilled discipline and idealism in their students, thus making them vulnerable to exploitation. The better-educated nurses constantly sought to separate nursing education from hospital ward service, and in so doing clashed with hospital nursing schools, who tended to place hospital work ahead of education. As late as 1925, almost three-quarters of hospital nursing schools relied upon students for ward nursing service. Moreover, within the nursing associations the majority of members were far more concerned with pay and working conditions than with raising educational standards. In 1948 a report commissioned by the Russell Sage Foundation, *Nursing for the Future*, recommended that nursing education should require a college degree. Although the requirement became the basis for a new program, neither the American Nurses Association nor the National League of Nursing Education put the recommendations to a vote of the membership. And as late as 1965 only 14 percent of new nurses had academic degrees.[36]

A second issue that divided nurses was the concept of nursing as a womanly service. As Susan Reverby wrote, the dilemma in contemporary American nursing is "the order to care in a society that refuses to value caring." The advocates of making nursing a profession could scarcely argue against the womanly virtues of nurturing, motherhood, and Christian service. The medical profession has always stressed its dedication to humanity, without, however, permitting this dedication to interfere with its economic welfare. Yet these same physicians expected the idealism and dedication of women nurses and teachers to more than compensate them for low pay and long hours of hard work. Nursing leaders responded to the concept of womanly duty by emphasizing that nursing also needed technical expertise.[37]

The emergence of visiting nurses in the early twentieth century greatly helped the public image of the profession. Visiting nursing began around the turn of the century when philanthropic women, appalled at conditions in the slum areas, began to visit the homes of the sick poor or employed nurses to do so. The success of the early visiting nurses encouraged dozens of community and philanthropic organizations to adopt similar nurse programs. At the same time, health departments and school boards were beginning to send physicians and nurses into the schools to examine the children for infectious diseases. The visiting nurse movement grew rapidly at first and spread throughout the United States. The New York City Health Department was one of the earliest municipal agencies to employ visiting nurses, but voluntary organizations were the mainstay of visiting nurses. In 1909 some 58 organizations sent 372 visiting nurses into the tenement areas of New York City.[38]

The single organization that gave the most support to visiting nurses was the Metropolitan Life Insurance Company. Recognizing that maintaining the health of its policy holders was both a humanitarian aim and sound economics, in 1909 the company organized the Metropolitan Visiting Nurses Association and contracted with visiting nurse associations in over seven thousand cities. The program was quite successful for many years. With the entrance of the federal government into the health area in the late 1930s the company gradually began to reduce the budget of its social welfare program. As late as 1940, however, the company was still funding its nursing service at the rate of five million dollars a year. Faced with the rising cost of nursing services and convinced that the program was no longer economically beneficial, in 1953 the Metropolitan ended its program.[39]

The introduction of visiting nurses in the last decade of the nineteenth century coincided with the institutionalization of public health. These were years, too, when advances in medical knowledge were beginning to solve the major problems of community hygiene, such as those relating to food, water, and the disposal of sewage and garbage. In consequence, the emphasis on health was shifting from community health to personal hygiene. Visiting nurses found themselves becoming health educators rather than nurses to the sick. Meanwhile, health departments, which had earlier enjoyed strong support from the medical profession, had discovered that the medical problems of infants, school-children, and mothers went far beyond what had been anticipated.

Since the lower-paid working class could not afford physicians, health departments expanded their dispensaries and established specialized clinics to provide medical care. These actions brought down the wrath of the medical profession, and health departments responded by closing their clinics and transforming their visiting nurses into public health nurses, nurses whose chief function was to educate the public in health matters. The steady expansion of state and local health departments in the next forty years led them to take on many of the responsibilities formerly handled by visiting nurses. As government assumed more responsibility for health, the private organizations that had supported visiting nurses gradually disappeared or withdrew from the field.

The number of visiting nurses grew slowly, since they were largely dependent upon charitable organizations. They were also troubled about their role. Should it be nursing the sick or serving as health educators? While visiting nurses were debating this question, the entire nursing profession was in the doldrums. Graduate nurses in the early years of the century had almost no choice but to join a visiting nurse association or a public health department, or to serve as private duty nurses, since hospitals continued to rely largely on nursing students, practical nurses, and nurses' aides. The economic position of registered nurses improved somewhat during the 1930s, when the Great Depression closed many nursing schools and forced hospitals to employ more R.N.'s. In the same years, nurses, despairing of the American Nurses Association (ANA), joined unions and resorted to the threat of strikes. The result of these tactics was a gradual improvement in pay and working conditions. Incidentally, it is a commentary on the divisions among nurses that the ANA did not formally sanction collective bargaining until 1946.[40]

The Civil War had given an impetus to nursing, and this was true of succeeding wars. Some 1,700 contract nurses were employed during the Spanish-American War, the majority of whom were women. In August of 1898 an Army Nurses Corps Division of the Surgeon General's Office was established. The excellent work performed by women nurses in the Spanish-American War led Congress in 1901 to give the Army Nursing Corps permanent status. During World War I the corps was expanded to a total of 22,000 and was supplemented by another 11,000 Red Cross nurses.[41] In the postwar years interest in nursing waned, and the number of students in nursing schools dropped sharply. The outbreak of World War II once again brought a great demand for nurses, and the Public Health Service organized a program of nursing education in conjunction with junior and community colleges. In addition, by 1946 many of the better hospital nursing schools had strengthened their ties with universities, and over ninety of these institutions had developed five-year nursing programs. More significantly, several universities had established separate schools of nursing offering a choice of a four- or five-year curriculum.

The professionalization of nursing, however, carried with it a high degree of specialization. Increasingly nurses were performing functions formerly handled by physicians, and, as medicine specialized, it brought with it a corresponding change in nursing services. Surgical, pediatric, obstetrical, and psychiatric nurses, to name a few, now began working with physicians and surgeons. The need for trained nurses in psychiatric wards pointed up the shortage of males in the nursing field. The domination of nursing by women is reflected in the relative percentages of male and female graduate nurses. As of 1940 males represented only 2.3 percent of all graduate nurses. In the postwar years the emergence of professional schools for nursing encouraged the entrance of men into the profession, but progress has been slow. As of 1984 men represented only 3.3 percent of the registered nurses working in their profession. The percentage of men admitted to nursing school programs in 1988, however, was 7.3.[42]

Despite the growing number of graduate nurses, the expanding demand for medical services following World War II led to a continuing shortage of nurses. The result was that licensed practical nurses, medical technicians, and orderlies increasingly assumed many of the duties formerly performed by R.N.'s. The effect of the shortage was to raise the status of graduate nurses. One major development stemming from the professionalization of nursing is the gradual decline of the autocratic and hierarchical tradition in nursing introduced by the early British nurses and reinforced by the pioneer nurses to gain acceptance by male physicians. Nurses are assuming broader responsibilities and becoming less subservient to physicians.

Much of this change has occurred since the 1960s, a time when nurses were still expected to make any of their recommendations appear to have come from the physician. A major factor encouraging nurses to fight for coequal status is the increasing number with academic training. As of 1990 approximately 65 percent of hospital staff nurses have received some college training or hold college degrees. Other factors are the growing number of male nurses, the nursing shortage, and the recognition that physicians are no longer infallible. The emergence of health maintenance organizations (HMOs) in which nurses are given greater responsibility for screening patients and the licensing of nurse practitioners have helped to raise the status of nurses.[43] Just over a decade ago Barbara Milosh argued that nursing could never become a profession because its autonomy is constrained by the dominance of the medical profession. Nonetheless, nurses today are beginning to insist that nursing is an autonomous health profession with a well-defined area of expertise.[44]

CHAPTER 19

Minorities in Medicine

AN AREA OF HISTORY that has been sadly neglected is the role of blacks in medicine. Possibly the earliest African American physician on record is a Dr. James Derham or Durham. Although a somewhat nebulous figure, he is firmly enshrined in black history. A journal article in 1916 spoke of him as "the most distinguished physician in New Orleans." A more recent historian described him as "a man of liberal education," "a superb linguist," and "an authority on the relationship of disease to climate."[1] The truth is that a slave named Derham was sold to Dr. John Kearsley, Jr., of Philadelphia. Kearsley taught him to compound drugs and "perform many of the menial duties of our profession." Eventually Derham ended up in the hands of a Dr. Robert Dove of New Orleans, who according to legend, completed his medical training and freed him to practice in New Orleans.[2]

Unfortunately, Derham was not a well-known physician in New Orleans. The Spanish authorities required all physicians to obtain licenses and kept complete records of all licenses granted. After a careful search of all official records in New Orleans, I have found only two blacks mentioned. One was a black phlebotomist named Domingo, and the other was a free black called Derum. In 1801 the Cabildo, noting that five practitioners were practicing medicine without a license, ordered them to cease and desist until they had passed the required examination. Mention was also made of "a free negro Derum . . . having the right only to cure throat disease and no other." Nothing was said of licensing him, and presumably he was allowed to carry on with his limited practice.

The "Dr. Robert Dove" mention earlier was undoubtedly Dr. Robert Dow, a Scottish physician who was a leading practitioner in the city. New Orleans had many visitors in those days, and it is odd that none of them mentioned Derham. A former slave with an extensive practice among whites would certainly have aroused their interest, and it is inconceivable that Derham, had he been a prominent physician, would not have been mentioned in the official records, newspapers, travel accounts, or descriptions of New Orleans. There is no question that a former slave with that name had contact with Dr. Benjamin Rush and practiced on a limited scale in New Orleans, but he was not a distinguished physician.[3]

The accomplishments of African Americans in the face of enormous handicaps during the nineteenth century are real and do not need to be bolstered artificially. A number of free blacks in the years before the Civil War did manage to acquire medical skills and engage in practice. Some were self-taught, others learned medicine through an apprenticeship, and a few earned medical degrees from American schools in the decade or so before the Civil War. Several of the more fortunate ones studied abroad. Dr. James McCune Smith, who received a medical degree from the University of Glasgow in 1837, was probably the first of these. It is likely that some of the free black men in New Orleans may have obtained medical degrees in France. An editorial in a New Orleans newspaper on the death of Dr. L. C. Roudanez (1826–90) described him as a "worthy and intelligent representative of the colored element that was free before the war — a man of undoubted skill in his profession and great popularity in this city."[4] In the North the abolition movement led several medical schools to open their doors to African Americans, but only a handful of degrees were awarded in the pre–Civil War period. One of these was earned by Dr. R. B. Leach of Cleveland. Leach began his career by nursing the sick on Great Lakes steamers and in 1858 graduated from the Cleveland Homeopathic Medical College.[5]

Despite widespread racial prejudice, during the Civil War eight black physicians were appointed to the Army Medical Corps. The highest-ranking black medical officer was Dr. Alexander T. Augusta, a graduate of Trinity Medical College in Toronto, Canada, who was raised to a lieutenant-colonel in March 1865. The most beneficial effect of the war, however, was to eliminate slavery and thus enhance opportunities for blacks in all areas.[6]

A wartime agency that contributed most directly to helping African

Americans was the Freedman's Bureau. Although its main purpose was to provide food and shelter, it did promote education and encourage blacks to enter the professions. In light of the refusal of most medical schools to accept black students, the prospective black doctors' best hope lay in the establishment of special medical schools. The first of these was Howard University, an institution founded under the auspices of the first Congregational Church of Washington, D.C., to educate both whites and blacks, males and females. With the help of General Oliver Otis Howard of the Freedman's Bureau the school opened in 1867, and its medical department was established the following year. Despite many difficulties, including active opposition from the faculty of the Medical College of Georgetown, Howard managed to survive. The second black medical school, Meharry Medical College of Nashville, was founded by the Methodist Episcopal Church in 1876, and, like Howard, continues to make a significant contribution to medical education. Other black medical schools came into existence in the succeeding years, but all had relatively brief careers. By the time Flexner made his survey in 1909, he found only seven black medical schools: Flint Medical College (New Orleans), Howard (Washington, D.C.), Knoxville (Tennessee), Leonard (Raleigh, North Carolina), Louisville (Kentucky), Meharry (Nashville), and the University of West Tennessee Medical Department in Memphis. All but Howard and Meharry soon disappeared.[7]

Although those institutions accepting African American medical students were willing to accept women, few black females acquired medical degrees. According to M. O. Bousfield, only about ninety had graduated from American medical schools up to 1923, and sixty-four of these were products of Meharry and Howard.[8]

The rising standards of medical education, to which the Flexner report, the Rockefeller Foundation, and the AMA's Council on Medical Education contributed, eliminated many of the weaker medical schools, including all of the black schools except Howard and Meharry. It was not by intention, since both Flexner and the foundation favored maintaining separate schools for blacks. In 1913 Flexner criticized the AMA Council on Medical Education for its condemnation of substandard southern medical schools. He felt that the AMA council needed to be more flexible and should follow his own policy of allowing for special circumstances. In giving Meharry Medical College an "A" rating, Flexner wrote, he was judging it in terms of other schools in "their respective section."[9] Nevertheless, Howard and Meharry were the only two black medical schools to survive the early twentieth-century reform years.

Despite support from the Rockefeller Foundation, relatively little progress was made in opening the medical profession to blacks. Most white schools in the North officially admitted them, but in practice they accepted a mere token number. Before 1940 only about twenty black physicians a year were produced by the approximately fifty-five white schools willing to admit black applicants, leaving the chief responsibility for producing black physicians to Howard and Meharry. Unfortunately, academic standards at the two schools were low, and a high percentage of their graduates were unable to pass the medical board examinations. In the late 1920s and the 1930s the Julius Rosenwald Fund, the Duke Endowment, and the Rockefeller General Education Board began programs to train black physicians and improve the health of blacks.[10] The decisive factor, however, was the changing climate of opinion after World War II and the action of the federal government, which through supreme court decisions and congressional legislation literally forced the acceptance of black students. The threat of losing federal funding was far more effective in persuading southern medical schools to integrate than any appeals based on morality and the democratic principle of human equality.

While medical schools for blacks were designed to facilitate entrance into medicine, black medical societies arose out of sheer necessity. For example, when three able black physicians, two of whom were members of the Howard faculty, were proposed for membership in the Medical Society of the District of Columbia in 1869, all three applications were rejected. In consequence, the following year Howard faculty members founded the National Medical Society of the District of Columbia, an organization for both white and black physicians. Since the American Medical Association, on one pretext or another, refused to support membership for blacks, local black medical societies gradually appeared as the century drew on. By 1895 these organizations were able to fuse into the National Medical Association. Shortly before this, in 1892, Dr. Miles Vandahurst Lynk of Jackson, Tennessee, founded the first black medical journal, the *Medical and Surgical Observer.* It was followed in 1909 by the appearance of the *Journal of the National Medical Association* under the editorship of Dr. Charles V. Roman.[11]

The late nineteenth century also witnessed the growth of black hospitals. Here again they arose out of necessity, since the majority of hospitals either refused to accept blacks or else provided them miserable accommodations. The need for hospitals was even worse in the case of black physicians, who were rigidly excluded from practicing in most institutions. By 1910 almost 100 black hospitals were in existence, and by 1929 the number had reached 129. Aside from providing better care for patients and facilities for black physicians, the hospitals contributed to medical education by increasing the number of internships and residencies open to blacks. The black hospitals in the South were particularly weak, and most black interns were forced to go north. Even in the North their opportunities were restricted. Cleveland City Hospital did not hire its first black physician until 1927, and the first black intern was not appointed until three black councilmen forced the issue in 1931.[12]

Even among public health workers, the most liberal members of the health professions, discrimination against blacks was common. In 1933, Dr. Midian Othello Bousfield, president of the National Medical Association, became the first black to speak before the American Public Health Association. In no uncertain terms he charged that health officers in the North and South paid little attention to the health of blacks. It was Bousfield, Peter M. Murray, and other northern black physicians who led the struggle in the pre–World War II years to raise professional standards of southern blacks and to improve the quality of their hospitals.[13]

While a few blacks such as Bousfield were able to overcome both the direct and subtle handicaps facing them because of their race, blacks' entrance into the medical profession continued to be difficult during the first half of the twentieth century. As medical education became more stringent and expensive, blacks, whose collective economic status was well below that of whites, were caught in an economic squeeze. The Great Depression aggravated the situation, and the number of black medical graduates, which had increased rapidly between 1890 and 1910, declined to around seventy per year by the late 1930s. In the years from 1910 to 1942, despite a considerable increase in the population, the number of black physicians in the country rose by only 400, from 3,409 to 3,810.[14]

The World War II era, however, marked the beginning of a renewed effort by blacks to gain their rightful place in society. Whereas only 156 blacks were commissioned as medical officers during World War I, in

World War II the figure was around 600. A mere token number of black nurses were allowed to enlist in World War I, but approximately 500 were accepted in World War II. In the postwar years, led by Dr. Montague Cobb, editor of the *Journal of the NMA*, blacks steadily pressed for entrance into white medical societies and hospitals, and with the help of the government, they were able to force southern and border-state medical schools to admit them.[15]

Nonetheless, segregation barriers still impeded the entrance of blacks into medicine and hindered their progress within the profession until the 1960s signaled a renewed drive for equal rights. Aided by the formation of the biracial Medical Committee for Civil Rights and its successor, the Medical Committee for Human Rights, black and white liberal physicians and other medical personnel began a more militant quest for justice. Their first victory came in 1954 when the Veterans Administration ordered an end to segregation in all of its hospitals. The reformers next turned their attention to the Hill-Burton Act of 1946, which had permitted federal funds to subsidize the building of some 104 segregated hospitals. Successful legal action in 1963 led to a ruling by the Supreme Court that the "separate but equal" clause in the Hill-Burton Act was unconstitutional. In August the following year Congress took the further step of requiring equal health opportunities in all federally aided hospitals. Ironically, the only losers from these reforms were the black hospitals. Their financial position had always been precarious, and they received only limited help from the Hill-Burton Act. To make matters worse, desegregation resulted in a mass exodus of both white and black physicians from black hospitals. By 1987 only ten black hospitals were in operation and those were struggling to survive.[16]

Although the Nixon administration that took over in 1968 was scarcely enthusiastic about minority rights, the momentum of the 1960s has continued to the present. The 1970s saw a determined effort by the federal government and responsible citizens to guarantee that blacks and other minorities have an equal opportunity to enter professional schools. In 1988 some 6.3 percent of students entering medical schools were blacks, yet they still constituted only about a quarter of the 24.4 percent total of minority students. In 1990 the percentage of entering black students was 7.1, of which 3.2 were men and 3.7 women. The number of African American physicians is slowly increasing. In 1970 approximately 6,100 blacks were practicing medicine; by 1985 the figure had increased to 15,600.[17] The number of blacks in medical and paramedical fields today is still not representative of the total black population, but the gap is gradually closing.

Jews and Catholics

Discrimination in medical schools has not been restricted to blacks and women. Two other groups have also experienced some difficulties in gaining entrance to the medical profession—Jews and Catholics. In restricting certain minorities, medical schools were reflecting prejudices that were all too common in the United States in the 1920s, prejudices that remain latent today. For Catholics the problem has never been acute since the existence of their own schools and hospitals guaranteed them access to education and clinical experience. Yet in certain geographic areas a subtle discrimination has been practiced against them. A five-year study by the Philadelphia Fellowship Commission published in 1957 showed that Protestant premedical students from Temple University and the University of Pennsylvania had a better chance for acceptance into medical schools than Catholics, who, in turn, fared better than Jews.[18]

Insofar as Jews are concerned, only a limited measure of discrimination existed within the medical field before World War I, but the next thirty or more years witnessed both official and unofficial discrimination against Jewish applicants to medical schools. So long as medical schools were largely proprietary institutions vying for students, white males had little difficulty in gaining acceptance. Moreover, Jews constituted a relatively small percentage of the population, and as such they represented no economic threat to practicing physicians. By the 1920s both of these factors had altered radically. The efforts of organized medicine to raise educational standards and to limit entrance into the profession greatly reduced the available places for medical students. At the same time, children of the relatively large numbers of Eastern European Jews who had entered America around the turn of the century were beginning to enter the professions. In a day and age when college, particularly in the East, was still largely a gentleman's prerogative, these highly motivated and intelligent young Jews in the eastern cities represented a serious threat to the relaxed, "gentlemanly" college way of life.

As early as 1910 four Jewish professors were dismissed from the Medical Department of Washington University under circumstances that indicate prejudice, but discrimination against Jews in the medical area did not peak until the 1920s and 1930s. Shortly after World War I, Harvard University appointed a "Sifting Committee," which placed a quota on Jews in order to maintain what it felt was a proper balance within the student body. Whereas Harvard openly limited Jewish students, most other institutions resorted to subterfuge to achieve the same ends. An article in the *Nation* in June 1922 pointed out that within a short period Columbia and New York University had reduced the percentage of Jewish students by over 50 percent.[19]

In most schools, admissions committees and officers quickly and unofficially limited the entrance of Jewish applicants. Where quota systems were more or less official, it was argued that admitting students on a competitive basis to the private eastern schools might result in a 50 percent Jewish enrollment, a situation thought to be socially unacceptable.[20] Although periodic protests led to occasional investigations, discrimination against Jewish students continued at all levels in colleges and universities during the 1920s and 1930s. It was particularly acute in medicine, since the AMA's fight to reduce the number of doctors was proving all too successful.

In 1930 Dr. Frank Gavin of the General Theological Seminary asserted that it was three times as hard for a Jewish male student to enter medical school than for other male applicants, and he denounced the application of a quota system in an area "where the best competence and ability must be secured for the public good." In response, a revealing article in the *Literary Digest* maintained that there was little point to admitting Jewish students since non-Jews would not consult Jewish physicians. Four years later, in 1934, *School and Society*, citing the high percentage of Jewish applicants to medical schools and the restrictions placed on them by foreign governments and state legislatures, advised Jewish premedical students to seek fields other than medicine.[21] All too aware of this discrimination, Jewish medical students fled overseas, with most of them attending British medical schools. Scottish medical schools attracted the great majority of Jewish American students in Great Britain. In 1938, for example, over five hundred American medical students, nearly all Jewish, were enrolled in the medical schools of Glasgow and Edinburgh.[22]

The rise of Hitler, rather than shocking Americans into an awareness of the full implications of anti-Semitism, gave an added stimulus to it. Since American Jews were concentrated in the northeastern cities, policies that restricted the number of admissions from large cities, certain geographic areas, or out of state all served to keep the number of Jewish students to a minimum. School officials who disclaimed the anti-Semitism implicit in their actions resorted to sophistry by arguing that a disproportionate number of Jews in medicine and law would breed resentment; thus, they claimed, the quota system was in the best interest of Jews.[23]

As the full horror of the consequences of German anti-Semitism was revealed in the mid-1940s, overt discrimination began to fade. Nonetheless, studies conducted by the New York Department of Education and the State Board of Regents in 1950 and 1952 still showed some discrimination. Within a few years, however, almost 50 percent of students in the state's nine medical schools were Jewish.[24] By the 1960s the quota system generally had been abandoned throughout America, and, although far too much latent anti-Semitism still exists, discrimination against Jewish applicants to medical schools today has been significantly reduced.

CHAPTER 20

The Medical Profession in the Twentieth Century

FOR MOST OF THEIR HISTORY Americans had emphasized practicality as against "book learning," but the new
age of science and industry gave respectability to specialized knowledge. In consequence the twentieth century witnessed a general rise of
professionalism as dozens of new professions were added to the three
traditional ones of theology, medicine, and law. Medicine benefited
from this development, as well as from the rising standard of living,
but it also strengthened its prestige by claiming for itself the mantle
of science. In addition to these basic factors, the medical profession
contributed notably to improving its social and economic position by
successful drives to improve the quality of medical education and to
limit entrance into the profession.

A major effect of all these changes has been an enormous improvement in the level of medical care for the average patient. Physicians of
today are far better trained than their predecessors at the turn of the
century and have a great many more, and far better, medical therapeutics at their command. Their comprehension of all forms of disease
is infinitely greater, and their diagnostic ability is now supported by
a host of technological devices and medical techniques undreamed of
a hundred years ago. Specialization has broadened medical knowledge
and vastly improved medical and surgical techniques. Whereas drugs
were formerly discovered by trial and error, today pharmacologists and
other scientists literally tailor them to combat specific medical conditions. Within the lifetime of the author the life expectancy of diabetics

was fifteen years, tuberculosis was viewed with horror, and pneumonia was referred to as the friend of the aged. Our medical care system is far from perfect, but few of us would want to return to the health care of 1900.

As the foregoing shows, higher professional standards contributed notably to raising the level of health care in the long run, but their immediate effect was limited. Although stronger licensing regulations curtailed the number of individuals entering the profession, thousands of poorly trained doctors continued to practice. Richard H. Shryock, who spent a good part of his life studying the history of American medicine, estimated that the ratio of physicians to population was excessive at least until 1910.[1] As weaker medical schools were eliminated and the number of medical graduates was reduced, physicians' incomes slowly rose, only to fall again with the onset of the Great Depression. The prosperity engendered by the New Deal and World War II steadily increased the demand for medical services. The families of factory workers, clerks, and other lower-income groups who had formerly seen doctors only in emergencies were now beginning to visit physicians for checkups, minor ailments, and vaccinations. By the late 1930s physicians' incomes began to rise at a rate well in excess of rising prices, and by the 1950s medicine was at least one of the highest paid professions, a position it maintains today. Although the AMA and its constituent societies fought against Medicare and Medicaid, these two federal programs have proven a boon to the medical profession. Along with the growth of for-profit and nonprofit health insurance organizations, they have increased the demand for medical services and eliminated much of the need for charitable work.

Following the major drive to establish licensure laws in the late nineteenth and early twentieth centuries, the licensing system has made only slight gains, largely as a result of higher requirements for medical degrees. Medical licensure boards have not been receptive to changes. For example, they failed to meet the challenge raised by the multiplication of specialties. Fortunately, specialists, led by the ophthalmologists, who established a national examining board in 1916, took the initiative and began certifying those qualified to practice. State examining boards also neglected still another important consideration, the need for busy practitioners to keep abreast of the constant changes in medicine. In this instance medical schools stepped in and provided refresher courses. Since these courses are optional, they are only a partial answer.

In the past—and even today—those physicians most in need of additional training are frequently the ones least interested and least willing to spare the time.[2]

The problem of quackery has been and still is a difficult one for medical licensing boards, although the boards are only partially to blame. Prosecution depends upon the willingness of patients, local authorities, and district attorneys to press charges, and even when charges are brought, a complicated legal fight often ensues. In the 1920s several newspapers and magazines ran exposés on diploma mills, revealing the weaknesses of licensing boards. Two states, Connecticut and Missouri, were notorious for issuing bogus medical degrees and licenses. A reporter for the St. Louis *Star* in 1923 applied to a diploma mill posing as a coal salesman looking for an easier job. For $25 he obtained a high school diploma and for $1,200 he was given a medical diploma.[3] Missouri, which had a long history of disreputable medical schools, was ranked at the bottom by the AMA's Council on Medical Education.

Another major weakness of American medical licensing laws has always been their diversity. Even today licensing is handled by fifty-five separate jurisdictions. The AMA sought to standardize qualifications for medical practice in 1915 by establishing a National Board of Medical Examiners. The board, which included representatives of the AMA, the Association of American Medical Colleges, the American College of Surgeons, and the Federation of State Medical Boards, began giving examinations on a voluntary basis the following year. In the first five years the examinations were taken by only 325 students, of whom 269 passed. As the better schools recognized the value of the program, more students applied. By 1940 about one-fourth of all medical students were taking the examinations, and the concept of national board examinations was gradually gaining acceptance. As of 1989 medical board examinations of one type or another were administered to students from 120 of the 127 medical schools in the United States. Not only do they serve to evaluate students, but they are also useful in judging the relevance of the curriculum.[4]

The licensing of physicians is far better today than it was at the beginning of the century, but much remains to be done. One of the more serious problems is the failure in far too many cases of state licensing boards to discipline physicians guilty of crimes of moral turpitude or malpractice. The boards are generally dominated by physicians and tend to hold their sessions behind closed doors. Aside from the fact that physicians, who are constantly making value judgments, are reluctant to criticize their colleagues, licensing boards generally have only limited budgets and seldom have the personnel necessary to make a case strong enough to stand up in court. In 1982 a newspaper reporter checking on the Healing Arts Commission, the agency responsible for regulating physicians in the District of Columbia, discovered that it had revoked only two doctors' licenses in the previous five years, one of which subsequently had been restored. In defense of its record, the chairman of the commission stated that lack of staff made it impossible to act even on cases involving criminal actions.[5]

A 1988 investigation of the Maryland Commission on Medical Discipline found a comparable situation. In 1986 a gynecologist was convicted of raping a patient. The Maryland Commission took up the case seven months later and voted to allow him to practice gynecology as long as a chaperone was present. An examination of the 157 formal disciplinary actions taken by the commission during the previous twenty years showed that Maryland physicians rarely lost their licenses, even when convicted of crimes of moral turpitude or found to be incompetent.[6] Moreover, licensing boards seldom revoke licenses for negligence or incompetence. The executive director of the Louisiana Board of Medical Examiners stated in September 1990 that the state board sometimes requires doctors with malpractice histories to take continuing education or to participate in risk management programs, but that those physicians do not usually face formal sanctions. Reflecting the limited budget and staff shortages characteristic of so many state boards, the director added that the state board was hiring a medical consultant and director of investigations to help in its oversight of the medical profession.[7]

Hospital review boards exercise some control over medical practice through peer review, but they are reluctant to revoke the privileges of physicians providing substandard care since a decision to do so could involve the hospital in a costly lawsuit. Federal guidelines effective in 1990 require hospitals to report any actions against physicians both to federal authorities and to state boards. These guidelines, however, do nothing about the threat of court action against a hospital that revokes the privileges of one of its physicians, nor will notifying state boards have much effect unless the boards are made far more effective. An equally serious problem is that even when a physician loses his or her license, the individual need only move to another state and reapply. The differing state licensing requirements create still another problem. America is a mobile society, but since licensing is a state prerogative and certain states do not offer reciprocity, the movement of physicians around the country is somewhat limited.[8] Until standardized state licensing laws are enacted or a national qualifying board is created, these problems will remain.

By 1920 the reorganized AMA had become an effective organization and a powerful lobby. It had already flexed its muscles by gaining victories over quackery and harmful proprietary drugs. The first success came when it joined forces with Harvey W. Wiley, Samuel Hopkins Adams, and other progressives to pass the 1906 Food and Drugs Act, a relatively weak measure but one marking the first broad federal action in the area. Assisted by state and federal drug officials, the AMA continued the struggle to expose quackery and strengthen the drug laws. Although some progress was made, it took a national drug scandal in the 1930s over "Elixir Sulfanilamide," a mixture of the new wonder drug with a poisonous solvent that brought a horrible death to at least 107 individuals, to bring about a major revision of the 1906 act. This tragedy, in conjunction with agitation by the Food and Drug Administration, women's organizations, and other interested individuals and groups, resulted in passage of the Food, Drug, and Cosmetic Act of 1938, a much stronger law.[9]

In the late 1950s Senator Estes Kefauver of Tennessee began hearings on the profits of the drug industry, but he was also interested in the danger inherent in the distribution of new and powerful drugs. His campaign for stronger control over drugs was strengthened by another major tragedy, the thalidomide affair. This drug was submitted to the Food and Drug Administration for clearance as a sleeping tablet, sedative, and anti-emetic in pregnancy. Dr. Frances O. Kelsey of the FDA had doubts about the drug and refused to give it clearance until she had made a thorough check. In the meantime the drug company distributed thousands of samples to physicians for clinical testing. Upon hearing of the birth of deformed babies to women in England and Germany who had taken thalidomide, Dr. Kelsey issued public warnings about the drug. Thanks to Dr. Kelsey, the drug was never officially placed on the market, but the samples that were distributed may have resulted in a number of deformed infants. At a time when Kefauver's campaign against the drug industry was losing headway, the thalidomide incident revived public interest, and on October 10, 1962, the Kefauver-Harris

Drug Amendments unanimously passed both houses of Congress. The result was to strengthen the Food and Drug Administration's control over the licensing of new drugs and to aid in its fight against quackery.[10]

The optimism shared by drug reformers in the late 1960s did not last long. The past twenty years have seen the cultural climate become receptive to a wide variety of health fads and quackery. In these same years the AMA, one of the early watchdogs against quackery, abolished its quackery committee and closed its Department of Investigation. Insofar as the federal government was concerned, the Reagan administration's policy of deregulation worked all too well. The Federal Trade Commission virtually made no effort to restrain false advertising related to health, and the Food and Drug Administration, faced with new responsibilities and limited budgets, reduced its spending to combat health fraud to an absolute minimum. Consequently, the problem of quackery, if anything, is larger than ever. In 1990 estimates of the cost of quackery placed the figure at somewhere between twenty and thirty billion dollars.

The FDA's struggle with Laetrile, a quack cancer cure, illustrates public suspicion both of the medical profession and the federal government in the 1970s and 1980s. Led by members of the extreme right, Laetrile's supporters battled in the courts, state legislatures, and Congress to legalize this so-called cure, and by the early 1980s they had managed to secure laws giving it special status in half the states. In the meantime the FDA was subjected to barrages of bitter criticism in the news media and legislative halls. The public gradually lost interest in Laetrile, but it quickly turned to other forms of quackery. The new cancer quacks emphasize the need to avoid "unnatural" treatments such as surgery and radiation and offer a multiple approach through diet, internal irrigation, natural drugs, and mind control.[11]

One major piece of progressive legislation that aroused the interest of the AMA was health insurance. Several European countries had already established some form of compulsory health insurance, when the Progressive Party in 1912 espoused the concept. Despite the disappearance of the party after the election, health insurance became a significant political issue. The AMA's journal and its national officers were at first supportive, and several state societies formally endorsed compulsory health insurance. Beginning about 1917 this favorable climate of opinion shifted drastically. Precisely why this occurred is still a matter of debate. James G. Burrow, in his history of the AMA, attributes it to the end of Progressivism, preoccupation with World War I and the League of Nations, and the general conservative reaction that followed. Ronald L. Numbers in his account of the affair adds additional factors, for he believes that the rising income of physicians between 1916 and 1919 made health insurance far less attractive. For example, the taxable income of physicians in Wisconsin rose 41 percent between 1916 and 1919. Another reason for this shift in opinion, according to Numbers, is that most physicians, having watched the movement sweep through Europe, felt at first that health insurance was inevitable, but, as Progressivism waned in the United States and private medicine became more lucrative, they became reluctant to try an unknown system. Whatever the case, the majority of physicians rejected compulsory insurance, and their views were soon reflected in the AMA journal. In 1920 the AMA officially went on record as opposing any plan of compulsory health insurance—a view that it maintained until recent years.[12]

A medical profession by its nature must be conservative. In dealing with life-and-death situations, one can scarcely undertake experiments lightly. Yet in health and social concerns organized medicine in the nineteenth and early twentieth centuries generally supported the liberal viewpoint. Physicians individually and collectively advocated sanitary measures, public health laws, regulation of food and drugs, and the collection of vital statistics. In addition, they helped establish and support hospitals, clinics, and dispensaries—nearly all of which provided free medical care for the lower-income groups. At the turn of the century physicians began having doubts about making medical care too readily available for the working poor. As educational qualifications gradually restricted the practice of medicine to the middle and upper classes, the profession turned against all forms of social legislation except for those relating directly to the quality of medical care. In the 1920s the AMA fought against the Sheppard-Towner Act, which provided federal subsidies to encourage states to establish maternal and child health programs. It opposed the law establishing Veterans Hospitals in 1924 on the grounds that the bill proposed to offer medical care for non-service-connected disabilities. As group hospitalization plans developed in the 1920s, the AMA first expressed qualms about them, and, as they began to succeed, by 1930 was denouncing them as socialistic and unworkable.[13]

The Great Depression forced the AMA to modify its views somewhat. Although accepting most of the principles embodied in the Social

Security legislation of the 1930s, it constantly warned about the danger of governmental encroachment upon medical care. It also deplored the relatively large sums voted for maternal and child care and for aid to dependent children. The social and economic problems of the Depression created a public awareness of health, since economic, social, and health problems are inextricably entwined. The idea of compulsory health insurance again came to the fore, and the AMA promptly launched a counterattack. One of its main themes was the purported failure of the British system, a theme that disregarded favorable reports by many individuals and such organizations as the American College of Dentists and the Michigan State Medical Society.[14]

In response to accumulating evidence that a high percentage of Americans received little or no medical care, the AMA conducted its own survey and declared that the only citizens receiving inferior care were those under the jurisdiction of government agencies. In 1938, a time when Mississippi's physician-to-population ratio was half the national average and the state's per capita income was only about two hundred dollars, an AMA report concluded "that there is practically no one in Mississippi who cannot secure medical care regardless of the ability to pay." The report did concede that hospital facilities for blacks were limited.[15] As political pressure began to build in support of a national health bill in the late 1930s, the AMA softened its earlier opposition to voluntary health insurance programs, recognizing that these programs offered the only alternative to a compulsory one.

By this time the United States was involved in World War II, and the AMA performed creditably in helping mobilize medical resources. One of its major contributions was to insist on medical deferments for medical students. At the end of the war it advocated refresher courses and other means to assist physicians returning to civilian practice. While doubtful about proposals to increase the number of medical schools, the AMA did support passage of the Hill-Burton Act in 1946, which provided subsidies for hospital construction. When the Cold War raised prospects of attacks on the American mainland, the AMA helped organize an emergency medical service program. It was also instrumental in helping to weed out corruption and inefficiency in the Veterans Administration in the postwar years. On the international scene it gave active support to the World Medical Association and the World Health Organization.

The end of the World War II once more brought the issue of health care to the fore, and again the AMA rallied its forces to fight socialized medicine. The basic problem, as Rosemary Stevens perceptively observed some twenty years ago, is that while the private fee-for-service practice was suitable for a simpler age, the medical profession failed to realize that the growth of specialism, the expansion of new health professions, and social changes in the twentieth century required structural adjustments in the medical care system. Throughout this century far too many physicians have continued to envision medical care in terms of the classic picture of the physician by the bedside of the patient. By the mid-sixties, physicians represented a minority of those providing medical care, since for every physician there were approximately four other health professionals. Had physicians been more realistic, Stevens suggested, they could have emerged as the skilled manager of a medical care team, one that included social workers, consultants, and technicians. Instead, by refusing to face the social facts of medicine, physicians may have placed their professional authority in even greater danger.[16]

Paul Starr asserts that the expansion of hospitals between 1940 and 1960 was mutually beneficial to both physicians and hospitals. From the physicians' standpoint, hospital practice enabled them to improve their financial position by seeing far more patients. The expansion of hospitals also created a demand for more interns at a time when medical enrollments were decreasing. To attract interns, unaffiliated community hospitals sought medical school connections. This in turn led to the emergence of medical school empires in which the chairpersons of major departments assumed control of policy making. In more recent years the emergence of corporate medicine in the form of multihospital systems, investor-owned chains, and HMOs now threatens the power of both independent hospitals and physicians. According to Starr, the medical profession, which still fears government regulation, faces its real threat today from the rise of corporate medicine.[17]

Starting with the Wagner-Murray-Dingell Bill in 1943, national health insurance was pushed strongly for the next few years. When Truman proposed a national health insurance program in 1945, he was careful to assure the public that his program was not socialized medicine, insisting that no change would be involved in medical and hospital services. Despite his efforts to appease physicians, the AMA denounced his proposal in the bitterest terms. The AMA's reaction was even stronger when Truman made health insurance an issue in the 1948 election. It promptly employed a public relations agency and began a full-scale campaign involving speakers' bureaus, pamphlets, press releases, and a variety of other methods to defeat the program. It continued to resist all similar bills throughout the 1950s, although it reluctantly accepted, as the lesser of evils, the Kerr-Mills bill providing limited federal funds to help states pay for medical costs of the aged.[18]

The Democratic victory in 1960 renewed the drive for a national health program. The AMA once again issued a call to arms and fought a rearguard battle against rising public support for a federal program to provide medical care for the aged. Although unsuccessful in stopping the proposed legislation, it did manage to modify the laws in accordance with its own views. In consequence, in 1965 the Social Security laws were amended to include Medicare and Medicaid. Medicare, which became effective in 1966, provides hospital and medical services to members of the Social Security system who have reached the age of sixty-five and who pay a small monthly fee. Medicaid allocates federal assistance to state medical programs for the indigent. Although Medicare made no attempt at a major revision of the medical care system, it demonstrated that the public would henceforth have a voice in determining the nation's health policy.[19]

Even though many health programs opposed by organized medicine have been enacted in the past sixty years, the AMA has played a decisive role in shaping them. Throughout these changes it has successfully preserved a large measure of private practice and the fee system; yet it has not been able to prevent encroachments by government, institutions, and corporations. Members of the armed forces, millions of veterans, and other groups are already receiving direct medical care under government auspices, and the number of group practices, health maintenance organizations, and corporate medical industries is growing. Judging by recent articles in medical journals, today's physicians, unlike their predecessors, recognize that there are serious problems with the American health care system, and that the multiplicity of overlapping government and private agencies engaged in health care is not only wasteful but does not provide adequate medical care for over thirty to forty million Americans.

In 1987 an article in the *New England Journal of Medicine* declared that the entire medical system was in need of drastic reform. The following year a series of letters in the same journal debated the issue of a national medical system. By 1990 the articles and letters in *JAMA* and the *New England Journal of Medicine* no longer debated whether to reform the medical care system, but how best to do it. Among the articles citing weaknesses in the present system was one, based on a study of some 600,000 patients in representative hospitals, that demonstrated that uninsured patients were far less likely to undergo each of five high-cost or high-discretion procedures than those with insurance. Another study estimated that health care administrative costs in the United States were 60 percent higher than in Canada and 97 percent higher than in Great Britain. Two other authors compared the Canadian and American medical systems and reported that although American physicians' fees were three times higher than those of Canadian physicians, their income was only one-third higher. They ascribed the difference to a much greater overhead and a lower workload for American physicians. In May 1991, *JAMA* devoted an entire issue to discussing various options for reforming or replacing the present method of health care. An editorial in the same issue declared that a survey made by *JAMA* showed most people favoring some type of universal medical care. There was no general agreement, however, on what form it should take.[20]

In terms of prestige the American medical profession probably reached its zenith around 1960. The picture of the white-coated physician had come to represent the epitome of science, and the profession was still basking in the glory arising from the discovery of "miracle" drugs and other medical advances of the previous twenty or so years. Ironically these same advances were, and still are, responsible in part for the continuing rise in medical costs. The development of sophisticated diagnostic, supportive, and therapeutic devices is an expensive process, and their operation and maintenance necessitates highly specialized technicians and paraprofessionals. Delicate and elaborate surgical procedures require not only years of training on the part of surgeons but also a large supportive cast, such as surgical nurses and anesthetists, and the present radiation and chemotherapy procedures are far removed from the simple prescriptions of fifty or sixty years ago. Thus, the medical advances that have done so much to improve health and extend life have also raised the cost of medical care.

By the 1970s the rising cost of medicine, along with the corrosive effect of the Vietnam War and the economic problems it created, tended to throw the affluence of the medical profession into sharp focus. At the same time the refusal of organized medicine to recognize that the American health care system did not adequately provide for millions of

Americans and its consistent opposition to all government measures to provide direct health care caused it to lose some of its prestige. Another development that has tarnished the image of the medical profession has been the escalation of malpractice suits. These suits have also added significantly to the rising cost of medicine. To the average American juror, insurance companies are vague conglomerations of wealth, and he or she has little compunction about distributing this wealth to individual citizens. The increasing affluence of physicians and the steady rise in medical fees undoubtedly predisposes the ordinary juror to favor the plaintiff in malpractice cases. Insurance companies, too, have added to the rash of suits by their willingness to settle many unjustifiable ones out of court, thus encouraging the filing of "nuisance" suits. And since insurance companies traditionally have passed on additional costs to their clients, they have had little incentive to minimize either the cost or number of suits.

While insurance companies share part of the blame, an even greater share can be attributed to the legal profession. The ratio of lawyers to population is several times higher in the United States than any other country, and it is more than a coincidence that our ratio of malpractice suits is also much greater. The contingency fee system, which allows lawyers to collect 30 to 40 percent of the settlement, has also encouraged a small number of lawyers to institute many unnecessary and unwarranted suits.

A basic reason for the growth of malpractice suits probably results from fundamental changes in health delivery. Despite the medical profession's constant emphasis upon the doctor-patient relationship, the close personal contact between the physician and patient is steadily diminishing. Urban society by its nature is impersonal, and the patient who may see his surgeon for a few minutes before surgery and his physician only occasionally, in the course of an office visit, scarcely has the same relationship that existed when family doctors regularly visited the homes of their patients. Moreover, heavy caseloads, combined with the use of laboratory tests and paramedical personnel, have tended to make office visits merely brief encounters. The high degree of specialization has also furthered the impersonalization of medicine. The dermatologists, urologists, or other specialists who constantly see new patients can scarcely develop a close personal identification with them. The nature of the specialists' training, too, tends to make them see cases rather than individuals.

The multiplication of specialists may have increased the possibility for discovering cases of malpractice. In the days when the family practitioner took major responsibility for medical care, if a patient died or suffered complications it was assumed that the physician had done all that was possible and there the matter rested. Whereas the family doctor was a close friend and advisor, the practitioner today is too often simply another professional for whom the patient has limited regard.

Had the medical profession been more zealous in policing its membership, the malpractice situation may not have become so acute. Unscrupulous and incompetent individuals exist in every profession, but the nature of medicine requires that this number be kept to an absolute minimum. Unfortunately, by permitting the existence of a few incompetents, the profession has opened the way to both justifiable and unwarranted malpractice suits. Before criticizing the medical profession, one should examine other professions. The public's apparent concern about the ethics of lawyers can scarcely be without some foundation. The American Association of University Professors has never dropped anyone from membership because of bad teaching, nor, judging by the many business frauds, have accountants and chambers of commerce paid much attention to the ethics of business. In justification of the medical profession, it should be pointed out that despite all scientific developments and the use of sophisticated instruments and laboratory techniques, medicine is still an art, and much of what a physician does is a matter of judgment. While cases of gross negligence or flagrant incompetence are fairly clearcut, defining the line between good and bad judgment is a matter of judgment itself. Precisely because physicians are constantly making judgments themselves, they are hesitant to question those of their fellow practitioners. Unfortunately, this attitude has only increased public suspicion of the profession.

Aside from the direct costs of malpractice suits, the indirect costs may be almost as large. In the first place they have forced physicians to practice defensive medicine. Expensive biopsies and other laboratory tests are frequently ordered by physicians in routine cases simply as a matter of protection. A second cost to society is that malpractice insurance rates in a field such as obstetrics are at a point where many obstetricians are giving up the practice, and general practitioners can scarcely afford the risk of delivering babies, creating acute problems for many prospective mothers. A final social cost is the loss of the services of many first-rate older physicians who would normally practice on a part-time basis, but who can no longer do so because of the expense of malpractice insurance.

The affluence of physicians, particularly in the past twenty years, has enabled many of them to invest in a wide variety of health care entities, such as clinical laboratories, diagnostic imaging centers, radiation and physical therapy centers, and ambulatory surgical facilities. Federal and state studies have demonstrated that joint ventures—facilities owned by physicians or those in which they share ownership—tend to have higher charges and that the physician owners order far more tests. For example, a recent study by the Office of the Inspector General involving four thousand physicians in seven states found that Medicare patients of physicians with financial interests in freestanding clinical laboratories underwent 34 percent more tests than the general population of Medicare patients. A similar two-year study by the Florida State Health Care Cost Containment Board showed that Medicare patients of physicians involved in joint ventures received 40 percent more tests. Moreover, it is not a question of a few greedy individuals ordering such evaluations, since the Florida study showed that over 40 percent of the state's doctors had financial interests in health care facilities.[21] Somewhat belatedly, the AMA has questioned the ethics of joint ventures, but it has not proscribed them. Aside from contributing to raising medical costs, this situation has heightened public hostility to the medical profession.

Despite these factors, the medical profession still ranks among the most prestigious of all occupations. Its status rests in part on developments in the biomedical sciences. Without doubt the quality of medical care provided by physicians is far better today than that provided even sixty years ago and many times improved over that of a hundred years ago. Physicians are highly trained and have a greater level of competence than their predecessors earlier in the century. While specialism may have helped to impersonalize medicine, it has also guaranteed a higher level of medical care. The profession's armamentarium in terms of drug therapy, medical devices, and surgical technique has grown explosively, and with it has come a corresponding improvement in medical care.

The medical profession is conservative, but the public perception of it as ultraconservative has been conditioned largely by the policies of the AMA. A major turning point in the attitude of the profession came with the adoption of Medicare. A poll taken in New York shortly before congressional action on the Medicare bill showed only 38 percent of physicians supporting it; five years later 92 percent of physicians polled voted in favor of the program. Recent surveys show that the majority of physicians accept group practice, peer review, HMOs, and a system incorporating nurse-practitioners, midwives, and physicians' assistants.[22] Whereas the AMA during the Great Depression, in the face of all evidence to the contrary, consistently maintained that medical care was available to everyone and continued to oppose all government health insurance proposals as late as the 1970s and 1980s, today the AMA is proposing a comprehensive program called Health Access America. Dr. James Todd, acting top executive of the AMA, concedes that physician price controls ("practice parameters") will be necessary under any major government health program, but he feels that the membership will reluctantly accept them. The AMA, however, no longer speaks with authority for the medical profession, since its membership has fallen from 73 percent of American physicians in the 1960s to only 43 percent in 1990.[23] Yet in its willingness to recognize that the traditional system of private practice leaves far too many Americans without adequate medical care it may well be speaking for the profession.

The medical profession has made remarkable gains in the course of the twentieth century. From an impoverished and barely respectable group, it has moved into preeminence among the professions in terms of affluence and prestige. This success has tended to make it politically and socially conservative, and for the past seventy years the organized medical profession has had a record of opposing virtually every piece of progressive legislation. Since the word "progressive" tends to connote the assumption of government responsibility for health, education, and welfare, one can argue that the medical profession may well be fighting for traditional American values with their emphasis on individual responsibility and initiative. Historically, as societies became more complex, life became more regulated. Every new development spawns a multitude of laws, regulations, ordinances, and administrative rulings, and medical care can scarcely escape such effects.

CHAPTER 21

The Community's Health

FROM EARLIEST COLONIAL DAYS American communities have taken measures to promote the health of their citizens. For the first three centuries health laws fell into three main categories: sanitation, quarantine, and the regulation of food supplies and markets. The motive for sanitary laws was a mixture of esthetics and a wish to promote health. It had become evident early in history that dirt and crowding were conducive to sickness, and it was even more clear that the presence of garbage, dead animals, and overflowing privies were offensive to the senses. In the second category were the quarantine laws. Until the bacteriological revolution in the late nineteenth century, pestilences were strange and unaccountable phenomena. A number of theories were posited to explain them, but the public was convinced that epidemics spread from person to person, and that disease could be kept out through quarantine laws or avoided by isolating the sick. Consequently, beginning in the late seventeenth century, colonial legislatures enacted a series of quarantine measures. The third category of health laws, those relating to the food supply, included town ordinances prohibiting the sale of "blowne" meat or putrid fish, regulating the price and weight of loaves of bread, and measures to keep the public markets in a sanitary condition.

Fortunately towns and cities in the colonial period were never as crowded and dirty as their European counterparts, and as a result the colonists enjoyed relatively good health. The immediate post-Revolutionary years saw a rapid increase in urban population and an even greater increase in sanitary problems. More important in terms of public health was the series of devastating yellow fever outbreaks that occurred in every American port from New England to Georgia during the years from 1793 to 1806. These repeated attacks led to the formation of the first temporary boards of health and the appointment of the first permanent health officers. The latter consisted usually of a health (quarantine) officer of the port and a port physician. In addition to the usual quarantine and sanitary measures, civic officials, reflecting the paternalism of colonial days, went to great lengths to provide medical care for the sick and food and shelter for their families. Once yellow fever was no longer a threat, the health boards ceased to exist, most of the laws fell into abeyance, and the two health offices became political plums. In the South, where the yellow fever attacks intensified, the port health officers were under constant pressure to minimize any restrictions on shipping.[1]

The rise of the industrial revolution in the early nineteenth century brought with it the concept of rugged individualism, one that emphasized a minimum role for government. In America its effects were exaggerated by the rise of Jacksonian democracy with its anti-intellectual and antimonopolistic spirit. The industrial revolution also brought large numbers of rural Americans and immigrants into towns and cities ill-prepared to handle the influx. Jammed into old and dilapidated housing and forced to rely on shallow water wells or hydrants located a block or two away, these poorly paid workers, living in incredibly brutal conditions, became a class apart from the middle and upper groups. Conscious of their own rectitude, the latter blamed the high morbidity and mortality rates among the poor upon their intemperance and filthy living conditions.

Little was done about the deplorable state of the city slums except on the occasional appearance of a deadly epidemic disorder. Two major Asiatic cholera outbreaks swept through the United States, one in 1832–33 and the second in 1849–50. In each case civic officials reacted by appointing temporary boards of health and instituting large-scale programs to cleanse their cities and eliminate the worst sanitary abuses. Once the danger was past, the abuses quickly reappeared. The second cholera epidemic, which coincided with the beginning of the sanitary movement, did provide the sanitary reformers with ammunition, and for the rest of the century the threat of cholera continued to give an impetus to sanitary reform.[2]

The first step to improve health conditions was to determine the level of health in the community, and this required the collection of vital statistics. A group of New Yorkers in 1836 took the initiative by founding the New York Statistical Society. The society survived only briefly, but its work was picked up by Lemual Shattuck, Dr. Edward Jarvis, and other Boston reformers. They organized the American Statistical Society, and Jarvis and Shattuck then joined forces to pressure the state legislature into passing the Massachusetts Registration Act of 1842. The law established a system for registering vital statistics, and Shattuck played a major role in shaping both the law and the resulting system. Shattuck's method for collecting vital statistics in Massachusetts set the pattern for registration systems in other states.[3]

By the mid-nineteenth century a number of American physicians— men such as Jarvis of Massachusetts, John H. Griscom and Elisha Harris of New York, Edwin M. Snow of Rhode Island, and Edward Barton and J. C. Simonds of New Orleans—were beginning to call attention to the deplorable living conditions of the workers and the desperate need for sanitary reform. Along with cholera, a series of major yellow fever epidemics in the 1850s had ravaged the southern port cities and threatened the entire East Coast. The ever-present danger of these diseases induced another of the sanitarians, Dr. Wilson Jewell of Philadelphia, to call for a national sanitary convention in 1857. The original purpose of the meetings was to standardize the quarantine laws, but in the successive meetings it became clear that the majority of delegates were convinced that the best defense against epidemic diseases was an effective sanitary program. The outbreak of the Civil War in 1861 ended these national meetings and temporarily delayed the movement for reform.[4]

The enormous amount of sickness among both Northern and Southern troops and the success achieved in reducing this sickness through enforcing sanitary regulations in army camps gave renewed strength to the sanitary movement. A major agency promoting camp sanitation during the war was the United States Sanitary Commission, a group of civilian reformers who aided the Union army in many ways, but whose most lasting contribution was to help spread the doctrine of community sanitation and personal hygiene.

By the 1870s the sanitary movement in America was in full swing. New York City in 1866 had created the first permanent board of health and in so doing provided a model for several other major cities. In 1872 the American Public Health Association came into existence, foreshadowing the establishment of public health as a discipline of its own. In response to a series of yellow fever epidemics and the threat of cholera the first national quarantine law was passed in 1878. This same year a major yellow fever outbreak that spread far up the Mississippi Valley prompted Congress to establish the first National Board of Health. Organized in the spring of 1879, the board was essentially a quarantine agency, although its members envisioned a wider purpose. Unfortunately it fell afoul of state and local health officials who were jealous of its authority, and of the United States Marine Hospital Service, whose officials also saw the National Board as a potential threat. Moreover the idea of the federal government dabbling in social concerns was counter to the spirit of the day. The result was that the board, although officially in existence until 1893, ran out of funds in 1883 and to all intents and purposes disappeared.[5]

At the state and local level the sanitary reformers were making steady progress. Louisiana had established the first state board of health in 1855, although it was essentially a health board for the City of New Orleans. In 1869 Massachusetts took the lead in establishing an effective board of health with statewide authority.[6] Most of the remaining states quickly followed suit. The majority of state health boards functioned primarily in an advisory capacity, since they had virtually no funding and very little authority. Most state boards accomplished little, but in a few states, where the health commissioner or president of the board was a strong individual, considerable progress was made in establishing public health programs at the city or town level. By the 1880s health officials were beginning to widen their concerns to include urban housing, air pollution, the health of infants and schoolchildren, and vital statistics. The first chemical laboratories appeared to test food and water, and health inspectors began checking on tenement housing, privies, plumbing, food-processing plants, and other possible sources of disease.

This cheerful picture of steady progress in community health had little to do with life in the United States in the nineteenth century. The rapid growth of urban areas had as its corollary a comparable increase in human misery. The well-to-do generally moved out of their old homes to new ones on the outskirts of the city, leaving their former residences to be occupied by an influx of workers seeking employment. As these houses overflowed, newcomers were forced to move into barns, stables, old factory buildings, and any other available type of shelter. In the second half of the century entrepreneurs began building multistory tenements, most of which had neither water nor any other amenities, and in which windows and ventilation were sadly deficient. It is a commentary on such conditions that New York, a relatively progressive city, passed a law in 1887 requiring new tenements to have one water closet or privy for every fifteen persons.[7]

There is scarcely an American city without its horror stories describing the squalid circumstances in which a good share of its inhabitants lived. In one small area of Chicago in the 1890s there were 811 sleeping rooms without outside windows and less than 3 percent of families had their own bathrooms. The *Weekly Medical Review* reported that the industrial workers were compelled to live in tainted tenements or "low fetid hovels, amidst poverty, hunger and dirt," where "in foulness, want and crime, crowded humanity suffers, and sickens, and perishes."[8] Dr. Joseph Jones, president of the Louisiana State Board of Health, declared in 1881: "One third of those dying in New Orleans die in poverty, and are buried at the public expense. One sixth of those who die in New Orleans, perish in silence and misery, with no kind companion, no efficient medicine, and no generous physician."[9] New Orleans at this date had no sewerage, a completely inadequate water system, and an inefficient city government.

New York City, which had one of the best municipal health departments, had only limited success in dealing with the health and social problems of its residents. Its teeming tenements produced so much garbage and human wastes that even under the best of conditions horses and wagons would have had difficulty removing them. The situation was compounded by the inefficiency and corruption that pervaded virtually all city governments. Street cleaning and the removal of the contents of privies was still a lucrative form of political patronage in American cities; the result was that in New York and elsewhere the streets and gutters were constantly filled with piles of garbage, dead animals, and the overflow from privies. To add to the distinctive urban atmosphere, dairy barns and stables accumulated huge manure piles, slaughterers let blood drain into the gutters and dumped offal outside their doors, and a host of other so-called "nuisance" industries befouled the atmosphere and created breeding grounds for a myriad of flies.

Nearly all early health leaders remarked on the enormous mortality among infants and children. Their comments were understandable, since the first few decades of the nineteenth century witnessed a steady rise in general urban mortality and an even greater rise in that of children under five years of age. The Boston City Registrar in 1865 compared the number of deaths of children below the age of five to deaths from all age groups and found that the percentage of children's deaths had shown a steady increase, rising from 23.0 percent in the years 1820–24 to a peak of 46.6 percent in 1855–59. Granting questions as to the accuracy of these statistics, infant mortality was on the rise in all major cities during these years and remained a major problem throughout the nineteenth century. The vital registrar of New York City, where the infant death rate was at least as high, in 1879 found it "gratifying, if not entirely satisfactory" that infant mortality had not risen significantly since the establishment of the Board of Health in 1866.[10]

Nothing indicates human degradation and the wastage of infant life better than the large numbers of foundlings picked off the streets of major cities. Foundlings in New York City were cared for by the female inmates of the almshouses and few lived beyond a year. In 1866 a special hospital was built for foundlings, but the infant mortality rate continued to average around 60 percent. In 1897 when the hospital was under attack, the Commissioner of Charities blandly stated that the 96 percent mortality rate was "not as bad as it looks," since many children were sick on arrival and others had been sent there to spare the parents the cost of a funeral. He further explained that limited funds compelled the institution to use women from the workhouse who mistreated the babies.[11]

In rural areas and small towns, health conditions were better for the lower income groups than in the cities. The environment could absorb the limited quantities of garbage and wastes, the water supply was usually safer, fresh air and sunshine were plentiful, and the food supply was generally — although not always — better. In the South, for example, the one-crop system tended to discourage the establishment of vegetable gardens, and tenant and small farmers who did raise chickens and vegetables often sold them for cash. While escaping some of the endemic disorders of the cities — smallpox, measles, mumps, scarlet fever, diphtheria, whooping cough, typhoid and other enteric infections — rural areas were subject to fatal and debilitating forms of malaria.

Scarcely any section of America avoided malaria at sometime in its history, and the disease moved westward with the frontier all the way to California. In 1874 the New Jersey State Health Commissioner declared that malaria was the state's principal medical problem, and it was 1890 before northern Illinois was free of the fever. Even New York City was recording almost 100 deaths annually from malaria as late as 1900, although the disease was usually contracted outside the city.[12] A number of states began antimosquito programs in the early years of the twentieth century, but it was not until the New Deal brought better housing, screening, improved medical care, and a higher standard of living in the 1930s that any real progress was made. The massing of troops in southern army camps in World War II forced the federal government to take decisive action against the threat of malaria. One of the most successful government agencies, the Atlanta-based Office for Malaria Control in War Areas, was largely responsible for the virtual elimination of malaria from the United States. At the end of the war, this agency was transformed into the present Centers for Disease Control.

By 1900 the two great dramatic pestilences that had aroused the most attention, yellow fever and cholera, were no longer a serious threat. One last outbreak of yellow fever occurred in New Orleans in 1905, but by this date the work of Walter Reed and his associates of the United States Marine Hospital Service had demonstrated the *Aedes aegypti* as the vector of the disease, and a massive campaign against mosquitoes soon ended the epidemic. The significance of these two disorders arises from the general fear they aroused. Their successive outbreaks supplied the impetus to the call for the National Sanitary Conventions in the 1850s, the establishment of the New York Metropolitan Board of Health, the first national quarantine law, and the National Board of Health. As late as 1892 the threat of cholera impelled the New York City Council to establish the city's first diagnostic laboratory.[13]

While these more dramatic pestilences drew most attention, a number of endemic disorders brought far more sickness and death. The leading cause of death was pulmonary tuberculosis. Known as consumption, its diagnosis was tantamount to a death sentence, and it was assumed that the only hope was to move to another climate. Koch's discovery of the bacillus in 1882 opened the way for treatment in the twentieth century, but as late as 1930 it was still a serious problem. Smallpox, which had been reduced to minor proportions in the early nineteenth century, began to flare up as the dreadful epidemics of earlier years faded from public memory and people grew careless about vaccination. Renewed drives for vaccination gradually brought it under control by the early twentieth century. In 1959 the World Health Organization began a drive to eliminate smallpox on a worldwide basis. Within approximately twenty years the program had succeeded, one of the great medical triumphs of this century.

Throughout the nineteenth century, diphtheria, scarlet fever, measles, and whooping cough constantly winnowed the ranks of infants and children. The most fatal disorder, diphtheria, showed a rising incidence in the latter part of the century. Fortunately, just as it reached a peak in the 1890s, advances in bacteriology made it possible to diagnose, treat, and finally prevent this fearful children's disease.

Although health conditions for all Americans left much to be desired, for African Americans and other minority groups the situation was far worse. As of 1900 life expectancy at birth for whites was 47.3 years, for nonwhites the figure was 33.0.[14] Some Native Americans were still fighting a hopeless battle to maintain their way of life, and the tribes who had given up the struggle found themselves in a netherland. The old values were gone, but they could not accept those of the whites; hence they eked out a bare living on reservations, beset by disease and alcohol abuse. The case of the blacks was little better. Free blacks in the antebellum area tended to be the lowest of economic classes, and as such were most subject to malnutrition and received the least medical care. The health of slaves in this era depended largely upon the beneficence and intelligence of their masters, but it is a reasonable assumption that it was below that of whites.[15]

The freedom blacks gained by the Civil War brought little if any improvement in their collective health, since any benefits were minimized for most of them by their economic dependence. Without capital or resources and with few skills, the majority were forced into economic peonage, either as free laborers or through the sharecropping system. Whereas most planters had felt some responsibility for the health and welfare of their slaves, they quickly shucked off this responsibility with emancipation. Many former slaves fled to towns and cities, where they encountered the endemic urban contagions and found their economic situation little better.

In the northern cities discrimination forced blacks into the lowest-paying jobs and compelled them to live in the worst slums. While some were able to fight their way out of the poverty cycle, the majority shared the abject misery of the poorest whites. Their economic condition was faithfully reflected in the vital statistics—everywhere their morbidity and mortality rates were far in excess of that of the general population.

Offsetting this grim picture of life in the last two decades of the nineteenth century, these same years saw the professionalization and institutionalization of public health. The American Public Health Association was organized in 1872, and the next thirty years witnessed the appearance of state and local health boards. In this period, too, the bacteriological revolution radically changed both medicine and public health. By the 1890s public health departments were establishing laboratories for diagnostic purposes and were beginning to make vaccines. They were also strengthening many of their existing programs and broadening their activities to include maternal and child health care, diagnostic services for physicians, dispensaries and clinics for the poor, and environmental concerns, and they were beginning to take an interest in occupational health. Health education, too, was becoming a significant part of public health work. The moves into new areas were helped by advances in technology and engineering that enabled health departments to spin off to separate government agencies functions such as garbage collection, water supplies, sewerage, and street cleaning, with health officials maintaining only minimal supervision.

One of the most important of the new fields was health education. Whereas health officials had formally campaigned for sanitary measures to prevent foul miasmas, they now concentrated on educational programs to eliminate pathogenic organisms. Stimulated by a drive against pulmonary tuberculosis, campaigns were organized against the common drinking cup and spitting in public. People were urged to cover their mouths when coughing and to eliminate flies and other insects capable of carrying disease. Health educators taught schoolchildren to brush their teeth and wash their hands and faces, and they emphasized the need for personal hygiene.

Until the twentieth century, public health was essentially an urban phenomenon, but the entrance of the automobile helped inaugurate a new era for rural health. Yet it was the railways that first brought health education to small towns and rural communities. The idea of using a train for health education purposes was first conceived by Dr. Oscar Dowling, president of the Louisiana State Board of Health. In 1910 he secured two cars from a local railway, one as an exhibit and demonstration car and the other to accommodate staff workers, and sent the train on an eight-month tour of the state. At the end of this time he reported that every town of 250 or more inhabitants had been visited.[16] The health train's success prompted a number of other states to follow suit.

Dr. Dowling's health-train tour coincided with the emergence of the first county health departments. The movement for rural public health grew out of the Rockefeller Sanitary Commission's efforts to eliminate hookworm in the South and was given further stimulus in 1914 by the Public Health Service's interest in pellagra and typhoid. As towns and cities began providing safe water, typhoid was becoming largely a rural problem. Both the commission and the health service recognized that any permanent solutions to the health problems in rural areas required the establishment of local health units. In the same decade, 1910–20, the National Tuberculosis Association, the Red Cross, and the United States Children's Bureau began sending public health nurses into rural areas and sponsoring a variety of health programs. Subsequently other foundations and agencies entered the picture. The number of county health units grew slowly, however, until the New Deal and World War II gave a sharp impetus to the rural health movement.

Although laypeople had taken a major role in the British and Continental sanitary movements, in America nearly all of the early leaders had been physicians. The successes gained in the second half of the century, however, had been made possible by the appearance of sanitary associations consisting of business and professional men and middle- and upper-class women. New Orleans depended on trade and commerce, and intelligent businesspersons in the 1880s and 1890s realized that the city's reputation for disease and pestilence was scarcely conducive to encouraging the influx of new capital or business enterprises. In consequence the more enlightened of them began to support the local sanitary association, pushed for expensive water and sewer systems, and generally advocated public health measures. In Memphis, which was devastated by the 1878 yellow fever epidemic and where conditions may have been even worse than in New Orleans, the business community initiated a complete overhaul of the municipal government and instituted major public health reforms.[17] Enlightened self-interest did not characterize all of the business community, but individual members contributed to the health reform movement throughout the country.

While individual physicians had led the public health movement, organized medicine played only a minor part. The leadership of the AMA supported many of the reforms, but the association itself had little political influence until its reorganization in the early years of the twentieth century. As indicated earlier, the reorganized AMA and its constituent societies strongly supported public health legislation so long as it did not interfere with private practice. For example, they co-operated with school medical inspection up to a point. When school nurses and medical inspectors began uncovering an alarming number of medical problems among poor children, health departments began setting up clinics to provide free health services. The medical profession, determined to keep the private fee-for-service system, reacted strongly and succeeded in closing most of these clinics. At the same time these physicians were equally successful in closing the many public dispensaries providing virtually free care to the lower income groups. In the case of the dispensaries, the changing nature of medicine would probably have brought their demise in any case.[18]

Since public health budgets depend upon politics, public health officials out of necessity cannot afford to offend any significant pressure group; hence, as the political power of the medical profession grew, health departments withdrew from the health care area and concentrated on such matters as health education, environmental conditions, inspection of food and water supplies, limited maternal and child programs, medical inspection of children, vaccination programs, and limited screening for diseases.

The federal government, which spent millions of dollars on diseases of farm animals, birds, and plants in the nineteenth century, spent almost nothing on the health of its citizens. The sum total of its contributions were the United States Marine Hospital Service, founded in 1798 to provide for sick seamen, the short-lived National Board of Health, and a weak national quarantine law. The first decade of the twentieth century saw the founding of the Hygienic Laboratory in 1901, the forerunner of the National Institutes of Health, and the passage of the Pure Food and Drug Law of 1906. The next federal action came in 1912 with the creation of the United States Children's Bureau and the transformation of the Marine Hospital Service into the Public Health Service. In this transformation, the Public Health Service was given responsibility for research and investigation of communicable diseases. World War I drew attention to venereal diseases, and a Federal Division of Venereal Diseases was established to assist cities and states in dealing with these infections. The first significant move by the federal government into the health care field came with the Sheppard-Towner Act of 1921. This measure broke new ground by providing grants-in-aid to states instituting maternal and child care programs. In part due to bitter opposition from the AMA, the program was allowed to lapse in 1929.[19]

The New Deal marked the first substantial efforts by the national government to enter the health care area. Almost every New Deal agency, temporary or permanent, made some contributions to health. As early as June 1933 the Federal Emergency Relief Administration authorized the use of its funds for medical care, nursing, and emergency dental work; Civilian Conservation Corps workers received medical care; the Civil Works Administration promoted rural sanitation and helped to control malaria and other diseases; and both the Works Progress Administration and the Public Works Administration built hospitals, health centers, and sewerage plants and contributed to other public health projects. In 1935 Titles V and VI of the Social Security Act authorized the use of federal funds for crippled children, maternal and child care, and the promotion of state and local public health agencies. As health sociologist Roy Lubove has pointed out, the Social Security Act is of special significance, since it established a permanent machinery for distributing federal funds for health purposes and recognized special needs in allocating these funds.[20]

The appropriation for health under the Social Security Administration grew rapidly in the late 1930s, aided by the results of a National Health Survey undertaken in 1935–36. This survey confirmed what earlier ones had shown, that the lowest economic groups suffered the greatest amount of sickness and disability and received the least medical care. Parenthetically, we might note that if all the money spent on rediscovering this fact in the past fifty years had been used for health care, it is quite possible that we would have fewer health problems today. Whatever the case, the survey showed that the average expenditures by states for public health amounted to only eleven cents per capita, and that municipal expenditures were not much higher. The bleak picture presented by this report provided further ammunition for reformers who had already made American health problems a significant political issue. In 1939 the Wagner Bill to establish a national health program was introduced into Congress. President Roosevelt's preoccupation with the war, the opposition of organized medicine, and other factors prevented its passage.

The decade of the 1940s saw limited progress in public health, although general health conditions improved steadily, largely as a result of the wartime and postwar prosperity. The billions of dollars spent on military camps and industries in the South raised the economic standard and health level of the entire region. Efforts to promote a national health program proved abortive, and the only significant steps by the federal government were the Hill-Burton Act of 1946 to promote the construction of hospitals and to start pouring funds into medical research. The tremendous expansion of the armed forces, however, meant that millions of Americans received medical and dental care—for many of them a relatively new experience. In addition, as veterans they were henceforth eligible for health benefits.

The 1950s saw the federal government support the construction of medical and public health schools, appropriate large sums for health research, and in 1953 establish a Department of Health, Education and Welfare. In these years federal spending for health-related services rose dramatically. As of 1960 annual federal expenditures amounted to almost three billion dollars, and by 1970 the figure had risen to approximately twenty billion. The purpose of the Hill-Burton Act was to facilitate the construction of hospitals in rural areas, but Congress steadily broadened the original act. States seeking funds were required to develop statewide hospital plans, but these plans proved meaningless. While the Hill-Burton Act did achieve some success in promoting hospitals in rural areas, the act failed woefully when it decentralized hospital policy and placed it in the hands of local and state leaders, which resulted in the continuing duplication of hospital facilities. Moreover, in response to public demand, Congress continued to enact more patchwork legislation relating to health, adding to the multiplicity of federal agencies involved in some aspect or aspects of health. By 1970 federal health programs were spread over 221 agencies or departments.[21]

The fight for direct health care remained in abeyance during the Republican years, 1952–60, and was not revived until the 1960s. The opening wedge was a bill to provide medical care for the aged—a group whose emotional appeal, while not quite on a par with motherhood, was still high—and, what was possibly more important, a group whose numbers and voting power were increasing. The first success came in 1962 with the passage of the Kerr-Mills Bill, which provided medical care for a limited group of the aged sick. The fight to extend these benefits culminated in the Medicare and Medicaid amendments to the Social Security laws in 1965. Essentially these amendments provided low-cost government subsidized medical insurance for Social Security recipients. In an interesting switch, the AMA and its allies sought to expand the benefits of the Medicare and Medicaid bill in hopes of killing it, while the liberals sought to minimize them in order to guarantee passage of the bill. The result was a far more generous program than the sponsors of the bill had envisioned. The past twenty-five years have seen Medicare and Medicaid steadily broadened to cover more individuals and provide greater benefits. By 1986 Medicare was providing coverage for over twenty-eight million Americans. In the process its budget grew from $4.7 billion in 1967 to $64.6 billion in 1984, and it still continues to grow.[22]

The concept of medical insurance in America dates back to the contract practice of medicine in the nineteenth century, but its present form is of more recent origin. In 1929 a group of teachers in Dallas, Texas, contracted with Baylor University Hospital to provide service benefits at a fixed fee per semester. The idea was picked up by the American Hospital Association in the early 1930s and led directly to the Blue Cross (hospital) and Blue Shield (medical and surgical) programs. As unions and corporations began negotiating health benefits, private corporations moved into the health insurance business. In the succeeding years voluntary health insurance experienced an explosive growth, encouraged in part by the medical profession's acceptance of it.

Growing alongside health insurance came another form of medical care somewhat akin to the former contract practice, the prepaid group practice. Two of the most successful of these are the Kaiser Foundation Health Plan organized in California in 1942 and the Health Insurance Plan of Greater New York dating back to 1947. By 1960 each of these plans was providing complete medical care to over half a million subscribers. Physicians participating in these early health maintenance organizations (HMOs) were subject to considerable pressure from the AMA and local medical societies, but the steady growth of HMOs has forced the medical profession to accept them.[23] Today they supply health care to over thirty million Americans.

A major factor in the rise of HMOs has been the impact of business corporations. The enactment of the Coal Mine Health and Safety Act of 1969 and the more comprehensive Occupational Health and Safety Act of 1970 made companies liable for the health of their employees and led them into health planning. Unions had long been pressing for health benefits, and by 1984 industry was providing health care coverage for about forty million Americans. As the cost of health care to industry escalated, corporations began turning first to HMOs as a method of restructuring and rationalizing health care. In more recent years, as a result of their studies of the entire health care system, a number of industrial leaders appear to be moving toward a comprehensive system of health insurance at the state or national level.[24]

The momentum developing in the 1960s may well have led to a national health insurance program in the 1970s had it not been for an economic recession and the Watergate scandal leading to the resignation of President Nixon. The rapidly increasing cost of medical care in the 1980s, however, once again brought national health insurance to the fore as a means for bringing health expenditures under control. In 1989 Walter B. Maher, director of employee benefits for Chrysler Corporation, described the United States health care system as "broke, both literally and figuratively." Adding that health costs had become a major competitive problem for American businesses, he declared the time is right for a fundamental change. Echoing his views, Jack Shelton, manager of employee insurance for the Ford Motor Company, declared that the problem was too large to be handled at the company level and there "needs to be some national strategy to respond to it." [25]

American medical care today is provided by or paid for through a variety of methods and agencies—Blue Cross and Blue Shield, commercial insurance, government-subsidized health insurance, and various forms of group practice. In addition, the government provides direct medical care to millions of individuals through the armed services, the Veterans Administration, the Public Health Service, the Indian Health Service, and a wide range of other agencies. Through outright grants and matching funds the federal government also subsidizes medical care for millions of other Americans.

Every major city has at least one municipal hospital and various clinics, dispensaries, and health care centers offering outpatient and inpatient services to those who cannot afford private medicine. In addition, state and county agencies supplement these services with a number of medical institutions and programs. Paralleling the state and government services are those offered by voluntary associations that concentrate upon specific medical problems or problem areas such as cancer and mental health. While voluntary groups tend to place their major efforts upon health education and raising funds for research, they also provide some diagnostic and treatment facilities.

The effect of government participation in health care has been to make medical service available to many individuals who formerly seldom visited a physician except in dire emergencies. Medicare and Medicaid have been of great help to the aged, but Medicare, although intended originally to help aged workers, has become a major benefit for senior members of the middle class, while Medicaid, a joint federal-state program intended to provide coverage for the poor, has been under-funded and supplies only second-class medical care. Moreover, some thirty-five million or more individuals in the lower income brackets ineligible for Medicare are neither covered by employer insurance nor able to afford personal health insurance. Hence any type of serious illness or injury becomes both a personal and economic catastrophe.

Aside from excessive duplication, the health care system has led to a maldistribution of physicians. For both financial and professional rea-sons, physicians tend to avoid urban ghettos and rural areas. In an effort to deal with this problem, beginning in the 1960s the federal govern-ment offered scholarship loans to medical students with the proviso that most of the loan would be canceled if the recipient practiced in an underserved area for a limited time. Another program, the National Health Service Corps, offered physicians a choice of military service or practicing in an area short of physicians. Individual states, too, subsi-dize medical students on a similar basis. Programs such as these are of help, but the same factors that draw physicians into affluent urban and suburban centers still operate once these physicians have served their time. The best program developed so far is the Area Health Education Centers. These centers are designed to attract young physicians into areas where they are needed and at the same time provide continuing education for local health professionals.[26]

With business leaders, unions, and large segments of the public beginning to demand some type of comprehensive medical program, what can Americans expect for the future? Unlike the older Western countries, philanthropy and volunteerism are firmly embedded in the American tradition, and the association of the word "socialist" with the British national health program makes it unlikely that it would appeal to Americans. All efforts in the past to provide some form of federal health insurance have included the principle of decentralization and minimum federal interference. Unfortunately there is need to restruc-ture medical services, and health insurance in itself cannot do so; in fact, it may merely compound the problems.

The Canadian medical system has been the subject of considerable discussion in recent medical and lay publications. Whatever the advantages or disadvantages of the British and Canadian systems, both of them provide the average citizen with at least as good care as he or she receives in the United States and at a lower cost. A possible harbinger of the future is the recently adopted Massachusetts universal health insurance plan, which in effect requires employers to offer health insurance to all full-time employees and sets up a state fund financed by a payroll tax to enable the unemployed to buy insurance. Among the proposed health plans currently under consideration is one to extend the Massachusetts program to the national level.

Whether or not the United States adopts some type of comprehensive medical care system, group practice is here to stay, and the traditional fee-for-service system is obviously coming under constraints. The development of Peer Review Organizations (PROS), designed to prevent questionable hospital admissions, and Diagnosis Related Groups (DRGs), intended to serve as a check on the expanding costs of Medicare, are indicative of the trend toward government regulation of medicine. In addition, government and private insurance companies are beginning to place limits on fees or at least are requiring physicians to justify them.

No one can predict what the future holds, but the present trend is clearly toward more government involvement in medical care. While many physicians still feel that medical care is a privilege, public opinion is beginning to consider it a right. Congress seldom provides leadership, but it does respond to public pressure. A national health law of some type seems almost inevitable; whether or not it is a sound one will depend on the willingness of the medical profession to face up to social and political realities and assist in writing a good measure.

CHAPTER 22

Whither Medicine?

SINCE EVERY MAJOR SCIENTIFIC DISCOVERY or technological breakthrough tends to speed up the rate of the
accumulation of knowledge, medical science is now advancing at such
an accelerating pace that it poses a challenge to our social and economic
institutions. Scarcely a week goes by without a dramatic announcement
of some development in gene therapy, chemotherapeutics, or medical
technology. While many of them are premature and others prove illu-
sory, most of them represent further advances in our understanding of
human physiology and disease processes. In August 1990 the National
Cancer Institute announced the first implantation of a nonhuman gene
into patients, in this instance a special marker gene attached to certain cancer-fighting cells. This achievement may well open the way to
a new era of gene transplants for therapeutic purposes. In the same
month a Johns Hopkins research group reported inhibiting the growth
of colon cancer cells in a test tube by replacing the damaged gene with
a normal one.

Meanwhile the Human Genome Initiative, the mapping of the
human genetic system that started in 1990, is steadily moving forward, and researchers are increasingly finding links between genes and
specific disease entities. Recently one has been made between osteo-
arthritis and genetic mutations. Among developments in 1990 was the
successful culturing of human brain cells in laboratory dishes by a team
of neuroscientists at Johns Hopkins. The ability to culture various
human cells has been responsible for a number of discoveries, ranging
from the Salk vaccine for polio to the identification of the AIDS virus,
and the work of these Johns Hopkins scientists offers new hope for

patients with brain disorders. Another significant announcement in this same year concerned a prototype Lyme disease vaccine. Mice injected with a genetically engineered protein lifted from the outer coat of the Lyme disease bacterium demonstrated a strong immune response. On the technological front a cochlear implant, a miniature hearing aid, has demonstrated its value, and experiments are being conducted on microelectrodes that may someday give vision to the blind. Laser and fiber optics are rapidly developing as major aids to diagnosis and treatment and have been particularly useful in connection with peripheral vascular disease and ophthalmology.

The vast amount of money invested in biological research undoubtedly has led to considerable duplication and has raised the argument that the returns to society might be greater if some of the money were spent on applying what is already known. Obviously the gap between medical knowledge and its application should not be too wide, and the decision as to where to use available resources rests on the level of health care in any given society. A question that does lend itself to an answer concerns the direction that medical research should take. Some twenty years ago Dr. Lewis Thomas, then of the Yale School of Medicine, in a thoughtful essay defined three categories of medical research and suggested that society needs to establish priorities among them.[1]

The first and highest level of medical research is the one seeking to understand human physiology and pathological processes and to find relatively simple ways to prevent or alleviate disorders. Prime examples of this type of research have been the development of vaccines against a wide variety of bacterial and virus diseases, the use of hormones to treat endocrine disturbances, and the current genome program. The time and money spent in mapping the human genetic system and identifying and replacing defective genes holds tremendous promise. The cost of this research is high, but the payoff may be much greater. The benefits of basic research have been shown in the case of tuberculosis, poliomyelitis, and a host of other diseases now virtually banished. Aside from the loss of human life, the expense of caring for thousands of cases of these disorders would be almost prohibitive in terms of today's medical costs. Nothing illustrates the huge savings arising from basic research better than the hundreds of iron lungs relegated to storage now that polio is no longer a serious threat. In a more recent article Dr. Thomas pointed out that had AIDS appeared ten or fifteen years ago before the research technologies of molecular biology had developed recombinant DNA, we would know nothing about the disease.[2]

The second category Dr. Thomas calls "halfway technology" and concerns itself precisely with the development of devices such as iron lungs, kidney machines, pacemakers, and other medical devices or procedures designed to alleviate or compensate for damage caused by little-understood disease processes. If we can discover the factors responsible for the destruction of the capillaries in the kidneys and prevent this process, then the intelligence, creativity, and material resources devoted to devising kidney machines and improving transplant techniques can be turned to more productive purposes, and the highly skilled manpower and equipment used to support these halfway measures can be released for other services. The same situation holds true in the case of atherosclerosis and cancer. The elimination or reduction of costly coronary care units and complicated surgical procedures would make available a wide range of medical resources. Aside from the human suffering and death caused by cancer, its victims often require exceedingly expensive care. Radical surgery, irradiation, and chemotherapy have proved effective in dealing with many forms of cancer, but the real solution lies in preventing the formation of cancerous cells. Once an understanding of the various forms of cancer can be found through basic research, these costly, painful, and mutilating methods for dealing with it will be relegated to a minor role.

The third category, which Dr. Thomas calls "nontechnology," is the supportive care provided for patients with terminal or incurable diseases for which little can be done other than to alleviate pain and discomfort and provide reassurance. While not requiring as great an expenditure as "halfway technology," this care does take a great deal of valuable time on the part of physicians and other medical personnel. These last two categories are largely responsible for the soaring cost of American health care and make it essential that medical research be concentrated on understanding human physiology and its relationship to disease rather than mitigating or relieving the results of disease. Angioscopy, angioplasty, atherectomy, pacemakers, and all the other devices and procedures are a credit to modern science, but a better understanding of irreversible muscle or valve disease would reduce the need for them.

The problem of understanding a disease process is an exceedingly difficult one, since the pathway or pathways to the solution usually include many blind alleys. Cancer research is a fine example. Vast sums have been invested in it, yet the survival rate for patients with the most serious forms of the disease has not improved commensurate with time and money invested. Moreover, in the earlier years much of the improvement in survival rates resulted from antibiotics, transfusion techniques, and other aids to surgery. What happened was that more people began surviving cancer operations.

The difficulties of knowing where to concentrate research can be shown by glancing at the past. In the late eighteenth and nineteenth centuries physicians were generally convinced that disease arose from climate and environmental conditions, and medical journals were filled with meteorological studies seeking to relate temperature, humidity, and other factors to epidemic disease. In the case of cancer, scientists have looked in many directions. Until quite recently virologists claimed a major share of cancer research funds. Emphasis then began to shift toward nutrition and environmental factors such as cigarettes, industrial chemicals, and solar and cosmic radiation. Today much research is concentrating on immunological and genetic factors. In common with all other fields of human endeavor, research has its vested interests, and the line between innovative ideas and absurd theories is ill defined. Virology, which could offer a quick and simple answer and possibly a Nobel Prize, is much more attractive than the slow, dogged, and collective work necessary to identify a wide range of environmental factors. Today, while scientists are following many possible leads, the emphasis would appear to be on genetics and immunology.

The enormous strides made by medical science in the twentieth century have had the effect of drastically raising the cost of medical care. While developments in medicine and medical technology contributed to this situation, social and economic factors are equally responsible. One such factor that is seldom recognized is the steadily upward movement of wages and salaries for ancillary workers. Hospital and clinic employees, nurses and receptionists, and many other individuals involved in medical or related fields were for many years among the lowest-paid workers. The ten- or twenty-dollar daily hospital charges of former years were predicated on virtual starvation wages for orderlies, nurses, and other staff employees, while interns and residents were expected to put in six or seven long days a week for room, board, and a nominal cash income. Minimum wage laws, stronger nursing associations, and rebellions by interns and residents have rectified a good share of these abuses, but the consequence has been a major increase in hospital and clinic budgets. The improved standard of living for hospital workers was part of the general rise in living standards that has dramatically raised the demand for medical services. This increased demand, combined with Medicare, Medicaid, and the growth of private and nonprofit health insurance organizations, has enabled hospitals to accede to the wage demands of their employees by simply charging higher rates.

Hospital trustees and administrators also share some of the blame for making medical care almost prohibitive for those without health insurance. Since many of them manage nonprofit institutions, they have made little effort to watch expenses, contenting themselves with meeting their growing budgets by increasing rates. Not infrequently hospitals have added expensive units such as machines for dialysis and coronary care centers simply as prestige items, in many cases duplicating similar facilities in adjacent institutions. In some instances these installations have been acquired purely for the convenience of the attending physicians or as a matter of local pride. All too often hospitals are built when existing ones have more capacity than the community needs. Recognition of the problem of excess hospital beds and the duplication of facilities has led to the creation of regional health planning boards, but, since virtually all of these planning boards to date have depended largely upon voluntary compliance, they have had limited success.

Paul Starr in his excellent study of the medical profession argues that the major factor in accelerating medical costs is the third-party payment system. Both private and government insurers insulate patients and providers from the true costs. Medicare and Medicaid have raised these costs even further by encouraging both physicians and hospitals to increase their charges. By reimbursing hospitals on the basis of their costs, hospital administrators have been encouraged to maximize them. The net effect of health insurance has been to create huge health care conglomerates and what Starr calls a "medical-industrial complex." [3]

It is true that the introduction of a third party between the physician and patient has been a significant factor in raising the cost of medicine and that the application, or misapplication, of Medicare and Medicaid has added a further burden. Yet medicine would have taken a larger share of the nation's productivity in any event. What private and government health insurance did was to accelerate changes that were already underway before the 1960s.

Whatever the case, multiplying health costs have drawn attention to the cumbersome, expensive, and inefficient method of health care delivery in the United States and added to the skepticism about the medical profession. The public attitude toward the profession has always been ambivalent, and this still holds true. It is characterized today by a faith in scientific medicine and individual physicians, but by a skepticism about the profession as a whole.

Since health is too closely related to cultural, social, and economic factors to be left exclusively to doctors, American laypeople have always engaged in do-it-yourself medicine, resorted to irregulars and quacks, and supported health movements. As a result of the current fad for physical fitness, our streets are beset by sweat-suited individuals of all ages doggedly jogging their way to health and long life. In addition, stores selling "natural" foods are flourishing, physical fitness salons have become a major business, and antismoking and weight-loss clinics and workshops are attracting thousands of individuals bent on leading cleaner and leaner lives. And those for whom physical activity in itself is not enough are seeking physical and mental well-being through faith healing, yoga, and a host of major and minor gurus.

When neither mental effort nor physical exercise can solve medical problems, the skeptics of modern medicine can always turn to the irregulars. A recent estimate places the number of Americans who have relied on an irregular practitioner at some time in their lives at sixty million, and, aided by the high cost of orthodox medicine, irregular medical practice appears to be on the rise. Most of the homeopaths were absorbed into orthodox medicine in the first half of the twentieth century, and their numbers dwindled in the succeeding years. In recent years, however, interest in homeopathy has revived, and lay homeopathic groups are currently seeking to reestablish homeopathic licensing boards. Osteopathy is also flourishing, but, as with homeopathy, many of its practitioners were absorbed into orthodox medicine early in the century. As a result of modifying the curricula in osteopathic schools, some thirty-eight states now grant doctors of osteopathy unlimited licenses. Hence osteopaths scarcely can be classified as irregulars.[4] The chiropractors, whose early success was predicated on the inability of the orthodox profession to deal with spinal problems, lost much of their raison d'être with advances in neurology and orthopedics, but they have survived strong attacks by organized medicine. Just as the early homeopaths flourished in reaction to the excessive drugging of nineteenth-century physicians, chiropractic is reviving today based in part on practicing a drugless form of physical therapy. Chiropractors had been nearly driven out of business by the 1950s, but by 1975 they had gained the right to practice in every state. As of 1980 chiropractic claimed to have 25,000 practitioners and over 7,000 students in 15 chiropractic schools.[5]

There can be no question that faith healing, by whatever name, can play a significant role in physical well-being. A major aspect of the doctor-patient relationship is a feeling of confidence or faith on the part of the patient, and even when this faith is placed in a witch doctor, medicine man, guru, or Christian faith healer, it can have beneficial effects. Yoga has long demonstrated, and recent studies have given further proof, that with training an individual can learn to control at least some of the involuntary muscles. Certain individuals appear to have been able to reduce their blood pressure by using the mind to relax the vascular system. Moreover, as Hippocrates recognized five centuries before Christ, worry and anxiety do cause disease. Hence a religion or philosophy that can promote inner peace and tranquility obviously is beneficial to health. Yet faith healing has its limitations. While it can ease pain temporarily through the placebo effect, it cannot cure serious diseases. Spontaneous remission of disease may occur with any patient, and some of the faith-healing victories undoubtedly belong in this category. As with patients treated by quacks, only those who survive are around to testify.

Although the economic consequences of the advancing front of medicine are great, of equal importance are the fundamental ethical issues arising from these developments. The success achieved in transplanting organs has raised the question of priorities — when the supply of organs is limited, to whom do they go? The situation is particularly acute in the case of heart patients, but it holds true for all patients needing transplants. The growing use of respirators, dialysis machines, and other mechanical devices to maintain life also involves the matter of priorities. Should life-support equipment be taken from a terminally ill patient for the benefit of one with a better chance for survival?[6]

More important is the fact that our ability to preserve life is forcing a redefinition of death. Sophisticated life-support devices can now ventilate, feed, filter the blood, and provide elimination for patients who are little more than vegetables. Young persons classified as brain dead or the terminally ill senile can be maintained alive for months or years. Aside from the enormous medical cost (it has been estimated that one-third of medical expenditures are spent in the final year of life), the survival of these individuals results in an immense emotional drain on their families. And this brings up the subject of euthanasia. Since euthanasia involves killing those individuals suffering from terminal illnesses or hopeless injuries as an act of mercy, it was relatively simple for Christian society to apply the commandment "Thou shalt not kill" and condemn the practice. Euthanasia under such circumstances was an act of commission and as such was forbidden by medical ethics and society's moral code.

With today's medical technology the distinction between life and death has become blurred. The physician's obligation to preserve life was predicated on the assumption that his efforts were largely supportive. When he and the patient's family agreed that no hope remained, the physician, by an act of omission, simply permitted the patient to die. Formerly most patients died in their homes, but now seriously ill patients almost invariably end up in a hospital where their medical care involves a large number of professionals and paraprofessionals. It is possible now to prolong life in elderly senile patients who are no longer thinking, conscious human beings, or to preserve life in the bodies of younger patients long after irreversible brain damage has guaranteed that they will never again be aware of the world around them. The life-or-death decision often involves deliberately cutting off the power supply to a mechanical respirator or some other device or by deciding not to use a specific life-preserving piece of equipment.

Whereas formerly decisions about suffering, terminally ill patients were made by physicians in conference with the patients' families, now the decisions have become a matter of public record. Actions taken by attending physicians are subject to hospital review boards, and the existence of detailed case records, which can be made available for malpractice suits or criminal action, necessarily makes doctors reluctant to withhold any form of life preserving technology. The advent of life-supporting mechanical devices has thrown the whole problem of euthanasia into sharper focus. When these devices are in use, euthanasia is no longer the result of an act of omission but rather one of commission or direct action. Conflicting court decisions as to whether or not physicians and hospitals must maintain life in hopeless cases—

even over the objection of the patient's family—indicate the public's ambivalence about the issue. If the medical profession can no longer use its judgment, then society must redefine the ground rules.

Just as medical advances have complicated the question of euthanasia, they have also raised new questions in connection with contraception and abortion. Dating back to primitive societies in which fertility rates were low and infant mortality high, abortion has rarely received social sanction, although it appears to have been practiced to some extent in early civilizations. A vastly improved understanding of the physiology involved from conception to birth has made abortion a much simpler and safer form of medical intervention. In consequence, abortions to save the life or health of the mother have gradually gained social acceptance, but the effect has been to make abortion available to all who could afford it. Physicians who believe in a woman's right to make her own decisions and doctors attracted by financial considerations are all willing to perform abortions. Regardless of the legal aspects, middle- and upper-class women seeking abortions have no difficulty in having them performed under safe medical supervision. The only effect of legal restrictions has been to raise the cost and effectively exclude poor and lower-income women from resorting to reputable physicians. Consequently these women have had to turn to empirics, quacks, and folk practitioners, subjecting themselves to the possibility of serious pelvic infections and other complications that occasionally bring death.

There is a measure of irony in the fact that the research directed toward helping women conceive has also contributed to more effective birth control and contraception. One might well ask whether facilitating conception and birth is any more of an interference with nature than preventing them. There has been, and still is, a movement to prevent in vitro fertilization of human ova, and the federal government has banned the cultivation of fetal cells for research purposes. Proponents of in vitro fertilization point out that this research is essential if we are to understand gestation and make progress toward the elimination of birth defects. Testing of fetal cells for defective genes is already underway, a development that holds the possibility for preventing the birth of defective children or for correcting abnormalities before birth. If abortion can be performed legally for the health of the mother, then in vitro fertilization for scientific purposes has a far more legitimate claim.

A number of major ethical questions have been raised by the breaking of the genetic code. Bioengineering, a recently developed field, is already altering and creating new forms of bacteria, modifying the genetic structure of plants, and applying the same techniques to farm animals. Experiments with gene transplants in humans are already underway, and the public is beset by a stream of reports claiming to have identified a specific gene that either causes or makes individuals susceptible to a particular disorder.

The selective manipulation of genes in plants and animals has made it possible to do the same for humans and brings into question the whole nature of human beings. The possibility of human genetic selection is some time in the future, but the ethics of doing so deserves serious thought. Parenthetically, it should be noted that the current scene with respect to genes is reminiscent of the years from 1880 to 1920 when scientific journals were full of reports claiming to have identified the specific bacteria responsible for diseases such as malaria, yellow fever, and pellagra. One can only hope that those scientists rushing into print today have thoroughly checked their findings.

As noted earlier, the past fifty years have seen medical research and public health shift from an emphasis on infectious diseases to the chronic and degenerative disorders. The wholesale prescribing of penicillin in the 1950s led public health departments to close their venereal disease clinics, assuming that venereal disorders were no longer a significant problem. By the 1960s and 1970s, aided by the sexual revolution, the incidence of syphilis and gonorrhea began to rise, and genital herpes and other sexual infections emerged as problems. In more recent years new diseases, or acute forms of old ones, such as Legionnaire's disease, Lyme disease, and AIDS have disrupted the trend away from infectious disorders. They have also, particularly in the case of AIDS, raised the question of the distribution of funds for health purposes. The allocation of government funds for research has always been subject to pressure groups and public opinion. Elected officials, as in the case of the amended Coal Mine Health and Safety Act of 1972, may even define what constitutes disease.[7] The intense lobbying on behalf of AIDS, however, has brought to the fore the whole question of political pressure determining the distribution of medical research funds. Moreover, this same pressure has also forced the FDA into relaxing its standards and simplifying the entire drug approval process. The lesson is clear; advances in medical science and public health in a democratic society require an informed public.

AIDS, as Allan M. Brandt states, "makes explicit, as few diseases could, the complex interaction of social, cultural, and biological forces." As a new and fatal disorder, its victims arouse fear and hostility, and its association with sexuality arouses deep cultural anxieties. As with venereal diseases, drug addiction, and mental illness, the public tends to blame AIDS on socially marginal groups, the poor, and foreigners. Ordinarily diseases equated with what is presumed to be sinfulness or lack of moral fiber receive minimal government funding. AIDS, however, seizes many of its victims from among members of the world of the arts, a highly articulate group. In consequence, funding for AIDS research has been far higher than if it had been restricted to a poor minority.[8]

Medicine has made great strides in the past one hundred years, and the explosion of biomedical knowledge in the twentieth century has been accompanied by a comparable improvement in community health and life expectancy. From a medical standpoint, the major factor in this change during the first half of the century has been the sharp decline in infectious diseases. Disorders such as typhoid, tuberculosis, measles, scarlet fever and streptococcal sore throat, and malaria were either virtually banished or drastically reduced. The vaccines, antitoxins, and isolation policies derived from the bacteriological revolution of the late nineteenth century contributed much to reducing the incidence of these infections, but the rising standard of living and the emphasis upon sanitary measures and personal hygiene may have had at least as great an effect. For example, the mortality rate from measles was declining well before the introduction of a measles vaccine, falling from 13.3 deaths per 100,000 population in 1900 to 0.3 in 1955.[9] Typhoid, a traditional killer disease, is no longer a threat, largely as a result of community sanitary measures. And improved living standards combined with the isolation of patients in sanatoriums contributed to reducing the incidence of tuberculosis long before an effective therapy was found in the 1940s.

Meanwhile steady progress in physiology and the basic sciences prepared the way for a general advance in all medical fields beginning around the World War II era. In the last forty years molecular biology gave an impetus to all areas of medicine, immunology and genetics have made major gains, and the use of microscopes and microscopic instruments have revolutionized surgery. The increase in life expectancy during the first half of the twentieth century was made possible primarily by eliminating childhood disease and reducing infant and child mortality. The last forty years have seen a steady improvement in the life expectancy of older people. An individual of fifty today can expect not only to live longer but to enjoy a much better quality of life than his forebears. In all probability biology has placed a limit on human life; the test confronting America today is to guarantee that the benefits of medicine are made available to all citizens.

Notes

Chapter 1: The Beginnings of American Medicine

1. The Indians did suffer from chronic complaints such as eye infections, arthritis, and rheumatism. For a discussion of these see Robert Fortuine, *Chills and Fever: Health and Disease in the Early History of Alaska* (Fairbanks, Alaska, 1989).

2. John Duffy, "Medicine and Medical Practices among Aboriginal Indians," in *History of American Medicine: A Symposium*, ed. Felix Marti-Ibanez (New York, 1959), 15–33.

3. Virgil J. Vogel, *American Indian Medicine* (Norman, Okla., 1977); see also Calvin Tomkins, *Keepers of the Game* (Berkeley, 1978).

4. P. M. Ashburn, *The Ranks of Death* (New York, 1947), 18–27. A recent excellent study on the impact of the coming of whites is Russell Thornton, *American Indian Holocaust and Survival: A Population History since 1492* (Norman, Okla., 1987).

5. Count Frontenac to the King, Quebec, November 6, 1679, in *Documents Relative to the Colonial History of New York*, vol. 9, ed. E. B. O'Callaghan (Albany, New York, 1855), 129; Mrs. Afra Coming to Sister, March 6, 1699, quoted in Edward McCurdy, *The History of South Carolina under the Proprietary Government, 1670–1719* (New York, 1897), 308.

6. "Communications," *Mississippi Valley Historical Review* 41 (1954–55): 762.

7. John Duffy, "The Passage to the Colonies," *Mississippi Valley Historical Review* 38 (1951–52): 21–38.

8. Wyndham B. Blanton, *Medicine in Virginia in the Seventeenth Century* (Richmond, 1930), 62–69.

9. Henry R. Viets, *A Brief History of Medicine in Massachusetts* (Boston, 1930), 13–14; John Duffy, *Epidemics in Colonial America* (Baton Rouge, La., 1953), 13.

10. For a summary of the impact of disease upon colonial America, see Duffy, *Epidemics in Colonial America*.

11. Alfred W. Crosby, Jr., "Virgin Soil Epidemics as a Factor in the Aboriginal Depopulation in America," *William and Mary College Quarterly*, ser. 3, 33 (1976): 289–99.

12. Roger Price to Secretary, Boston, April 3, 1752, Society for the Propagation of the Gospel in Foreign Parts MSS, Library of Congress Phototranscripts, London Letters, B20, fp. 46 (hereafter cited as SPG MSS).

13. Noah Webster, *A Brief History of Epidemic and Pestilential Diseases* . . . (Hartford, Conn., 1799), 1:233.

14. Eric H. Christianson, "Medicine in New England," in *Medicine in the New World: New Spain, New France, and New England*, ed. Ronald L. Numbers (Knoxville, 1987), 103–12.

15. Fielding H. Garrison, *An Introduction to the History of Medicine* . . . (4th ed., Philadelphia, 1929), 239, 394.

16. Lester S. King in *The Medical World of the Eighteenth Century* (Chicago, 1958), chapter 1, gives an excellent picture of the relations between the apothecaries and physicians.

17. The medical role of early ministers is discussed fully in Patricia Ann Watson, *The Angelic Conjunction: The Preacher-Physicians of Colonial New England* (Knoxville, 1991).

18. Viets, *Brief History of Medicine in Massachusetts*, 8–24.

19. Joseph M. Toner, *Contributions to the Annals of Medical Progress and Medical Education* . . . (Washington, D.C., 1874), 19–21.

20. Viets, *Brief History of Medicine in Massachusetts*, 36–37; Samuel A. Green, *History of Medicine in Massachusetts* (Boston, 1881), 30–31.

21. Blanton, *Medicine in Virginia in the Seventeenth Century*, 8–24.

22. James J. Walsh, *A History of Medicine in New York: Three Centuries of Medical Progress*, 3 vols. (New York, 1919), 1:18, 31.

23. Ibid., 23–25, 35–36; Adriaen van der Donck, *Remonstrance of New Netherland, and the Occurrences There, Addressed to the High and Mighty Lord States General of the United Netherlands, on the 28th July, 1649*, trans. E. B. O'Callaghan (Albany, 1856), 7–8.

24. Walsh, *History of Medicine in New York*, 1:35–36.

25. John B. Blake, *Public Health in the Town of Boston, 1630–1822* (Cambridge, Mass., 1959), 8–9; Isaac N. Stokes, *The Iconography of Manhattan Island*, 6 vols. (New York, 1915–28), 4:280.

26. Daniel J. Boorstin, *The Americans: The Colonial Experience* (New York, 1958), 233–38.

27. J. Worth Estes and David M. Goodman, *The Changing Humors of Portsmouth: The Medical Biography of an American Town, 1623–1983* (Boston, 1986), 16.

Chapter 2: The Eighteenth Century

1. William Douglass, *A Summary, historical and political, of the first planting, progressive improvements, and present state of British Settlements in North America*, 2 vols. (London, 1760), 2:351–52.

2. J. Worth Estes, "Patterns of Drug Usage in Colonial America," in *Early American Medicine: A Symposium*, ed. Robert I. Goler and P.J. Imperato (New York: Fraunces Tavern Museum, 1987), 33.

3. Ibid., 32–37. For a good picture of colonial medicine see Philip Cash, E. H. Christianson, and J. Worth Estes, eds., *Medicine in Colonial Massachusetts, 1620–1820* (Charlottesville, Va., 1981).

4. *Papers of the Lloyd Family of the Manor of Queens Village, Lloyd's Neck, Long Island, New York, 1654–1826*, 1:309–10, New York Historical Society *Collections* 59 (1926).

5. Cotton Mather, *The Angel of Bethesda*, introduction by Gordon W. Jones (Barre, Mass.: American Antiquarian Society and Barre Publishers, 1972), 250.

6. Mr. Bradford to Secretary, New York, September 12, 1709, in SPG MSS, A 5, film pages 141–50.

7. Whitfield J. Bell, Jr., "A Portrait of the Colonial Physician," *Bulletin of the History of Medicine* (hereafter cited as *Bull. Hist. Med.*) 44 (1970): 501–2; William Smith, *The History of the Province of New York* (London, 1776), 272–73.

8. Wyndham B. Blanton, *Medicine in Virginia in the Eighteenth Century* (Richmond, 1931), 214–15.

9. Elizabeth G. Gartrell, "Women Healers and Domestic Remedies in 18th-Century America: The Recipe Book of Elizabeth Coates Paschall," in *Early American Medicine: A Symposium*, ed. Goler and Imperato, 15–16; Elizabeth Drinker's Diary, 1758–75, Pennsylvania Historical Society MS.

10. Gartrell, "Women Healers," 16–20.

11. Joseph I. Waring, *A History of Medicine in South Carolina, 1670–1825* (Columbia, S.C., 1964), 36.

12. David L. Cowen, *Medicine and Health in New Jersey: A History* (Princeton, 1964), 11–12.

13. Bell, "Portrait of the Colonial Physician," 501–6.

14. *New York Gazette*, May 20, 1751.

15. Henry Lucas to Secretary, Newbury, New England, July 24, 1716, in SPG MSS, A 11–12, fp. 311.

16. Bell, "Portrait of the Colonial Physician," 505.

17. Cotton Mather, *A Letter about a Good Management under the Distemper of the Measles, etc.* (Boston, 1739).

18. Duffy, *Epidemics in Colonial America*, 23ff.

19. Worthington C. Ford, ed., *Diary of Cotton Mather*, 2 vols. (New York, n.d.), 2:634.

20. William Douglass to Cadwallader Colden, Boston, May 1, 1722, in "Letters from Dr. William Douglas[s] to Dr. Cadwallader Colden of New York," ed. Jared Sparks, Massachusetts Historical Society *Collections* (hereafter cited as Mass. Hist. Soc. *Colls.*) ser. 4, 2 (1854): 170; Edmund Massey, *A Sermon against the Dangerous and Sinful Practice of Inoculation . . .* (London, 1722), 24.

21. Duffy, *Epidemics in Colonial America*, 32.

22. Mary C. Gillett, *The Army Medical Department, 1775–1818* (Washington, D.C., 1981), 75.

23. Otho T. Beall, Jr., and Richard H. Shryock, *Cotton Mather, First Significant Figure in American Medicine* (Baltimore, 1954), 87–92, 149–54.

24. Jabez Fitch, *An Account of the Numbers that have died . . . within the Province of New Hampshire* (Boston, 1736); Jonathan Dickinson, *Observations on that Terrible Disease, Vulgarly called the Throat Distemper, with Advices as to the Method of Cure* (Boston, 1740).

25. Cowen, *Medicine and Health in New Jersey*, 6.

26. William Pepper, *The Medical Side of Benjamin Franklin* (Philadelphia, 1910), 11, 28.

27. Ibid., 20–21, 45, 72, 81.

28. Benjamin Franklin, *Some Account of the Pennsylvania Hospital*, introduction by I. B. Cohen (Baltimore, 1954).

29. For an excellent account of the physician-naturalists, see Brooke Hindle, *The Pursuit of Science in Revolutionary America, 1735–1789* (Chapel Hill, N.C., 1956), 36–58.

30. John Duffy, *A History of Public Health in New York City, 1625–1866* (New York, 1968), 42–44.

31. Ibid., 44–46.

32. Hindle, *Pursuit of Science in Revolutionary America*, 51; Waring, *History of Medicine in South Carolina, 1670–1825*, 254–60.

33. Claude E. Heaton, "Medicine in New York during the English Colonial Period, 1664–1775," *Bull. Hist. Med.* 17 (1945): 36–37.

34. The best biography of Morgan is Whitfield J. Bell, Jr., *John Morgan, Continental Doctor* (Philadelphia, 1965).

Chapter 3: The Medical Profession

1. John Z. Bowers and Elizabeth F. Purcell, eds., *Advances in American Medicine: Essays at the Bicentennial*, 2 vols. (New York, 1976), 1:4.

2. John E. Lane, "Daniel Turner and the First Degree of Doctor Conferred in the English Colonies of North America by Yale College in 1723," *Annals of Medical History* 2 (1919): 367.

3. Bell, *John Morgan*, 118–24.

4. Whitfield J. Bell, Jr., *Early American Science* (Williamsburg, Va., 1955), 25; Francis R. Packard, *History of Medicine in the United States*, 2 vols. (New York, 1931), 1:342–66; Genevieve Miller, "Medical Schools in the Colonies," *Ciba Symposia* 8 (1947): 522–32.

5. Walsh, *History of Medicine in New York*, 1:46, 48–49, 52.

6. Ibid., 48; Peter Middleton, *A Medical Discourse* (New York, 1769), 51; Field-

ing H. Garrison, *Contributions to the History of Medicine from the Bulletin of the New York Academy of Medicine, 1925–1935* (New York, 1966), 808.

7. Frederick Waite, "Medicinal Degrees Conferred in the American Colonies and in the United States in the 18th Century," *Annals of Medical History*, n.s., 9 (1937): 317–18.

8. Blanton, *Medicine in Virginia in the Seventeenth Century*, 149–50; John E. Ransom, "The Beginnings of Hospitals in the United States," *Bull. Hist. Med.* 13 (1943): 521; E. B. O'Callaghan, ed., *Register of New Netherland: 1626 to 1674* (Albany, N.Y., 1865), 128.

9. Samuel Wilson, Jr., "An Architectural History of the Royal Hospital and the Ursuline Convent of New Orleans," *Louisiana Historical Quarterly* 29 (1946): 559–60; John Duffy, ed., *The Rudolph Matas History of Medicine in Louisiana*, 2 vols. (Baton Rouge, La., 1958–62), 1:82–103.

10. Will of Jean Louis, November 16, 1735, Document 5948 (A 35/85), Cabildo Archives, New Orleans, Louisiana; Duffy, *Matas History of Medicine in Louisiana*, 1:103–11.

11. Robert J. Hunter, "Benjamin Franklin and the Rise of Free Treatment of the Poor by the Medical Profession of Philadelphia," *Bull. Hist. Med.* 31 (1957): 137.

12. Claude E. Heaton, "Three Hundred Years of Medicine in New York City," *Bull. Hist. Med.* 32 (1958): 520; Joseph I. Waring, "St. Philips Hospital in Charleston in Carolina," *Annals of Medical History*, n.s., 4 (1932): 284.

13. *Minutes of the Common Council of New York, 1675–1776* (New York, 1905), 6:211, 369–70.

14. Franklin, *Some Account of the Pennsylvania Hospital*, 25.

15. Ibid., 27.

16. Ibid., 29; Hunter, "Benjamin Franklin and the Rise of Free Treatment of the Poor," 138–40.

17. Franklin, *Some Account of the Pennsylvania Hospital*, 36.

18. Garrison, *Contributions to the History of Medicine*, 806–10; Hindle, *Pursuit of Science in Revolutionary America*, 118–19; James Hardie, *The Description of the City of New York* (New York, 1827), 256–57.

19. Richard H. Shryock, *Medical Licensing in America, 1650–1965* (Baltimore, 1967), 3–4.

20. Edward Ingle, "Regulating Physicians in Colonial Virginia," *Annals of Medical History* 4 (1922): 248–50; Blanton, *Medicine in Virginia in the Eighteenth Century*, 399–401.

21. Shryock, *Medical Licensing in America*, 16.

22. Walsh, *History of Medicine in New York*, 1:76, 78–79; *Report of a Committee of the Medical Society of New York, on the Subject of Medical Education* (Albany, N.Y., 1840), 3–4; Charles B. Coventary, "History of Medical Legislation in the State of New York," *New-York Journal of Medicine and the Collateral Sciences* 4 (1845): 152.

23. Christianson, "Medicine in New England," 127–37.

24. Gertrude L. Annan, "The Academy of Medicine of New York, 1825–1830, and Its Contemporary, the New York Academy of Medicine," *Bulletin of the Medical Library Association* 36 (1948): 117–23; Walsh, *History of Medicine in New York*, 1:57, 73; Heaton, "Three Hundred Years of Medicine in New York City," 520.

25. Waring, *History of Medicine in South Carolina, 1670–1825*, 65–66.

26. Joseph I. Waring, "Lionel Chalmers, Medical Author," *Bull. Hist. Med.* 32 (1958): 353–54.

27. Hindle, *Pursuit of Science in Revolutionary America*, 111–12, 127–28.

28. Cowen, *Medicine and Health in New Jersey*, 10–12.

29. Ibid., 11–12, 19.

30. Shryock, *Medical Licensing in America*, 18–19.

31. Estes and Goodman, *Changing Humors of Portsmouth*, 13, 16.

32. Christianson, "Medicine in New England," 119.

33. James J. Walsh, *History of the Medical Society of the State of New York* (Brooklyn, 1907), 33.

34. John Oldmixon, *The British Empire in America*, 2 vols. (London, 1741), 1:429; New York Historical Society *Collections*, vol. 61 (New York, 1928), 198, 254–55.

35. "William Byrd to Sir Hans Sloane, Virginia, April 20, 1706," *William and Mary College Quarterly*, ser. 2, 1 (1921): 186. For a discussion of the professions in America, see John Duffy, "American Perceptions of the Medical, Legal, and Theological Professions," *Bull. Hist. Med.* 58 (1984): 1–15.

36. Estes and Goodman, *Changing Humors of Portsmouth*, 11–12.

37. Christianson, "Medicine in New England," 139.

38. Bell, "Portrait of the Colonial Physician," 516–17.

39. Thomas C. Parramore, "The Saga of 'The Bear' and the 'Evil Genius,'" *Bull. Hist. Med.* 42 (1968): 321–22.

Chapter 4: Medicine in the Revolutionary Years

1. For a definitive account of these five physicians, see George E. Gifford, Jr., ed., *Physician Signers of the Declaration of Independence* (New York, 1976).

2. Philip Cash, *Medical Men at the Siege of Boston, April, 1775–April, 1776* (Philadelphia, 1973), 27, 82.

3. Louis C. Duncan, *Medical Men in the American Revolution, 1775–1783* (Carlisle Barracks, Pa., 1931), 153, 212; James Thacher, *A Military Journal during the American Revolutionary War, 1775–1783* . . . (Boston, 1823), 426.

4. Howard H. Peckham, ed., *The Toll of Independence: Engagements and Battle Casualties of the American Revolution* (Chicago, 1974), 130–33.

5. James Tilton, *Economical Observations on Military Hospitals and the Prevention of Diseases Incident to an Army* (Wilmington, Del., 1813), 34.

6. *American Archives*, ser. 4, 5:1036–39, 1083; Hugh Thursfield, "Smallpox and

the American War of Independence," *Annals of Medical History*, ser. 3, 2 (1940): 312–15.

7. Blanton, *Medicine in Virginia in the Eighteenth Century*, 257–59; Thacher, *A Military Journal*, 343; *American Archives*, ser. 5, 2:1363.

8. John C. Fitzpatrick, ed., *The Writings of George Washington* (Washington, 1931), 3:433; Cash, *Medical Men at the Siege of Boston*, 34–36.

9. Waring, *History of Medicine in South Carolina, 1670–1825*, 98–99.

10. Joseph M. Toner, *Medical Men of the Revolution, with a Brief History of the Medical Department of the Continental Army. . . .* (Philadelphia, 1876), 14 n. 2.

11. Duncan, *Medical Men in the American Revolution*, 60–64.

12. Bell, *John Morgan*, 208.

13. Cash, *Medical Men at the Siege of Boston*, 118–25.

14. John Morgan, *A Vindication of His Public Character in the Situation of Director-General* (Boston, 1777), 54–59; Genevieve Miller, "Dr. John Morgan's Report to General Washington, March 3, 1776," *Bull. Hist. Med.* 19 (1946): 450–54; *American Archives*, ser. 4, 5:1015–16.

15. Morgan, *A Vindication of His Public Character*, 103; Thacher, *A Military Journal*, 63, 306.

16. Bell, *John Morgan*, 188–90.

17. David Freeman Hawke, *Benjamin Rush, Revolutionary Gadfly* (Indianapolis, 1971), 186–87; Duncan, *Medical Men in the American Revolution*, 192–98; Bell, *John Morgan*, 222–23.

18. For an excellent history of the origins of the Army Medical Department, see Gillett, *Army Medical Department, 1775–1818*, chapters 2–5.

19. Ibid., 39–42.

20. Hawke, *Benjamin Rush*, 206–23.

21. Gillett, *Army Medical Department, 1775–1818*, 41–49; Duncan, *Medical Men in the American Revolution*, 333–46.

22. Waring, *History of Medicine in South Carolina, 1670–1825*, 107.

23. Benjamin Rush, "An Account of the Influence of the Military and Political Events of the American Revolution Upon the Human Body," *Medical Inquiries and Observations*, vol. 1 (Philadelphia, 1818), 128–32. Reprinted in *Bulletin of the New York Academy of Medicine* 46 (1970): 558–61.

24. Hawke, *Benjamin Rush*, 192–93.

25. Hindle, *Pursuit of Science in Revolutionary America*, chapters 12–13.

26. No American physician has received as much attention by historians as Dr. Benjamin Rush. Genevieve Miller's *Bibliography of the History of Medicine of the United States and Canada, 1939–1960* (Baltimore, 1964) lists fifty-eight books and articles on Rush published in a twenty-one-year period. Among the most perceptive works are those by Lyman H. Butterfield, George W. Corner, and Richard H. Shryock.

27. J. H. Powell, *Bring Out Your Dead* (Philadelphia, 1949), 77–78.

28. Genevieve Miller, "Benjamin Rush's Criticism of Hippocrates," *Communication au XVIIe Congrés International d'Histoire de la Médicine, Extrait du Tome I du Congrés* (Athens, 1960), 1:128–31.

29. King, *Medical World of the Eighteenth Century*, 147–50.

30. Powell, *Bring Out Your Dead*, 73–75, 82–84.

Chapter 5: Early Nineteenth-Century Medicine

1. Charles E. Rosenberg, "The Therapeutic Revolution," in *The Therapeutic Revolution: Essays in the History of American Medicine*, ed. Morris J. Vogel and Charles E. Rosenberg (Philadelphia, 1979), 1–9.

2. For an excellent account of nineteenth-century medicine, see John S. Haller, Jr., *American Medicine in Transition, 1840–1910* (Urbana, 1981), chapters 1–3; see also Duffy, *Matas History of Medicine in Louisiana*, 1:269–79.

3. Duffy, *Matas History of Medicine in Louisiana*, 2:5–6; David L. Cowen, "Nineteenth-Century Drug Therapy: Computer Analysis of the 1854 Prescription File of a Burlington Pharmacy," *Journal of the Medical Society of New Jersey* 78 (1981): 758–61.

4. Duffy, *Matas History of Medicine in Louisiana*, 1:269–75.

5. A. A. Gros and N. V. A. Gerardin, *Rapport fait à la Société Médicale sur la Fièvre Jaune qui a regné d'une Manière Épidémique pendant l'Été de 1817* (New Orleans, 1818), 20–21.

6. M. L. Haynie, "Observations on the Fever of Tropical Climates, and the Use of Mercury as a Remedy," *Medical Repository*, n.s., 1 (1813): 218–20.

7. Russell M. Jones, "American Doctors and the Parisian Medical World, 1830–1840," *Bull. Hist. Med.* 47 (1973): 40–65; Irving A. Beck, "An Early American Journal Keyed to Medical Students: A Pioneer Contribution of Elisha Bartlett," *Bull. Hist. Med.* 40 (1966): 124–34.

8. Joseph F. Kett, *The Formation of the American Medical Profession: The Role of Institutions, 1780–1860* (New Haven, 1968), 157–58; Bowers and Purcell, eds., *Advances in American Medicine*, 1:105.

9. For a good account of Washington's death, see Blanton, *Medicine in Virginia in the Eighteenth Century*, 305–12, and Owen H. Wangensteen and Sarah D. Wangensteen, *The Rise of Surgery from Empiric Craft to Scientific Discipline* (Minneapolis, 1978), 249.

10. Blanton, *Medicine in Virginia in the Eighteenth Century*, 305–7.

11. Jabez W. Heustis, *Physical Observations, and Medical Tracts and Researches, on the Topography and Diseases of Louisiana* (New York, 1817), 117–18.

12. Edward H. Barton, *The Application of Physiological Medicine to the Diseases of Louisiana* (Philadelphia, 1832), 38.

13. "Health in the Country," *New Orleans Medical Journal* 1 (1844): 247–48.

14. *New Orleans Medical and Surgical Journal* (hereafter cited as *New Orleans Med. Surg. J.*) 10 (1853–54): 279.

15. The best account of the cholera epidemics can be found in Charles E. Rosenberg, *The Cholera Years: The United States in 1832, 1849, and 1866* (Chicago, 1962).

16. *The Cholera Bulletin*, July 23, 1832, 57–60.

17. Warren Stone, "Cholera and Its Treatment," *New Orleans Med. Surg. J.* 19 (1866–67): 18, 25–26.

18. Donald D. Vogt, "Trends in 19th-Century American Cholera Therapy," *Pharmacy in History* 16 (1974): 43–44.

19. An excellent account of this institution can be found in Norman Dain, *Disordered Minds: The First Century of Eastern State Hospital in Williamsburg, Virginia, 1766–1866* (Williamsburg, Va., 1971).

20. For a good treatment of this subject, see Norman Dain, *Concepts of Insanity in the United States, 1789–1865* (New Brunswick, N.J., 1964), and Gerald N. Grob, *The State and the Mentally Ill: A History of the Worcester State Hospital in Massachusetts, 1830–1920* (Chapel Hill, N.C., 1966).

21. Dain, *Concepts of Insanity*, 175–77.

22. Ellen Dwyer, *Homes for the Mad: Life Inside Two Nineteenth-Century Asylums* (New Brunswick, N.J., 1987), 8–12, 215ff.

Chapter 6: The Irregulars and Domestic Medicine

1. Paul Starr, *The Social Transformation of American Medicine: The Rise of a Sovereign Profession and the Making of a Vast Industry* (New York, 1982), 65–71.

2. Samuel Thomson, *New Guide to Health; or Botanic Family Physician . . . to which is prefixed, A Narrative of the Life and Medical Discoveries of the Author*, 2d ed. (Boston, 1825).

3. Kett, *Formation of the American Medical Profession*, 108–16.

4. The best source for Thomsonianism is Thomson's *New Guide to Health*, but excellent brief accounts of the movement can be found in Kett, *Formation of the American Medical Profession*; William G. Rothstein, *American Physicians in the Nineteenth Century: From Sects to Science* (Baltimore, 1972); and James Harvey Young, *The Toadstool Millionaires: A Social History of Patent Medicine in America before Federal Regulation* (Princeton, 1961).

5. Kett, *Formation of the American Medical Profession*, 138–39.

6. *Code of Ethics of the American Medical Association, adopted May, 1847* (Philadelphia, 1848), 18–19. The best discussion of this and the following material can be found in Martin Kaufman, *Homeopathy in America: The Rise and Fall of Medical Heresy* (Baltimore, 1971), chapters 4–6.

7. Kaufman, *Homeopathy in America*, 63–74.

8. Richard H. Shryock, "Public Relations of the Medical Profession in Great Britain and the United States: 1600–1870 . . . ," *Annals of Medical History*, n.s., 2

(1930): 317. An excellent account of Neo-Thomsonianism can be found in Alex Berman, "Neo-Thomsonianism in the United States," *Journal of the History of Medicine and Allied Sciences* (hereafter cited as *J. Hist. Med. & All. Sci.*) 11 (1956): 133–55. See also Rothstein, *American Physicians in the Nineteenth Century*, 146.

9. For Graham's influence see Stephen Nissenbaum, *Sex, Diet, and Debility in Jacksonian America: Sylvester Graham and Health Reform* (Westport, Conn., 1980); for the early health movement see James C. Whorton, *Crusaders for Fitness: The History of American Health Reformers* (Princeton, 1982), chapters 1–4, and Harvey Green, *Fit for America: Health, Fitness, Sport and American Society* (New York, 1986).

10. Richard H. Shryock, *Medicine in America: Historical Essays* (Baltimore, 1966), 118.

11. Jane B. Donegan, *"Hydropathic Highway to Health": Women and Water-Cure in Antebellum America* (New York, 1986), 19–26; Norman Gevitz, ed., *Unorthodox Medicine in America* (Baltimore, 1988), 83–84.

12. Kitty Hamilton to Father, Biloxi, Miss., June 8, 13, 20, 1851, Hamilton (William S.) Papers, 1841–53, Louisiana State University Archives, MSS; Penelope Hamilton to Father, Biloxi, Miss., July 11, 19, 21, 1851, ibid.; Shryock, *Medicine in America*, 121–22; Donegan, *"Hydropathic Highway to Health,"* xiv.

13. Shryock, *Medicine in America*, 124.

14. John Duffy, *The Healers: The Rise of the Medical Establishment* (New York, 1976), 19, 48; Jane B. Donegan, *Women and Men Midwives: Medicine, Morality and Misogyny in Early America* (Westport, Conn., 1978), 134–35.

15. Laurel T. Ulrich, *A Midwife's Tale: The Life of Martha Ballard, Based on Her Diary, 1785–1812* (New York, 1990), 40, 61.

16. *Daily Pittsburgh Gazette*, November 9, 1837; *Pittsburgh Saturday Evening Visitor*, June 22, 1839, 5:49.

17. Young, *Toadstool Millionaires*, 17–18.

18. Henry Burnell Shafer, *The American Medical Profession, 1783–1850* (New York, 1936), 200–201; Jacques M. Quen, "Elisha Perkins, Physician, Nostrum-Vendor, or Charlatan?" *Bull. Hist. Med.* 37 (1963): 164.

19. Shryock, "Public Relations of the Medical Profession," 316.

20. Young, *Toadstool Millionaires*, covers the period up to 1906, and he continues his history into the twentieth century in *The Medical Messiahs: A Social History of Quackery in Twentieth-Century America* (Princeton, 1967; rev. paperback ed., Princeton, 1992) and *American Health Quackery* (Princeton, 1992).

21. Thomas Thacher, *A Brief Rule to Guide the Common People of New England how to order themselves and theirs in the Small Pocks, or Measles,* (Boston, 1677); John Wesley, *Primitive Physick, or an easy and natural Method of Curing most Diseases,* 12th ed. (printed by Andrew Stewart, Philadelphia, 1764).

22. Guenter B. Risse, R. L. Numbers, and J. W. Leavitt, eds., *Medicine without Doctors* (New York, 1977), consists of some fine essays on home health care.

23. James Ewell, *The Medical Companion, or Family Physician* (Washington, D.C., 1827), xv–xix.

24. John C. Gunn, *Gunn's Domestic Medicine, or Poor Man's Friend* (New York, 1853), 862–66.

25. J. Cam Massie, *Treatise on the Eclectic Southern Practice of Medicine* (Philadelphia, 1854), 5–8.

Chapter 7: The Foundations of American Surgery

1. Moses Hubbard, "Case of a Uterine Tumor — Removed by Operation," *Boston Medical and Surgical Journal* (hereafter cited as *Boston Med. Surg. J.*) 8 (1833): 69.

2. A.-A.-L.-M. Velpeau, *New Elements of Operative Surgery*, ed. Valentine Mott, translated by P. S. Townsend under the supervision of, and with notes and observations by, V. Mott (New York, 1847), 1:20.

3. L. R. C. Agnew and G. F. Shelden, "Philip Syng Physick (1768–1837): 'The Father of American Surgery,' " *Journal of Medical Education* 35 (1960): 545–46.

4. Duffy, *Matas History of Medicine in Louisiana*, 2:44.

5. Ibid., 55; "The New Orleans Charity Hospital," *Harper's Weekly* 3 (1859): 569–70.

6. Garrison, *Introduction to the History of Medicine*, 349; Emmet Field Horine, *Daniel Drake (1785–1852), Pioneer Physician of the Midwest* (Philadelphia, 1961), 71; Blanton, *Medicine in Virginia in the Eighteenth Century*, 17–18.

7. Samuel D. Gross, *Memorial Oration in Honor of Ephraim McDowell, "The Father of Ovariotomy"* (Louisville, 1879), 14ff.; Gross, *Lives of Eminent American Physicians and Surgeons of the Nineteenth Century* (Philadelphia, 1861), 207–30.

8. T. V. Woodring, *Pioneer Medicine and Early Physicians in Nashville* (n.d., n.p.), 11–14.

9. J. Marion Sims, *The Story of My Life* (New York, 1968), 115–16.

10. Ibid., 138, 226–46.

11. Wyndham B. Blanton in his *Medicine in Virginia in the Eighteenth Century* credits Dr. Jesse Bennett of Rockingham County, Virginia, with performing the first operation of this kind in America, reputedly operating on his wife in an emergency situation during 1794. In a paper entitled "The Legend of Jesse Bennet's 1794 Caesarean Section," which was delivered at the American Association of the History of Medicine's 1975 meeting in Philadelphia, Dr. Arthur G. King of Cincinnati completely demolished the Bennet story. Dr. King also has reservations about Prevost, but I think the evidence is fairly conclusive. See the St. Francisville [Louisiana] *Asylum*, February 7, 1825.

12. Rudolph Matas, "François Marie Prevost and the Early History of the Cesarean Section in Louisiana," *New Orleans Med. Surg. J.* 89 (1937): 606–25; Robert P. Harris, "A Record of Cesarean Operations that have been Performed in

the State of Louisiana during the Present Century," ibid., n.s., 6 (1878–79): 933–42; Harris, "Twenty Cesarean Operations, with 15 Women Saved, in Louisiana," ibid., n.s., 7 (1879–80): 456, 938–41; Duffy, *Matas History of Medicine in Louisiana,* 2:72–74.

13. Arthur G. King, "America's First Cesarean Section," *Obstetrics and Gynecology* 37 (1971): 797–802; Garrison, *Introduction to the History of Medicine,* 508.

14. Sir William Osler has an excellent account of the accident that opened the way for Beaumont's experiments in the introduction to a facsimile edition of Beaumont's book, *Experiments and Observations on the Gastric Juice and the Physiology of Digestion . . . Facsimile . . . with a Biographical Essay . . . by Sir William Osler* (New York, 1959); Victor Robinson, *The Story of Medicine* (New York, 1943), 466–68.

15. Jerome J. Bylebyl, "William Beaumont, Robley Dunglison and the Philadelphia Physiologists," *J. Hist. Med. & All. Sci.* 25 (1970): 3–21.

16. *Dictionary of American Biography,* 22 vols. (New York, 1946), 2:104–9.

17. Thomas E. Keys, *History of Surgical Anesthesia* (New York, 1963), 10–18.

18. Richard H. Shryock, *Development of Modern Medicine* (New York, 1969), 178–79; James E. Dexter, *A History of Dental and Oral Science in America* (Philadelphia, 1876), 12–13, 143–48, 180–81.

19. Keys, *History of Surgical Anesthesia,* 21–22.

20. Long's chief advocate is Frank K. Boland, *The First Anesthetic: The Story of Crawford Long* (Athens, Ga., 1950); James Harvey Young, "Crawford W. Long, M.D., a Georgia Innovator," *Bulletin of the New York Academy of Medicine,* 2d ser., 50 (1974): 421–37.

21. For two excellent studies of anesthesia, see Martin S. Pernick, *A Calculus of Suffering: Pain, Professionalism, and Anesthesia in Nineteenth-Century America* (New York, 1985), and Joseph C. Trent, "Surgical Anesthesia, 1846–1946," *J. Hist. Med. & All. Sci.* 1 (1946): 505–14.

22. Judith W. Leavitt, *Brought to Bed: Childbearing in America, 1750–1950* (New York, 1986), 199–200.

23. Henry Hayman, "The Economy of Pain," *Bibliotheca Sacra* 45 (1888): 7.

24. Charles D. Meigs, *Obstetrics: The Science and the Art* (Philadelphia, 1849), 316–19; A. D. Bundy, "Obstetrics in the Country," *Medical and Surgical Reporter* 56 (1887): 201.

25. For a discussion of obstetrical anesthesia, see John Duffy, "Anglo-American Reaction to Obstetrical Anesthesia," *Bull. Hist. Med.* 38 (1964): 32–44.

26. Ibid., 35–36.

27. *Dictionary of American Biography,* 19:640–41.

28. Boland, *First Anesthetic,* 120.

Chapter 8: Early Leaders in Medicine and Surgery

1. Edward D. Churchill, ed., *To Work in the Vineyard of Surgery: Reminiscences of J. Collins Warren (1842–1927)* (Cambridge, Mass., 1958), 1–18.

2. Christine Chapman Robbins, *David Hosack, Citizen of New York* (Philadelphia, 1964), 109, 134–36.

3. Horine, *Daniel Drake*, 96–100, 157–63, 380–81; Samuel D. Gross, *A Discourse on the Life, Character, and Services of Daniel Drake, M.D. . . . January 27, 1853* (Louisville, 1853), contains an excellent account of his life and work. It is especially useful if consulted in connection with Gross's *Lives*, 614–62.

4. Howard A. Kelly and Walter L. Burrage, *American Medical Biographies* (Baltimore, 1920), 470–73.

5. Oliver Wendell Holmes, "Report of Committee on Medical Literature, 1848," in *Medical America in the Nineteenth Century: Readings from the Literature*, ed. Gert H. Brieger (Baltimore, 1972), 50–54.

6. Oliver Wendell Holmes, "The Contagiousness of Puerperal Fever," *New England Quarterly Journal of Medicine and Surgery* 1 (1842–43): 503–30.

7. John B. Blake, *Benjamin Waterhouse and the Introduction of Vaccination: A Reappraisal* (Philadelphia, 1957).

8. John L. Riddell, "On the Binocular Microscope," *New Orleans Med. Surg. J.* 10 (1853–54): 321–27; *New Orleans Medical News and Hospital Gazette* 1 (1855–56): 118. See Duffy, *Matas History of Medicine in Louisiana*, 2:84–86, for further details.

Chapter 9: The Education, Licensing, and Status of Physicians

1. Hawke, *Benjamin Rush, Revolutionary Gadfly*, 84.

2. Robbins, *David Hosack*, 102–4.

3. Rothstein, *American Physicians in the Nineteenth Century*, 104–7.

4. J. W. Francis, *An Historical Sketch of the Origin, Progress, and Present State of the College of Physicians, of the University of the State of New-York* (New York, 1913), 8–16; Heaton, "Three Hundred Years of Medicine in New York City," 517–30; Fred B. Rogers, "Nicholas Romayne, 1756–1817: Stormy Petrel of the American Medical Profession," *Journal of Medical Education* 35 (1960): 258–60.

5. Carleton B. Chapman, *Dartmouth Medical School: The First 175 Years* (Hanover, N.H., 1973), 11–21.

6. Emmet F. Horine, "Early Medicine in Kentucky," *J. Hist. Med. & All. Sci.* 3 (1948): 265–68.

7. *The Medical Register of the City of New York, for the Year Commencing June 1, 1865* (New York, 1866), 195–97; Walsh, *History of Medicine in New York*, 1:53–54.

8. Chapman, *Dartmouth Medical School*, 19; George H. Callcott, *A History of the University of Maryland* (Baltimore, 1966), 20–22.

9. Wyndham B. Blanton, *Medicine in Virginia in the Nineteenth Century* (Richmond, 1933), 71.

10. Horace Montgomery, "A Body Snatcher Sponsors Pennsylvania's Anatomy Act," *J. Hist. Med. & All. Sci.* 21 (1966): 374–93.

11. Callcott, *History of the University of Maryland*, 23–28.

12. Shryock, *Medical Licensing in America*, 28; W. F. Norwood, *Medical Education in America before the Civil War* (Philadelphia, 1944), 430; N. S. Davis, *Medical Education and Medical Institutions in the United States of America, 1776–1876* (Washington, D.C., 1877), 41.

13. John Duffy, *The Tulane University Medical Center: One Hundred and Fifty Years of Medical Education* (Baton Rouge, La., 1984), 5–9.

14. John Duffy, ed., *Parson Clapp of the Strangers' Church of New Orleans* (Baton Rouge, La., 1957), 39–40.

15. Duffy, *Tulane University Medical Center*, 9–35.

16. Stanford E. Chaillé, *Historical Sketch of the Medical Department of the University of Louisiana* (New Orleans, 1861), 5–6.

17. For a good discussion of this topic see Kett, *Formation of the American Medical Profession*, 47ff.

18. Whitfield J. Bell, Jr., "The Medical Institution of Yale College, 1810–1885," *Yale Journal of Biology and Medicine* 33 (1960): 172.

19. Martin Kaufman, *American Medical Education: The Formative Years, 1765–1910* (Westport, Conn., 1976), 78–90.

20. *Proceedings of the National Medical Convention, Held in New York, May, 1846, and Philadelphia, May, 1847* (Philadelphia, 1847), 73–74.

21. Kaufman, *American Medical Education*, 102–3.

22. Shryock, *Medical Licensing in America*, 35.

23. A. E. Fossier, "History of Medical Education in New Orleans from Its Birth to the Civil War," *Annals of Medical History*, n.s., 6 (1934): 427–47; Duffy, *Matas History of Medicine in Louisiana*, 2:260–68, 529–30.

24. See Chapter 3.

25. Walsh, *History of Medicine in New York*, 1:81–82.

26. Duffy, *Matas History of Medicine in Louisiana*, 1:326–40.

27. Rothstein, *American Physicians in the Nineteenth Century*, 79–80.

28. Cowen, *Medicine and Health in New Jersey*, 69–70; Duffy, *Matas History of Medicine in Louisiana*, 2:114–15; Shryock, *Medical Licensing in America*, 30–31.

29. Horine, *Daniel Drake*, 76; T. V. Woodring, *Pioneer Medicine*, 16.

30. Estes and Goodman, *Changing Humors of Portsmouth*, 29–36.

31. Shafer, *American Medical Profession*, 157–61.

32. Ibid., 166–67.

33. Rothstein, *American Physicians in the Nineteenth Century*, 34; Barnes Riznik, "The Professional Lives of Early 19th Century New England Doctors," *J. Hist. Med. & All. Sci.* 19 (1964): 3–5.

34. Genevieve Miller, "One Hundred Years Ago," *Bull. Hist. Med.* 21 (1947), 488.

35. Philip M. Hamer, *The Centennial History of the Tennessee State Medical Association, 1830–1930* (Nashville, 1930), 22–23.

36. Genevieve Miller, "Medical Education One Hundred Years Ago—An Introductory Lecture," *Ohio Medical Journal* 54 (1958): 1578–82; ibid. 55 (1959): 40–41, 44.

37. Oliver S. Hayward and Elizabeth H. Thompson, *The Journal of William Tully, Medical Student at Dartmouth, 1808–1809* (New York, 1977), 51–52.

38. Gert H. Brieger, "Fit to Study Medicine: Notes for a History of Pre-medical Education in America," *Bull. Hist. Med.* 57 (1983): 21; Samuel Rezneck, "The Study of Medicine at the Vermont Academy of Medicine (1827–29) as Revealed in the *Journal of Asa Fitch*," *J. Hist. Med. & All. Sci.* 24 (1969): 418–20; Churchill, *To Work in the Vineyard of Surgery*, 27 n. 16.

39. John Harley Warner, *Medical Practice, Knowledge, and Identity in America, 1820–1885* (Cambridge, Mass., 1986), 1–2.

40. *Proceedings of the Physico-Medical Society of New Orleans in Relation to the Trial and Expulsion of Charles A. Luzenberg, with comments on the same: Published by Order of the Society* (New Orleans, 1838), 24–25.

41. See Duffy, *Matas History of Medicine in Louisiana*, 2:88–92.

42. New Orleans *Daily Delta*, August 28, September 10, 1859; New Orleans *Bee*, August 31, September 10, 1859.

43. Duffy, *Matas History of Medicine in Louisiana*, 2:95.

44. For a discussion of this, see Thomas N. Bonner, "The Social and Political Attitudes of Midwestern Physicians, 1840–1940: Chicago as a Case History," *J. Hist. Med. & All. Sci.* 13 (1953): 133–64; Bonner, *Medicine in Chicago, 1850–1950: A Chapter in the Social and Scientific Development of a City* (Madison, 1957), 10–11.

45. P. S. Townsend, *An Account of the Yellow Fever, as It Prevailed in the City of New York, in the Summer and Autumn of 1822* (New York, 1823), 235; Duffy, *Matas History of Medicine in Louisiana*, 2:172–73, 183.

46. *New-York Medical and Physical Journal* 7 (1828): 174–75; Genevieve Miller, "Dr. John Delameter, 'True Physician,'" *Journal of Medical Education* 34 (1959), 24–31; *Cincinnati Medical Observer* 2 (1857): 129.

47. New Orleans *Courier*, August 8, 1839; *Planters' Banner* (Franklin Parish, Louisiana), July 15, 1847; Shryock, *Medicine in America*, 150–51.

Chapter 10: Medicine in the Civil War

1. The two standard works for Civil War medicine are H. H. Cunningham, *Doctors in Gray: The Confederate Medical Service* (Baton Rouge, La., 1958), and George W. Adams, *Doctors in Blue: The Medical History of the Union Army in the Civil War* (New York, 1952). A recent excellent account of the Union Medical Ser-

vice can be found in Mary C. Gillett, *The Army Medical Department, 1818–1865* (Washington, D.C., 1987), chapters 8–13.

2. Cunningham, *Doctors in Gray*, 3, 6–7; James O. Breeden, *Joseph Jones, M.D., Scientist of the Old South* (Lexington, Ky., 1975), 152. Breeden's biography is particularly good for the Civil War years.

3. Gillett, *Army Medical Department, 1818–1865*, 153.

4. Ibid., 153–54; Adams, *Doctors in Blue*, 4.

5. The best account of the United States Sanitary Commission is the classic one by Charles J. Stillé, *History of the United States Sanitary Commission, Being the General Report of Its Work during the War of the Rebellion* (Philadelphia, 1866).

6. Jane Turner Censer, *The Papers of Frederick Law Olmsted*, vol. 4, *The Civil War and the U. S. Sanitary Commission* (Baltimore, 1986), 13.

7. *Daily Pittsburgh Gazette*, June 28, 1862, and July 6, 1863; *New York Times*, January 24, 1864.

8. Adams, *Doctors in Blue*, has a good account of Hammond's work. For Jonathon Letterman, see Gordon W. Jones, "The Medical History of the Fredericksburg Campaign: Course and Significance," *J. Hist. Med. & All. Sci.* 18 (1963): 241–56.

9. Gillett, *Army Medical Department, 1818–1865*, 295.

10. Joseph Jones, "The Medical History of the Confederate Army and Navy," *Southern Historical Society Papers* 20 (1892): 118.

11. Joseph Janvier Woodward, *Outlines of the Chief Camp Diseases of the United States Armies*, introduction by Saul Jarcho (New York, 1964), 267.

12. Ibid., 58–59, 74–75.

13. Alvin R. Sunseri, "The Organization and Administration of the Medical Department of the Confederate Army of Tennessee," reprint from *Journal of the Tennessee State Medical Association* 52–53 (Jan.–July 1960): 167.

14. For vivid descriptions of operating conditions in the field hospitals, see Adams, *Doctors in Blue*, 112–29, and "The School of Medicine and the Civil War," *Medical Affairs* 2 (Spring 1961).

15. Gillett, *Army Medical Department, 1818–1865*, 286.

16. Adams, *Doctors in Blue*, 129.

17. Mary Louise Marshall, "Medicine in the Confederacy," *Bulletin of the Medical Library Association* 3 (1942): 285; Blanton, *Medicine in Virginia in the Nineteenth Century*, 303.

18. An excellent picture of conditions confronting nurses can be found in Kate Cumming, *Kate: The Journal of a Confederate Nurse*, ed. Richard B. Harwell (Baton Rouge, La., 1959).

19. George W. Smith, *Medicines for the Union Army: The United States Army Laboratories during the Civil War* (Madison, Wis., 1962), 1.

20. Cunningham, *Doctors in Gray*, 148–49; see also Norman H. Franke, *Pharma-*

ceutical Conditions and Drug Supply in the Confederacy (Madison, Wis., 1955).

21. .Duffy, *Matas History of Medicine in Louisiana*, 2:312–16.

Chapter 11: The Emergence of Modern Medicine

1. John Duffy, "American Perceptions of the Medical, Legal and Theological Professions," *Bull. Hist. Med.* 58 (1984): 1–15.

2. Shryock, *Medicine in America*, 77–78

3. Thomas N. Bonner, *American Doctors and German Universities: A Chapter in International Intellectual Relations, 1870–1914* (Lincoln, Neb., 1963), 23.

4. For Welch's contributions see Donald Fleming, *William H. Welch and the Rise of Modern Medicine* (Boston, 1954), chapters 7–9.

5. Samuel D. Gross, *History of American Medical Literature from 1776 to the Present Time* (Philadelphia, 1876), 55–56; Fielding H. Garrison, *John Shaw Billings: A Memoir* (New York, 1915), 15–16, 213–27; John B. Blake, ed., *Centenary of Index Medicus, 1879–1979* (Bethesda, Md., 1980).

6. Charles E. Rosenberg, "The Cause of Cholera: Aspects of Etiological Thought in Nineteenth Century America," *Bull. Hist. Med.* 34 (1960): 338–51.

7. Phyllis Allen Richmond, "American Attitudes toward the Germ Theory of Disease (1860–1880)," *J. Hist. Med. & All. Sci.* 9 (1954): 428–43; "Minutes of the American Medical Association at its 34th Annual Session, . . . June 5–8, 1883," *JAMA* 1 (1883): 2.

8. George T. Harrell, "Osler's Practice," *Bull. Hist. Med.* 47 (1973): 550; Duffy, *Matas History of Medicine in Louisiana*, 2:341.

9. Richmond, "American Attitudes toward the Germ Theory," 445–51.

10. Paul F. Clark, "Theobald Smith, Student of Disease," *J. Hist. Med. & All. Sci.* 14 (1959): 490–514.

11. The best study of the Rockefeller Institute is George Corner's *A History of the Rockefeller Institute, 1901–1953* (New York, 1964). See also Richard H. Shryock, *American Medical Research, Past and Present* (New York, 1947).

12. John Duffy, *The Sanitarians: A History of American Public Health* (Urbana, 1990), 172, 241; Victoria A. Harden, *Inventing the NIH: Federal Biomedical Research Policy, 1887–1937* (Baltimore, 1986), 19–20.

13. The two standard histories of the United States Public Health Service are Ralph C. Williams, *The United States Public Health Service, 1798–1950* (Washington, 1951), and Bess Furman, *A Profile of the United States Public Health Service, 1798–1948* (Washington, n.d.).

14. For a short history of yellow fever, see John Duffy, "Yellow Fever in the Continental United States during the Nineteenth Century," in *Symposia in Clinical Tropical Medicine*, ed. Kevin M. Cahill, vol. 1 (New York, 1970). For the work of the Reed Commission, see John M. Gibson, *Soldier in White: The Life of General*

George Miller Sternberg (Durham, N.C., 1958), and William B. Bean, *Walter Reed: A Biography* (Charlottesville, Va., 1982).

15. François Delaporte, *The History of Yellow Fever: An Essay in the Birth of Tropical Medicine* (Cambridge, Mass., 1991).

16. Victoria A. Harden, *Rocky Mountain Spotted Fever: History of a Twentieth-Century Disease* (Baltimore, 1990), 23–71.

17. John Ettling, *The Germ of Laziness: Rockefeller Foundation and Public Health in the New South* (Cambridge, Mass., 1981), 208–20; Furman, *Profile of the United States Public Health Service*, 258–60; Raymond B. Fosdick, *The Story of the Rockefeller Foundation* (New York, 1952), 10, 24, 30ff.

18. The best account of Goldberger and pellagra can be found in Elizabeth W. Etheridge, *The Butterfly Caste: A Social History of Pellagra in the South* (Westport, Conn., 1972). See also Milton Terris, ed., *Goldberger on Pellagra* (Baton Rouge, La., 1964).

19. Austin Flint, "Conservative Medicine," in *Medical America in the Nineteenth Century*, ed. Brieger, 135–36.

20. James Harvey Young, *Pure Food: Securing the Pure Food and Drugs Act of 1906* (Princeton, 1989), 120; Warner, *Medical Practice*, 37, 55–57.

21. Warner, *Medical Practice*, 154ff.; Charles Rosenberg, "The Practice of Medicine in New York a Century Ago," *Bull. Hist. Med.* 41 (1967): 240–53.

22. Duffy, *Matas History of Medicine in Louisiana*, 2:350.

23. David F. Musto, *The American Disease: Origins of Narcotic Control* (New Haven, 1973), 2–3, 252 n. 5; John S. Haller, Jr., and Robin M. Haller, *The Physician and Sexuality in Victorian America* (Urbana, 1974), 275–77. See also David T. Courtwright, *Dark Paradise: Opium Addiction in America before 1940* (Cambridge, Mass., 1982).

24. Rothstein, *American Physicians in the Nineteenth Century*, 194–95.

25. Young, *Toadstool Millionaires*, 129.

26. Moritz Schuppert, "Blood-Letting and Kindred Questions," *New Orleans Med. Surg. J.*, n.s., 9 (1881–82): 247–56.

27. "Editorial," *New Orleans Med. Surg. J.*, n.s., 14 (1886–87): 231.

28. Rothstein, *American Physicians in the Nineteenth Century*, 182.

29. Charles E. Rosenberg, "Social Class and Medical Care in 19th-Century America: The Rise and Fall of the Dispensary," *J. Hist. Med. & All. Sci.* 29 (1974): 32–33; see also David Rosner, *A Once Charitable Enterprise: Hospitals and Health Care in Brooklyn and New York, 1885–1915* (Cambridge, 1982), chapter 6.

30. Starr, *Social Transformation of American Medicine*, chapter 4.

31. Morris J. Vogel, *The Invention of the Modern Hospital: Boston, 1870–1930* (Chicago, 1980), 2–4, 99.

32. Charles E. Rosenberg, *The Care of Strangers: The Rise of America's Hospital System* (New York, 1987), 9.

33. Stanley J. Reiser, *Medicine and the Reign of Technology* (Cambridge, 1978),

144–47; Irvine Loudon, "The Concept of the Family Doctor," *Bull. Hist. Med.* 58 (1984): 347–48.

34. The Pittsburgh *Daily Post* from December 7, 1867, to February 13, 1868, reported four doctors elected to office in this two-month period; *Daily Post*, February 19, 1868.

35. A wealth of literature on this topic has appeared in the past twenty years. Two excellent studies are Haller and Haller, *Physician and Sexuality in Victorian America*, and H. Tristram Engelhardt, Jr., "The Disease of Masturbation: Values and Concept of Disease," *Bull. Hist. Med.* 48 (1974): 234–48.

36. Samuel A. Cartwright, "Report on the Diseases and Peculiarities of the Negro Race," *New Orleans Med. Surg. J.* 7 (1851): 691–715; ibid., 8 (1851–52): 187–94; "White Supremacy," ibid., n.s., 61 (1908–9): 642–43.

37. Eugene F. Cordell, *The Medical Annals of Maryland, 1799–1899* (Baltimore, 1900), 173.

38. Rima D. Apple, ed., *Women, Health, and Medicine in America: A Handbook* (New York, 1990), presents a first-rate survey of its subject.

39. *New England Journal of Medicine* 270 (1964): 449.

Chapter 12: The Flowering of Surgery

1. Robert Weir "On the Antiseptic Treatment of Wounds, and Its Results," *New York Medical Journal* 26 (1877): 561.

2. Duffy, *Matas History of Medicine in Louisiana*, 2:364–67.

3. Mark M. Ravitch, *A Century of Surgery: The History of the American Surgical Association*, 2 vols. (Philadelphia, 1981), 1:28–32.

4. The best account of the introduction of rubber gloves into surgery can be found in William S. Halsted, "The Employment of Silk in Preference to Catgut . . . ," *JAMA* 60 (1913): 1119–26.

5. Vogel, *Invention of the Modern Hospital*, 65.

6. Rudolph Matas, "Post-Operative Thrombosis and Pulmonary Embolism before and after Lister, a Retrospect and Prospect," *University of Toronto Medical Bulletin* 10 (1932): 10–12.

7. Stewart A. Fish, "The Death of President Garfield," *Bull. Hist. Med.* 24 (1950): 378–92.

8. Brieger, ed., *Medical America in the Nineteenth Century*, 201, 209.

9. James Turner, *Animals, Pain, and Humanity in the Victorian Mind* (Baltimore, 1980), 108; Wangensteen and Wangensteen, *The Rise of Surgery*, 488.

10. Duffy, *Matas History of Medicine in Louisiana*, 2:369–75.

11. Walter C. Burket, ed., *Surgical Papers of William Stewart Halsted*, 2 vols. (Baltimore, 1952), 2:514; for a survey of Halsted's career, see "An Appreciation," 1:xv–xliii.

12. William L. Fox, *Dandy of Hopkins* (Baltimore, 1984), 43, 63; A. Scott Earle,

ed., *Surgery in America: From the Colonial Era to the Twentieth Century*, 2d ed. (New York, 1983), 289. The best source for brief biographies of medical leaders is Martin Kaufman, Stuart Galishoff, and Todd L. Savitt, eds., *Dictionary of American Medical Biography*, 2 vols. (Westport, Conn., 1984).

13. Richard H. Meade, *An Introduction to the History of General Surgery* (Philadelphia, 1968), 291–94; Earle, ed., *Surgery in America*, 289.

14. Keys, *History of Surgical Anesthesia*, 65–67; Duffy, *Matas History of Medicine in Louisiana*, 2:374–75.

15. Burket, ed., *Surgical Papers by William Stewart Halsted, 1852–1922*, 1:167–68.

16. I am indebted to one of my former students, Debra A. Lowe, for gathering this and other information from the *Annual Announcements of the Board of Visitors of the Baltimore College of Dental Surgery, 1840 to 1858*.

17. A good short history of dentistry in Maryland can be found in Ben Robinson, "The Foundations of Professional Dentistry," *Proceedings*, Dental Centenary Celebration, Baltimore, Maryland, March 18, 19, and 20, 1940 (Baltimore, 1940), 1000–1029.

18. Chapin A. Harris, *The Dental Art: A Practical Treatise on Dental Surgery* (Baltimore, 1839).

19. William Simon, *History of the Baltimore College of Dental Surgery* (n.p., 1904), 1–15; Robinson, "Foundations of Professional Dentistry," 1015–24; Cordell, *Medical Annals of Maryland*, 105.

20. Garrison, *Introduction to the History of Medicine*, 615; Duffy, *Matas History of Medicine in Louisiana*, 2:383–84.

21. Steven L. Schlossman, JoAnne Brown, and Michael Sedlak, *The Public School in American Dentistry*, Rand Publication Series (Santa Monica, Calif., 1986), v–viii, 64.

22. Ronald L. Kathren, "Early X-ray Protection in the United States," *Health Physics* 8 (1962): 503–11; Kathren, "William H. Rollins (1852–1929): X-ray Protection Pioneer," *J. Hist. Med. & All. Sci.* 19 (1964): 287–94.

23. Duffy, *Matas History of Medicine in Louisiana*, 2:382–83.

24. Ravitch, *Century of Surgery*, 44–45.

25. Meade, *Introduction to the History of General Surgery*, 341–42; Wangensteen and Wangensteen, *Rise of Surgery*, 527, 538, 540.

26. Francis D. Moore, "Surgery," in *Advances in American Medicine*, ed. Bowers and Purcell, 2:640–41; Meade, *Introduction to the History of General Surgery*, 100–101.

27. Meade, *Introduction to the History of General Surgery*, 297.

28. Duffy, *Matas History of Medicine in Louisiana*, 1:381.

29. E. Warren, *A Doctor's Experience on Three Continents* (Baltimore, 1885), reprinted in *Bulletin of the New York Academy of Medicine* 49 (1973): 1019–20.

30. Ravitch, *Century of Surgery*, 398.

31. Vogel, *Invention of the Modern Hospital*, 93.

32. Peter Olch, "Evarts A. Graham, the American College of Surgeons, and the American Board of Surgery," *J. Hist. Med. & All. Sci.* 27 (1972): 247–49.

Chapter 13: Medical Education

1. C. B. Burr, ed., *Medical History of Michigan*, 2 vols. (Minneapolis, 1930), 1:468.

2. Kaufman, *American Medical Education*, 157–58; William Pepper, *Higher Medical Education, the True Interest of the Public and of the Profession: Two Addresses Delivered before the Medical Department of the University of Pennsylvania on Oct. 1, 1877 and Oct. 2, 1893* (Philadelphia, 1894), 15–16.

3. Shryock, *Medical Licensing in America*, 60.

4. Martin Kaufman, "Edward H. Dixon and Medical Education in New York," *New York Historical Society Quarterly* 24 (1970): 405.

5. Charles McIntyre, "The Percentage of College-Bred Men in the Medical Profession," *Medical Record* 22 (December 16, 1882): 681–84.

6. Kaufman, *American Medical Education*, 127–28.

7. Ibid., 128–30; Kenneth M. Ludmerer, "Reform at Harvard Medical School, 1869–1909," *Bull. Hist. Med.* 55 (1981): 345–48.

8. The standard history is Alan M. Chesney, *The Johns Hopkins Hospital and the Johns Hopkins School of Medicine: A Chronicle*, 3 vols. (Baltimore, 1963), continued by Thomas B. Turner, *Heritage of Excellence: The Johns Hopkins Medical Institutions, 1914–1947* (Baltimore, 1974). An excellent analysis of Welch and his role at Hopkins can be found in Fleming, *William H. Welch and the Rise of Modern Medicine.*

9. John J. Byrne, "Lengthening Shadows," *New England Journal of Medicine* 305 (1981): 1051–59.

10. Kaufman, *American Medical Education*, 138–40.

11. Ibid., 154–55; Robert L. Hudson, "Abraham Flexner in Perspective: American Medical Education, 1865–1910," *Bull. Hist. Med.* 46 (1972): 551.

12. Kaufman, *American Medical Education*, 156–59.

13. American Medical Association, Council on Medical Education, *Report of the First Annual Conference, 1905* (Chicago, 1905), and *Report of the Second Annual Conference* (Chicago, 1906).

14. Abraham Flexner, *Medical Education in the United States and Canada: A Report to the Carnegie Foundation for the Advancement of Teaching* (New York, 1910).

15. Ibid., 233, 238.

16. Shryock, *American Medical Research*, 119–21.

17. Duffy, *Tulane University Medical Center*, 86–87.

18. Ludmerer, "Reform at Harvard Medical School," 352–53.

19. Duffy, *Tulane University Medical Center*, 108–9.

20. Abraham Flexner, "Medical Education, 1909–1924," *JAMA* 82 (1924): 834–35.

21. Hudson, "Abraham Flexner in Perspective," 545; Kenneth M. Ludmerer, *Learning to Heal: The Development of American Medical Education* (New York, 1985), 4–7.

22. E. Richard Brown, "He Who Pays the Piper: The Medical Profession and Medical Education," in *Health Care in America: Essays in Social History*, ed. Susan Reverby and David Rosner (Philadelphia, 1979), 132–54.

23. Daniel M. Fox, "Abraham Flexner's Unpublished Report: Foundations and Medical Education, 1909–1928," *Bull. Hist. Med.* 54 (1980): 490.

24. For an elaboration of this point, see Gerald E. Markowitz and David K. Rosner, "Doctors in Crisis: A Study of the Use of Medical Education Reform to Establish Modern Professional Elitism in Medicine," *American Quarterly* 25 (1973): 83–107, and John Duffy, "The American Medical Profession and Public Health: From Support to Ambivalence," *Bull. Hist. Med.* 53 (1979): 1–22.

Chapter 14: The Medical Profession Organizes

1. Rosenberg, "The Practice of Medicine in New York a Century Ago," 229.

2. "Meeting of February 12, 1898," *Proceedings of the Orleans Parish Medical Society, 1898* (New Orleans, 1898), 51–54; George Rosen, *Fees and Fee Bills: Some Economic Aspects of Medical Practice in Nineteenth Century America* (Baltimore, 1946), 88–89; see also, Jan Coombs, "Rural Medical Practice in the 1880s: A View from Central Wisconsin," *Bull. Hist. Med.* 64 (1990): 35–62.

3. New Orleans *Bee*, June 22, 1875; New Orleans *Daily Picayune*, June 29, 1875.

4. "Is Medicine a Science?," editorial, *The Sanitarian* 4 (1876): 339–40.

5. Haller, Jr., *American Medicine in Transition*, 281–82.

6. A. H. Smith, "The Family Physician of the Future," Anniversary Discourse, New York Academy of Medicine *Transactions*, 2d ser., 4 (1890): 49–50; Donald E. Konold, *A History of American Medical Ethics, 1847–1912* (Madison, Wis., 1962), 46–47.

7. Blanton, *Medicine in Virginia in the Nineteenth Century*, 91.

8. Stanford E. Chaillé, *Address on State Medical Organization* (New Orleans, 1879).

9. Charles A. Reed, "Presidential Address," *JAMA* 36 (1901): 1601.

10. Dorothy Long, ed., *Medicine in North Carolina: Essays in the History of Medical Science and Medical Service, 1524–1960*, 2 vols. (Raleigh, N.C., 1972), 1:215–22.

11. Joseph I. Waring, *History of Medicine in South Carolina, 1825–1900* (Columbia, S.C., 1967), 144–45.

12. Duffy, *Matas History of Medicine in Louisiana*, 2:403–12.

13. Kaufman, *American Medical Education*, 143–46.

14. Duffy, *Matas History of Medicine in Louisiana*, 2:409–10.

15. Shryock, *Medical Licensing in America*, 58–59.

16. Duffy, *Matas History of Medicine in Louisiana*, 2:355.

17. E. J. Doering, "Mutual Protection against Blackmail," *JAMA* 7 (1885): 115.

18. Konold, *History of American Medical Ethics*, 49–50.

19. Cowen, *Medicine and Health in New Jersey*, 72.

20. Kaufman, *Homeopathy in America*, 76–92, 126–34.

21. Morris Fishbein, *A History of the American Medical Association, 1847 to 1947* (Philadelphia 1969), 108–13, 201–13.

22. Rothstein, *American Physicians in the Nineteenth Century*, 317–18.

23. Ibid., 318–22.

24. The best account of McCormack's work can be found in James G. Burrow, *Organized Medicine in the Progressive Era: The Move toward Monopoly* (Baltimore, 1977), 16–28.

25. Burrow, *Organized Medicine*, chapter 6; Young, *Pure Food*, 187–88.

26. Duffy, *The Sanitarians*, 185. For swill milk, see Duffy, *History of Public Health in New York City, 1626–1866*, 427–37.

27. Starr, *Social Transformation of American Medicine*, 16, 112–40, 180–232.

Chapter 15: The Advancing Front of Medicine

1. For a brief summary of American physiology, see *A Century of American Physiology*, National Library of Medicine (Bethesda, Md.), 1987.

2. James Bordley, III, and A. McGehee Harvey, *Two Centuries of American Medicine, 1776–1976* (Philadelphia, 1976), 228ff. This is the best scientific and technological account of twentieth-century American medicine.

3. George W. Thorn, "Metabolism and Endocrinology," in *Advances in American Medicine*, ed. Bowers and Purcell, 1:157–59.

4. Michael Bliss, *The Discovery of Insulin* (Chicago, 1982), presents an excellent account of this development.

5. Kaufman et al., eds., *Dictionary of American Medical Biography*, 1:21–22.

6. Robert E. Kohler, "Medical Reform and Biomedical Science," in *The Therapeutic Revolution*, ed. Vogel and Rosenberg, 29–30. For the history of biochemistry see Kohler's *From Medical Chemistry to Biochemistry: The Making of a Biomedical Discipline* (Cambridge, 1982).

7. Kenneth J. Carpenter, *The History of Scurvy and Vitamin C* (Cambridge, 1986), 173ff.

8. Elizabeth W. Etheridge, *The Butterfly Caste: A Social History of Pellagra in the South* (Westport, Conn., 1972), 207.

9. Thorn, "Metabolism and Endocrinology," 161; Bordley and Harvey, *Two Centuries of American Medicine*, 477–78.

10. Elizabeth Fee, *Disease and Discovery: A History of the Johns Hopkins School of Hygiene and Public Health, 1916–1939* (Baltimore, 1987), 129–30; Bordley and Harvey, *Two Centuries of American Medicine*, 242–44.

11. *Scientific American* 161 (1939): 297; ibid. 164 (1939): 323.

12. Bordley and Harvey, *Two Centuries of American Medicine*, 250–56.

13. Maxwell M. Wintrobe, *Blood, Pure and Eloquent: A Story of Discovery, of People, and of Ideas* (New York, 1980), 23–25, 339–44, 359–60.

14. Bordley and Harvey, *Two Centuries of American Medicine*, 256–64.

15. Theobald Smith and F. L. Kilbourne, "Investigations into the Nature, Causation, and Prevention of Texas or Southern Cattle Fever," *Eighth and Ninth Annual Reports of the Bureau of Animal Industry for the Years 1891 and 1892* (Washington, D.C., 1893), 177–304.

16. A. P. Waterson and Lise Wilkinson, *An Introduction to the History of Virology* (London, 1978), 33–35.

17. For Rivers's work see Saul Benison, Oral History Memoir, *Tom Rivers: Reflections on a Life in Medicine and Science* (Cambridge, Mass., 1967).

18. Timothy C. Jacobson, *Making Medical Doctors: Science and Medicine in Vanderbilt since Flexner* (Tuscaloosa, Ala., 1987), 222–37.

19. Paul B. Beeson, "Infectious Diseases (Microbiology)," in *Advances in American Medicine*, ed. Bowers and Purcell, 1:140–41; Waterson and Wilkinson, *Introduction to the History of Virology*, 114, 138, 167.

20. James W. Fisher, "Origins of American Pharmacology," *Trends in Pharmacological Sciences* 7 (1986): 41–45; Hubert A. Lechevalier, "The Search for Antibiotics at Rutgers University," in *The History of Antibiotics: A Symposium*, ed. John Parascondola (Madison, Wis., 1980), 113–23.

21. Harry F. Dowling, *Fighting Infection: Conquests of the Twentieth Century* (Cambridge, Mass., 1977), 105–12, 123–57.

22. Ibid., 158–92; Henry Welch and Felix Marti-Ibanez, *The Antibiotic Saga* (New York, 1960), 75–98.

23. Robert P. Hudson, "Polypharmacy in Twentieth-Century America," *Clinical Pharmacology and Therapeutics* 9 (1968): 5.

24. Young, *Medical Messiahs*, 409–13.

25. Bordley and Harvey, *Two Centuries of American Medicine*, 307–9, 709–12.

26. Robert G. Frank, Louise H. Marshall, and H. W. Magoun, "The Neurosciences," in *Advances in American Medicine*, ed. Bowers and Purcell, 2:579–84.

27. Dowling, *Fighting Infection*, 91–92.

28. Geoffrey Marks and William K. Beatty, *The Story of Medicine in America* (New York, 1973), 303–5.

29. I am indebted for this information to Gerald N. Grob, who sent me a MS copy of chapter 1 of his book, *From Asylum to Community: Mental Health Policy in Modern America* (Princeton, 1991). An excellent account of psychiatry and mental hospitals can be found in his *Mental Illness and American Society, 1875–1940* (Princeton, 1983).

30. Harry A. Moore, *Public Health in the United States: An Outline with Historical Data* (New York, 1923), 114; Haven Emerson, "Public Health and Mental Hygiene," *Hospital Social Service* 19 (1929): 385.

31. E. Fuller Torrey, *Nowhere to Go: The Tragic Odyssey of the Homeless Mentally Ill* (New York, 1988), 55–58.

32. Gerald N. Grob, manuscript for *From Asylum to Community*, chapter 1.

33. Marks and Beatty, *Story of Medicine in America*, 305; Edwin Shorter, *The Health Century* (New York, 1987), 121–28.

34. Joint Commission on Mental Illness and Health, "Action for Mental Health," in *Health and the Community: Readings in the Philosophy and Sciences of Public Health*, ed. Alfred H. Katz and Jean S. Felton (New York, 1965), 549; E. Fuller Torrey, "Community Mental Health Policy—Tennis, Anyone?" *Wall Street Journal*, March 29, 1990.

35. Torrey, *Nowhere to Go*, 29–34, 97–98; Jon E. Guderman and Miles F. Shore, "Beyond Deinstitutionalization," *New England Journal of Medicine* 302 (1984): 832–33.

36. Torrey, "Community Mental Health Policy," *Wall Street Journal*, March 29, 1990.

37. "APA Issues Position Statement on Child, Adolescent Hospitalization," *Psychiatric News* 24 (July 7, 1989): 1, 18; Tim W. Ferguson, "Any Wonder Medical Premiums Are Rising Like Crazy?" *Wall Street Journal*, May 22, 1990.

38. Torrey, *Nowhere to Go*, 164, 214–15.

39. U.S. Congress, Office of Technology Assessment, *Biology, Medicine, and the Bill of Rights—Special Report*, OTA-/CIT-371 (Washington, D.C., 1988), 21–27; Bernard D. David, "The New Biology," unpublished manuscript, 1–3.

40. James V. Neel, "Human Genetics," in *Advances in American Medicine*, ed. Bowers and Purcell, 1:39–42, 90.

41. U.S. Congress, *Biology, Medicine, and the Bill of Rights*, 45–46.

42. Dowling, *Fighting Infection*, 4, 24, 193–94; Wesley W. Spink, *Infectious Diseases: Prevention and Treatment in the Nineteenth and Twentieth Centuries* (Minneapolis, 1978), 320, 328–32.

43. Waterson and Wilkinson, *Introduction to the History of Virology*, 61–62; Dowling, *Fighting Infection*, 208–18.

44. Waterson and Wilkinson, *Introduction to the History of Virology*, 65–66.

45. Dowling, *Fighting Infection*, 225–26.

46. Bordley and Harvey, *Two Centuries of American Medicine*, 628–34.

47. Michael B. Shimkin, "Neoplasia," in *Advances in American Medicine*, ed. Bowers and Purcell, 1:215–18.

48. Bordley and Harvey, *Two Centuries of American Medicine*, 677–81.

49. James T. Patterson, *The Dread Disease: Cancer and Modern American Culture* (Cambridge, Mass., 1987), viii–x, 188–90.

50. Shimkin, "Neoplasia," 223–35.

51. Stephen Rosenberg et al., "Gene Transfer in Humans—Immunotherapy of Patients with Advanced Melanoma . . . ," *New England Journal of Medicine* 323 (1990): 570–78. I am indebted to Dr. John E. Salvaggio for much of this and the following material on recent developments in cancer therapy.

52. For a discussion of other possible developments see Andrew Skolnik, "Molecular Biology Offers New Weapons Against Cancer," *JAMA* 263 (1990): 2289–90.

Chapter 16: Surgery and Medical Technology since World War I

1. Moore, "Surgery," 643–44.

2. Olch, "Evarts A. Graham," 247–48.

3. J. Rogers Hollingsworth, *A Political Economy of Medicine: Great Britain and the United States* (Baltimore, 1986), 102–3.

4. Olch, "Evarts A. Graham," 249–61.

5. *Introduction to the History of General Surgery*, 100–101.

6. Kaufman et al., *Dictionary of American Medical Biography*, 1:370–71.

7. Keys, *History of Surgical Anesthesia*, 58, 89–90.

8. Ravitch, *Century of Surgery*, 532.

9. Meade, *Introduction to the History of General Surgery*, 341.

10. Ravitch, *Century of Surgery*, 71–72.

11. Wangensteen and Wangensteen, *Rise of Surgery*, 164–65.

12. Ravitch, *Century of Surgery*, 403.

13. Moore, "Surgery," 651–52; Meade, *Introduction to the History of General Surgery*, 179–82.

14. Meade, *Introduction to the History of General Surgery*, 111.

15. Ibid., 189–90; Wangensteen and Wangensteen, *Rise of Surgery*, 270–72; A. McGehee Harvey, *Adventures in Medical Research: A Century of Discovery at Johns Hopkins* (Baltimore, 1974), 232–39.

16. Moore, "Surgery," 655–56.

17. Ravitch, *Century of Surgery*, 1071; Meade, *Introduction to the History of General Surgery*, 111–12.

18. Meade, *Introduction to the History of General Surgery*, 365–66.

19. Moore, "Surgery," 672.

20. Meade, *Introduction to the History of General Surgery*, 369–70.

21. Reiser, *Medicine and the Reign of Technology*, 158–59.

22. For a good survey of early developments in microsurgery see David L. Drotar, *Microsurgery: Revolution in the Operating Room* (New York, 1981).

23. Arthur J. Viseltear, "Joanna Stephens and the Eighteenth-Century Lithotriptics: A Misplaced Chapter in the History of Therapeutics," *Bull. Hist. Med.* 43 (1968): 199–220.

24. Hollingsworth, *Political Economy of Medicine*, 175–76.

25. *Newsweek*, January 26, 1987, 70–71.

26. Diana B. Dutton, *Worse than the Disease: Pitfalls of Medical Progress* (Cambridge, 1988), 91–126.

27. Hollingsworth, *Political Economy of Medicine*, 178–79.

28. Ronald Bayer and Arthur L. Caplan, *In Search of Equity: Health Needs and the Health Care System* (New York, 1983), 96; Bryan Jennett, *High Technology Medicine: Benefits and Burdens* (Oxford, 1986), 193, 249.

29. *Wall Street Journal*, February 21, 1992.

Chapter 17: Medical Education since Flexner

1. The emergence of medical specialties is well covered in Rosemary Stevens, *American Medicine and the Public Interest* (New Haven, 1971).

2. Edward C. Atwater, "Internal Medicine," in *The Education of American Physicians: Historical Essays*, ed. Ronald L. Numbers (Berkeley and Los Angeles, 1980), 168–74.

3. John H. Warner, "Physiology," in *The Education of American Physicians*, ed. Numbers, 70; John B. Blake, "Anatomy," ibid., 44.

4. Lawrence D. Longo, "Obstetrics and Gynecology," in *The Education of American Physicians*, ed. Numbers, 218–25.

5. Gert H. Brieger, "Surgery," in *The Education of American Physicians*, ed. Numbers, 200–204.

6. David L. Cowen, "Materia Medica and Pharmacology," in *The Education of American Physicians*, ed. Numbers, 112–21.

7. Duffy, *The Sanitarians*, 251; Judith W. Leavitt, "Public Health and Preventive Medicine," in *The Education of American Physicians*, ed. Numbers, 261–272.

8. Samuel A. Cartwright, "Address of Samuel A. Cartwright, M.D. . . , *New Orleans Med. Surg. J.* 2 (1845–46): 727–31.

9. Chester R. Burns, "Medical Ethics and Jurisprudence," in *The Education of American Physicians*, ed. Numbers, 283–89.

10. Martin Kaufman, "American Medical Education," in *The Education of American Physicians*, ed. Numbers, 72.

11. For an example, see Duffy, *Tulane University Medical Center*, chapter 10.

12. John A. D. Cooper, "Undergraduate Medical Education," in *Advances in American Medicine*, ed. Bowers and Purcell, 1:284; Kaufman, "American Medical Education," in *The Education of American Physicians*, ed. Numbers, 26–28

13. T. B. Turner, "The Medical Schools Twenty Years Afterward: The Impact of the Research Programs of the National Institutes of Health," *Journal of Medical Education* 42 (1967): 109–18.

14. William G. Rothstein, *American Medical Schools and the Practice of Medicine* (New York, 1987), 255, 334.

15. Ibid., 230–33, 246–47, 254–55, 288–89, 331.

Chapter 18: Women in Medicine

1. Lamar R. Murphy, *Enter the Physician: The Transformation of Domestic Medicine, 1760–1860* (Tuscaloosa, Ala., 1991), xiv–xviii.

2. John Duffy, *A History of Public Health in New York City, 1866–1966* (New York, 1974), 259, 462.

3. Frances E. Kobrin, "The American Midwife Controversy: A Crisis of Professionalization," in *Sickness and Health in America: Readings in the History of Medicine*

and Public Health, ed. Judith W. Leavitt and Ronald L. Numbers (Madison, Wis., 1978), 217–25; Duffy, *History of Public Health in New York City, 1866–1966*, 461–62.

4. John B. Blake, "Women and Medicine in Ante-Bellum America," *Bull. Hist. Med.* 39 (1965): 111–12.

5. Elizabeth Blackwell, *Pioneer Work in Opening the Medical Profession to Women: Autobiographical Sketches* (rpt., New York, 1970), 5, 46, 58ff.; *Boston Med. Surg. J.* 37 (1847): 405.

6. Kent L. Brown, ed., *Medicine in Cleveland and Cuyahoga County, 1810–1976* (Cleveland, 1977), 52–53; Gulielma F. Alsop, *History of the Woman's Medical College, Philadelphia, Pennsylvania, 1850–1950* (Philadelphia, 1950), 12–24.

7. Thomas A. Ashby, "Abstract of an Address on the Medical Education of Women . . . ," *Maryland Medical Journal* 9 (1882): 272.

8. Carol Lopate, *Women in Medicine* (Baltimore, 1968), 7.

9. Martin Kaufman, "John Stainback Wilson and Female Medical Education," *J. Hist. Med. & All. Sci.* 28 (1973): 397.

10. *Boston Med. Surg. J.* 41 (1850): 520–22; ibid. 48 (1853): 66; ibid. 53 (1855): 292–94; ibid. 54 (1856): 168–74.

11. Charles D. Meigs, *Females and Their Diseases* (Philadelphia, 1848), 47; Fishbein, *History of the American Medical Association*, 82–83; *Medical and Surgical Reporter* 2 (1859): 275–76.

12. *Medical and Surgical Reporter* 2 (1859): 295–96; ibid. 16 (1867): 335; *New Orleans Med. Surg. J.* 17 (1860): 908–11.

13. "The Discussion of the Female Physician Question . . . ," *Boston Med. Surg. J.* 84 (1870): 350–54; James R. Chadwick, "The Admission of Women to the Massachusetts Medical Society," ibid. 106 (1882): 547–49; "One Hundred and Third Annual Meeting of the Massachusetts Medical Society," ibid. 110 (1884): 584–87.

14. Fishbein, *History of the American Medical Association*, 91; "Annual Convention of the American Medical Association," *Boston Med. Surg. J.* 84 (1870): 334–36, 350–55; *Transactions of the American Medical Association* 22 (1871): 90; Lopate, *Women in Medicine*, 12–13, 17.

15. Ashby, "Abstract of an Address on the Medical Education of Women," 273–74.

16. "Women's Medical College of Chicago," *JAMA* 2 (1884): 488; "Domestic Correspondence," ibid. 5 (1885): 52; "The Higher Education of Women," ibid. 7 (1886): 267–69.

17. Gloria Moldow, *Women Doctors in Gilded-Age Washington: Race, Gender and Professionalization* (Urbana, 1987), 2–7, 77, 94–113, 167.

18. Ibid., 6, 15.

19. Ashby, "Abstract of an Address on the Medical Education of Women," 271–72; *Boston Med. Surg. J.* 100 (1879): 727–30, 789–91.

20. Regina Markell Morantz-Sanchez, *Sympathy and Science: Women Physicians and American Medicine* (New York, 1985), 86–87; Simon Flexner and James Thomas

Flexner, *William Henry Welch and the Heroic Age of American Medicine* (New York, 1941), 215–21.

21. Duffy, *Tulane University Medical Center*, 84–85, 134–36.

22. Lopate, *Women in Medicine*, 193; *Journal of Medical Education* 59 (1974): 303; "Undergraduate Medical Education," *JAMA* 264 (1990): 807.

23. Morantz-Sanchez, *Sympathy and Science*, 356. For an overview of medicine and women, see Elizabeth Fee, *Women and Health: The Politics of Medicine* (Farmingdale, N.Y., 1983).

24. S. Josephine Baker, *Fighting for Life* (New York, 1939).

25. Alice Hamilton, *Exploring the Dangerous Trades: The Autobiography of Alice Hamilton* (Boston, 1943); Barbara Sicherman, *Alice Hamilton: A Life in Letters* (Cambridge, Mass., 1984).

26. For an excellent picture of the obstacles encountered by women medical professors, see Harvey, *Adventures in Medical Research*, chapter 18.

27. Duffy, *History of Public Health in New York City, 1866–1966*, 408, 413–36.

28. Duffy, *Matas History of Medicine in Louisiana*, 1:89–91.

29. Lavinia L. Dock and Isabel M. Stewart, *A Short History of Nursing*, 4th ed. (New York, 1938), 148–49.

30. Ibid., 148–50.

31. Fishbein, *History of the American Medical Association*, 77–78.

32. Duffy, *History of Public Health in New York City, 1866–1966*, 187–88.

33. Susan B. Reverby, "The Search for the Hospital Yardstick: Nursing and the Rationalization of Hospital Work," in *Sickness and Health in America*, ed. Leavitt and Numbers, 207–208; Richard H. Shryock, *The History of Nursing: An Interpretation of the Social and Medical Factors Involved* (Philadelphia, 1959), 300.

34. Helen E. Marshall, *Mary Adelaide Nutting, Pioneer of Modern Nursing* (Baltimore, 1972), 33–39, 51.

35. Ibid., 135–36; Minnie Goodnow, *Nursing History in Brief* (Philadelphia, 1939), 229.

36. Barbara Milosh, *"The Physician's Hand": Work Culture and Conflict in American Nursing* (Philadelphia, 1982), 4–5, 37, 69, 159, 207–208; Susan B. Reverby, *Ordered to Care: The Dilemma of American Nursing, 1850–1945* (Cambridge, Mass., 1987), 1, 6, 58, 75.

37. Reverby, *Ordered to Care*, 1–2; Milosh, *"The Physician's Hand,"* 25.

38. Karen Buhler-Wilkerson, "Left Carrying the Bag: Experiments in Visiting Nursing," *Nursing Research* 36 (1987): 42–43.

39. Diane Hamilton, "The Metropolitan Visiting Nurse Service (1909–1953)," paper delivered at the annual meeting of the American Association for the History of Medicine, May 1, 1987.

40. Reverby, *Ordered to Care*, 3, 6, 142; Reverby, "The Search for the Hospital Yardstick," 212.

41. Mary C. Gillett, "The Army Medical Department, 1865–1917," chapters 5

and 12, MS, forthcoming; Goodnow, *Nursing History in Brief*, 133–34.

42. Shryock, *History of Nursing*, 309–15; *Facts About Nursing, '86–'87*, American Nurses' Association (Kansas City, Mo., 1887), 10; Peri Rosenfield, *Nursing Student Census, 1989* (New York, 1990), 59, 65.

43. L. I. Stein, D. T. Watts, and Timothy Howell, "Sounding Board: The Doctor-Nurse Game Revisited," *New England Journal of Medicine* 322 (1990): 546–49.

44. Milosh, *"The Physician's Hand,"* 20, 211.

Chapter 19: Minorities in Medicine

1. Kelly Miller, "The Historic Background of the Negro Physician," *Journal of Negro History* 1 (1916): 99–109; Harold E. Farmer, "An Account of the Earliest Colored Gentlemen in Medical Science in the United States," *Bull. Hist. Med.* 8 (1940): 599–618; M. O. Bousfield, "An Account of Physicians of Color in the United States," ibid. 17 (1945): 61–84; Herbert M. Morais, *The History of the Negro in Medicine* (New York, 1967), 8–10.

2. Lyman H. Butterfield, ed., *Letters of Benjamin Rush*, 2 vols. (Princeton, 1951), 1:497.

3. Duffy, *Matas History of Medicine in Louisiana*, 1:324–25.

4. New Orleans *Daily Picayune*, March 12, 1890.

5. Brown, ed., *Medicine in Cleveland and Cuyahoga County*, 71.

6. Morais, *History of the Negro in Medicine*, 36–37.

7. Henry A. Bullock, *A History of Negro Education in the South from 1619 to the Present* (Cambridge, Mass., 1967), 33–34; Flexner, *Medical Education in the United States and Canada*, 202, 230, 232, 280–81, 303–5, 307.

8. Bousfield, "An Account of Physicians of Color in the United States," 70.

9. Fox, "Abraham Flexner's Unpublished Report," 488–89.

10. Edward H. Beardsley, *A History of Neglect: Health Care for Blacks and Mill Workers in the Twentieth-Century South* (Knoxville, 1987), 77–78, 89.

11. L. A. Falk and N. A. Quaynor-Malm, "Early Afro-American Medical Education in the United States: The Origins of Meharry Medical College in the Nineteenth Century," *Proceedings* of the Twenty-third International Congress of the History of Medicine, London, September 2–9, 1972 (London, 1974), 1:346–56; Morais, *History of the Negro in Medicine*, 68–69; Todd L. Savitt, "Entering a White Profession: Black Physicians in the New South, 1880–1920," *Bull. Hist. Med.* 61 (1987): 507–40.

12. Vanessa N. Gamble, *The Black Community Hospital: Contemporary Dilemmas in Historical Perspective* (New York, 1989), 40; Brown, ed., *Medicine in Cleveland and Cuyahoga County*, 75–76.

13. Edward H. Beardsley, "Making Separate, Equal: Black Physicians and the

Problems of Medical Segregation in the Pre–World War II South," *Bull. Hist. Med.* 57 (1983): 390–93.

14. Bousfield, "An Account of Physicians of Color in the United States," 72–73; Morais, *History of the Negro in Medicine*, 85–86, 127.

15. Morais, *History of the Negro in Medicine*, 110, 128; Beardsley, *History of Neglect*, 249ff.

16. Gamble, *Black Community Hospital*, 53, 59, 66, 71–73; Beardsley, *History of Neglect*, 271.

17. Clay E. Simpson, Jr., and Remy Arnoff, "Factors Affecting the Supply of Minority Physicians in 2000," *Public Health Reports* 103 (1988): 179–80; Harry S. Jones et al., "Undergraduate Medical Education," *JAMA* 262 (1989): 1016; ibid., 264 (1990): 807.

18. Benjamin R. Epstein and Arnold Foster, *Some of My Best Friends* (New York, 1962), 178–79. For an excellent discussion of prejudice in this period see Saul Jarcho, "Medical Education in the United States—1920–1956," *Journal of the Mount Sinai Hospital* 26 (1959): 357–60.

19. Fox, "Abraham Flexner's Unpublished Report," 482–83; *New York Times*, June 23–24, 1922; "Harvard's Sifting Committee on Racial Proportion," *School and Society* 16 (1922): 12–13; Editorial, *Nation* 114 (1922): 108.

20. R. P. Boas, "Who Shall Go to College?" *Atlantic* 130 (1922): 441–48.

21. *Literary Digest* 105 (1930): 32; ibid. 106 (1930): 20; *School and Society* 40 (1934): 836.

22. Kenneth Collins, "American Jewish Medical Students in Scotland: 1925–1940," paper delivered at the annual meeting of the American Association for the History of Medicine, May 2, 1987.

23. See "Anti-Semitism at Dartmouth," *New Republic* 113 (1945): 208–9.

24. Nathan C. Belth, ed., *Barriers, Patterns of Discrimination Against Jews* (New York, 1958), 74–76.

Chapter 20: The Medical Profession in the Twentieth Century

1. Shryock, *Medical Licensing in America*, 30.

2. For the development of specialties in the nineteenth century, see Rothstein, *American Physicians in the Nineteenth Century*, and for the twentieth century, see Stevens, *American Medicine and the Public Interest*.

3. "Quack Doctors by the Thousands," *Literary Digest* 79 (1923), December 8: 11–12, December 22: 35–38; Editorial, "The Medical Diploma Scandal," *American Journal of Public Health* 14 (1924): 141–42.

4. Shryock, *Medical Licensing in America*, 80–83; Paul R. Kelley, "Evaluation Services to Medical Schools," *National Board of Medical Examiners, 75th Anniversary, Special Commemorative Annual Report* ([Philadelphia], 1990), 60–61.

5. *Washington Post,* March 31, 1982, C3.

6. Ibid., January 10, 1988, A1.

7. Baton Rouge *Sunday Advocate,* September 2, 1990, 8A.

8. Robert C. Derbyshire, *Medical Licensure and Discipline in the United States* (Baltimore, 1969), 163–68.

9. Young, *Medical Messiahs,* 184–88; James G. Burrow, *AMA: Voice of American Medicine* (Baltimore, 1963), 67ff.

10. Young, *Medical Messiahs,* 415–18.

11. This information appears in the expanded paperback edition of Young, *The Medical Messiahs: A Social History of Health Quackery in Twentieth-Century America* (Princeton, 1992), 436–37.

12. Burrow, *Organized Medicine,* 148–53; Ronald L. Numbers, *Almost Persuaded: American Physicians and Compulsory Health Insurance, 1912–1920* (Baltimore, 1978), 113–14.

13. Fishbein, *History of the American Medical Association,* 331; see also his section "The War Against Socialized Medicine — 1925–1929," 358–80.

14. Burrow, *AMA,* 198–90.

15. Ibid., 214–15.

16. Stevens, *American Medicine and the Public Interest,* 267–71, 418–21.

17. Starr, *Social Transformation of American Medicine,* 359–63, 428–30, 444–49.

18. Ibid., 280–83, 368–69.

19. Stevens, *American Medicine and the Public Interest,* 438–42.

20. *New England Journal of Medicine* 318 (1988): 1130–31; ibid. 323 (1990): 884–88, 991–92; ibid. 324 (1991): 1253–58; *JAMA* 265 (1991): 374, 2108–9, 2653–55; ibid. 266 (1991): 104–9.

21. State of Florida Health Care Cost Containment Board, "Joint Ventures among Health Care Providers in Florida" (Tallahassee, Fla., 1992), vol. 1, appendix B, 9–10; vol. 2, v, chapter 1, 12–13; vol. 3, 5, chapter 2, 3.

22. John Colombotos and Corinne Kirchner, *Physicians and Social Change* (New York, 1986), 138–43, 182–85, 196.

23. *Wall Street Journal,* April 10, 1990, A19.

Chapter 21: The Community's Health

1. For a more detailed account of public health in this period, see Duffy, *The Sanitarians,* chapters 1–3.

2. Ibid., chapters 4–7.

3. James H. Cassedy, *American Medicine and Statistical Thinking, 1800–1860* (Cambridge, Mass., 1984), 194–99.

4. Cavins, "National Quarantine and Sanitary Conventions," 404–26.

5. Peter W. Bruton, "The National Board of Health" (Ph.D. diss., University of Maryland, 1974), 54ff.

6. For an account of early public health in these two states, see Gordon E. Gillson, *Louisiana State Board of Health: The Formative Years* (n.d., n.p.), and Barbara G. Rosenkrantz, *Public Health and the State: Changing Views in Massachusetts, 1842–1936* (Cambridge, Mass., 1972).

7. Duffy, *A History of Public Health in New York City, 1866–1966*, chapter 6 and pp. 220–35; Duffy, *The Sanitarians*, 178.

8. Bonner, *Medicine in Chicago*, 20–21; *Annual Report of the Louisiana State Board of Health, 1881* (New Orleans, 1882), 242–44.

9. Duffy, *Matas History of Medicine in Louisiana*, 2:465–66.

10. Richard R. Meckel, *Save the Babies: American Public Health Reform and the Prevention of Infant Mortality, 1850–1929* (Baltimore, 1990), 29, 38.

11. Duffy, *History of Public Health in New York City, 1866–1966*, 208–11.

12. Stuart Galishoff, *Safeguarding the Public Health: Newark, 1895–1918* (Westport, Conn., 1975), 70; Duffy, *History of Public Health in New York City, 1866–1966*, 163.

13. Duffy, *History of Public Health in New York City, 1866–1966*, 94–95.

14. U.S. Department of Commerce, *Historical Statistics of the United States: Colonial Times to 1957, A Statistical Abstract Supplement* (U.S. Government Printing Office, Washington, 1960), 25.

15. Todd L. Savitt, *Medicine and Slavery: The Diseases and Health Care of Blacks in Virginia* (Urbana, 1978); John Duffy, "Slavery and Slave Health in Louisiana," *Bulletin of the Tulane University Medical Faculty* 26 (1967): 1–6.

16. Gordon E. Gillson, *Louisiana State Board of Health: The Progressive Years* (Baton Rouge, 1976), 216–22.

17. John H. Ellis, "Businessmen and Public Health in the Urban South during the Nineteenth Century, New Orleans, Memphis, and Atlanta," *Bull. Hist. Med.* 44 (1970): 197–212.

18. John Duffy, "The American Medical Profession and Public Health: From Support to Ambivalence," *Bull. Hist. Med.* 53 (1979): 8–9.

19. Duffy, *The Sanitarians*, 247–49.

20. Roy Lubove, "The New Deal and National Health," *Current History* 45 (August 1963): 77–86.

21. Stevens, *American Medicine and the Public Interest*, 500–503, 509–13; Daniel M. Fox, *Health Policies, Health Politics: The British and American Experience, 1911–1965* (Princeton, 1986), 130ff.

22. David Blumenthal, Mark Schlesinger, and Pamela D. Drumheller, eds., *Renewing the Promise: Medicare and Its Reform* (New York, 1988), 15–16.

23. Cecil G. Sheps and Daniel L. Drosness, "Medical Progress, Prepayment for Medical Care," *New England Journal of Medicine* 264 (1961): 390–96, 444–48, 494–99.

24. Betty Leyerle, *Moving and Shaking American Medicine: The Structure of a Socioeconomic Transformation* (Westport, Conn., 1984), 8–9, 79, 137.

25. *Wall Street Journal,* April 3, 1989.

26. Fitzhugh Mullan, "The National Health Service Corps and Health Personnel Innovations," in *Reforming Medicine: Lessons of the Last Quarter Century,* ed. Victor and Ruth Seidel (New York, 1984), 184–85.

Chapter 22: Whither Medicine?

1. Lewis Thomas, "Guessing and Knowing, Reflections on the Science and Technology of Medicine," *Saturday Review* 55 (December 23, 1972): 52–57.

2. Lewis Thomas, "AIDS: An Unknown Distance to Go," *Scientific American* 259 (1988): 152.

3. Starr, *Social Transformation of American Medicine,* 428–49.

4. Norman Gevitz, *The D.O.s: Osteopathic Medicine in America* (Baltimore, 1982), 86–87.

5. Gevitz, ed., *Unorthodox Medicine in America,* viii, 116–21, 139–40; Russell W. Gibbons, "Physician-Chiropractors — Medical Pressure on the Evolution of Chiropractic," *Bull. Hist. Med.* 55 (1981): 233–45. For a recent discussion of chiropractic see the work by Stephen Barrett and the editors of *Consumer Reports* titled *Health Schemes, Scams and Frauds* (Mount Vernon, N.Y., 1990), chapter 2.

6. In the past thirty years there has been a flood of literature on medical ethics, stimulated by the creation of a number of institutes devoted to the subject, such as the Hastings Center in Hastings, New York, and the Center for Ethics, Medicine and Public Issues in Houston. Among the better publications are William B. Bondeson et al., *New Knowledge in the Biomedical Sciences: Some Moral Implications of Its Acquisition, Possession, and Use* (Dordrecht, 1982); H. Tristram Englehardt, Jr., "The Philosophy of Medicine: A New Endeavor," *Texas Reports on Biology and Medicine* 31 (Fall 1973): 443–52; Carol Levine and Robert M. Beatch, eds., *Cases in Bioethics* (Hastings-on-Hudson, N.Y., 1982); Samuel Gorovitz, *Doctors' Dilemmas: Moral Conflict and Medical Care* (New York, 1982).

7. Daniel M. Fox and Judith F. Stone, "Black Lung: Miners' Militancy and Medical Uncertainty, 1968–72," *Bull. Hist. Med.* 54 (1980): 62–63.

8. Elizabeth Fee and Daniel M. Fox, eds., *AIDS, The Burden of History* (Berkeley and Los Angeles, 1988), 163.

9. *Historical Statistics of the United States: Colonial Times to 1957,* 26.

Bibliography

There is no definitive history of American medicine that treats the social, institutional, and scientific sides of medicine, although Geoffrey Marks and William K. Beatty, *The Story of Medicine in America* (New York, 1973), is a useful work, and Francis R. Packard's *History of Medicine in the United States*, 2 vols. (New York, 1931), although an older study, also has some good material. An excellent history with respect to the scientific and technological side of medicine is James Bordley III and A. McGehee Harvey, *Two Centuries of American Medicine, 1776–1976* (Philadelphia, 1976), and some valuable essays can be found in John Z. Bowers and Elizabeth F. Purcell, eds., *Advances in American Medicine: Essays at the Bicentennial*, 2 vols. (New York, 1976). The encyclopedic medical history by Fielding H. Garrison, *An Introduction to the History of Medicine*, 4th ed. (Philadelphia, 1929), is invaluable for details. A small work that contains a series of essays of varying quality is Felix Marti-Ibanez, ed., *History of American Medicine: A Symposium* (New York, 1958). The only history of surgery devoted to the United States is A. Scott Earle, ed., *Surgery in America: From the Colonial Era to the 20th Century* (New York, 1983), but American developments are treated in two good general histories of surgery: Owen H. Wangensteen and Sarah D. Wangensteen, *The Rise of Surgery from Empiric Craft to Scientific Discipline* (Minneapolis, 1978), and Richard H. Meade, *An Introduction to the History of General Surgery* (Philadelphia, 1968).

The primary sources for medical history can be found in a variety of places. Among the manuscript materials cited are items from the following: Society for the Propagation of the Gospel in Foreign Parts, Library of Congress Phototranscripts; Pennsylvania Historical Society MSS; Cabildo Archives, New Orleans; and the Hamilton Papers (William S.), Louisiana State University Archives. I have also consulted other source collections and annual reports such as: American Archives; E. B. O'Callaghan, ed., *Register of New Netherland: 1626 to 1674* (Albany, New York, 1865); *Minutes of the Common Council of New York, 1675–1776* (New York, 1905); *United States Public Health Reports; Annual Reports of the United States Bureau of Animal Industry*; and publications of the National Library of Medicine and the Congressional Office of Technology Assessment. The annual reports and other materials published by the American Medical Association, American Dental Association, American Nurses Association, and the major hospitals have contributed to this history.

Medical journals, such as the *Journal of the American Medical Association* and the many state and regional publications, are basic to any medical study. There are too many to be cited here, but the major ones, in addition to *JAMA*, include the *American Journal of Public Health, Boston Medical and Surgical Journal, Clinical Pharmacology and Therapeutics, Journal of Medical Education, Medical Affairs, Medical and Surgical Reporter, Medical Record, Medical Repository, New England Journal of Medicine, New York Journal of Medicine, New York Medical and Physical Journal, New Orleans Medical and Surgical Journal, Philadelphia Medical Journal, The Sanitarian,* and the *Yale Journal of Biology and Medicine.*

General historical sources are invaluable, and I have used many state and local historical collections, such as the New-York Historical Society *Collections* and the Massachusetts Historical Society *Collections.* An examination of the following journals of medical history is essential for any research in American medical history: *Bulletin of the History of Medicine* (1926–); *Journal of the History of Medicine and Allied Sciences* (1946–); *Annals of Medical History* (1917–42); *Pharmacy in History.*

I have consulted a number of newspapers, lay journals, pamphlets, and miscellaneous sources, which are cited in the notes but not listed here.

Books

Ackernecht, Erwin H. *Malaria in the Mississippi Valley, 1760–1900.* Baltimore, 1945.

Adams, George W. *Doctors in Blue: The Medical History of the Union Army in the Civil War.* New York, 1952.

Alcott, Louisa May. *Hospital Sketches.* New York, 1957.

Alsop, Gulielma F. *History of the Woman's Medical College, Philadelphia, Pennsylvania, 1850–1950.* Philadelphia, 1950.

Apple, Rima D., ed. *Women, Health and Medicine in America: A Historical Handbook.* New York, 1990.

Ashburn, P. M. *The Ranks of Death.* New York, 1947.

Baker, S. Josephine. *Fighting for Life.* New York, 1939.

Barrett, Stephen, and the editors of *Consumer Reports. Health Schemes, Scams and Frauds.* Mount Vernon, N.Y., 1990.

Barton, Edward H. *The Application of Physiological Medicine to the Diseases of Louisiana.* Philadelphia, 1832.

Bayer, Ronald, and Arthur L. Caplan. *In Search of Equity: Health Needs and the Health Care System.* New York, 1983.

Beall, Otho T., Jr., and Richard H. Shryock. *Cotton Mather, First Significant Figure in American Medicine.* Baltimore, 1954.

Bean, William B. *Walter Reed, A Biography.* Charlottesville, Va., 1982.

Beardsley, Edward H. *A History of Neglect: Health Care for Blacks and Mill Workers in the Twentieth-Century South.* Knoxville, 1987.

Beaumont, William. *Experiments and Observations on the Gastric Juice and Physiology of Digestion . . . Facsimile . . . with a Biographical Essay . . . by Sir William Osler.* New York, 1959.

Bell, Whitfield, Jr. *Early American Science.* Williamsburg, Va., 1955.

———. *John Morgan, Continental Doctor.* Philadelphia, 1965.

Belth, Nathan C., ed., *Barriers, Patterns of Discrimination Against Jews.* New York, 1958.

Benison, Saul. *Tom Rivers: Reflections on a Life in Medicine and Science.* Cambridge, Mass., 1967.

Blackwell, Elizabeth. *Pioneer Work in Opening the Medical Profession to Women: Autobiographical Sketches.* Reprint. New York, 1970.

Blake, John B. *Benjamin Waterhouse and the Introduction of Vaccination: A Reappraisal.* Philadelphia, 1957.

———. *Public Health in the Town of Boston, 1630–1822.* Cambridge, Mass., 1959.

———, ed. *Centenary of Index Medicus, 1879–1979.* Bethesda, Md., 1980.

Blanton, Wyndham B. *Medicine in Virginia in the Seventeenth Century.* Richmond, 1930.

———. *Medicine in Virginia in the Eighteenth Century.* Richmond, 1931.

———. *Medicine in Virginia in the Nineteenth Century.* Richmond, 1933.

Bliss, Michael. *The Discovery of Insulin.* Chicago, 1982.

Blumenthal, David, Mark Schlesinger, and Pamela D. Drumheller, eds. *Renewing the Promise: Medicare and Its Reform.* New York, 1988.

Boland, Frank K. *The First Anesthetic: The Story of Crawford Long.* Athens, Ga., 1950.

Bondeson, William B., et al. *New Knowledge in the Biomedical Sciences: Some Moral Implications of Its Acquisition, Possession, and Use.* Dordrecht, Holland, 1982.

Bonner, Thomas N. *Medicine in Chicago, 1850–1950: A Chapter in the Social and Scientific Development of a City.* Madison, Wis., 1957.

———. *The Kansas Doctor: A Century of Pioneering.* Lawrence, Kans., 1959.

———. *American Doctors and German Universities: A Chapter in International Intellectual Relations, 1870–1914.* Lincoln, Neb., 1963.

Boorstin, Daniel J. *The Americans: The Colonial Experience.* New York, 1958.

Breeden, James O. *Joseph Jones, M.D., Scientist of the Old South.* Lexington, Ky., 1975.

Brieger, Gert, ed. *Medical America in the Nineteenth Century: Readings from the Literature.* Baltimore, 1972.

Brown, Kent L., ed. *Medicine in Cleveland and Cuyahoga County, 1810–1976.* Cleveland, 1977.

Bullock, Henry A. *A History of Negro Education in the South from 1619 to the Present.* Cambridge, Mass., 1967.

Burket, Walter C., ed. *Surgical Papers of William Stewart Halsted.* 2 vols. Baltimore, 1952.

Burr, C. B., ed. *Medical History of Michigan.* 2 vols. Minneapolis, 1930.

Burrow, James G. *AMA: Voice of American Medicine*. Baltimore, 1963.

———. *Organized Medicine in the Progressive Era: The Move toward Monopoly*. Baltimore, 1977.

Butterfield, Lyman H., ed. *Letters of Benjamin Rush*. 2 vols. Princeton, 1951.

Cahill, Kevin M. *Symposia in Clinical Tropical Medicine*. 2 vols. New York, 1970.

Callcott, George H. *A History of the University of Maryland*. Baltimore, 1966.

Carpenter, Kenneth J. *The History of Scurvy and Vitamin C*. Cambridge, 1986.

Cash, Philip. *Medical Men at the Siege of Boston, April, 1775–April, 1776*. Philadelphia, 1973.

Cash, Philip, E. H. Christianson, and J. Worth Estes, eds. *Medicine in Colonial Massachusetts, 1620–1820*. Charlottesville, Va., 1981.

Cassedy, James H. *American Medicine and Statistical Thinking, 1800–1860*. Cambridge, Mass., 1984.

Censer, Jane T. *The Papers of Frederick Law Olmsted*. Vol. 4, *The Civil War and the U.S. Sanitary Commission*. Baltimore, 1986.

Chaillé, Stanford E. *Historical Sketch of the Medical Department of the University of Louisiana*. New Orleans, 1861.

———. *Address on State Medical Organization*. New Orleans, 1879.

Chapman, Carleton B. *Dartmouth Medical School: The First 175 Years*. Hanover, N.H., 1973.

Chesney, Alan M. *The Johns Hopkins Hospital and the Johns Hopkins School of Medicine: A Chronicle*. 3 vols. Baltimore, 1963.

Churchill, Edward D., ed. *To Work in the Vineyard of Surgery: Reminiscences of J. Collins Warren (1842–1927)*. Cambridge, Mass., 1958.

Colombotos, John, and Corinne Kirchner. *Physicians and Social Change*. New York, 1986.

Cordell, Eugene F. *The Medical Annals of Maryland, 1799–1899*. Baltimore, 1900.

Corner, George. *A History of the Rockefeller Institute, 1901–1953*. New York, 1964.

Courtwright, David T. *Dark Paradise: Opium Addiction in America before 1940*. Cambridge, Mass., 1982.

Cowen, David L. *Medicine and Health in New Jersey: A History*. Princeton, 1964.

Cumming, Kate. *The Journal of a Confederate Nurse*. Edited by Richard B. Harwell. Baton Rouge, La., 1959.

Cunningham, H. H. *Doctors in Gray: The Confederate Medical Service*. Baton Rouge, La., 1958.

Dain, Norman. *Disordered Minds: The First Century of Eastern State Hospital in Williamsburg, Virginia, 1766–1866*. Williamsburg, Va., 1971.

Davis, N. S. *Medical Education and Medical Institutions in the United States of America, 1776–1886*. Washington, 1877.

Delaporte, François. *The History of Yellow Fever: An Essay on the Birth of Tropical Medicine*. Cambridge, Mass., 1991.

Derbyshire, Robert C. *Medical Licensure and Discipline in the United States*. Baltimore, 1969.

Dexter, James E. *A History of Dental and Oral Science in America.* Philadelphia, 1876.

Dickinson, Jonathan. *Observations on that Terrible Disease, Vulgarly called the Throat Distemper, with Advices as to the Method of Cure.* Boston, 1740.

Dock, Lavinia L., and Isabel M. Stewart. *A Short History of Nursing.* 4th ed. New York and London, 1920.

Donegan, Jane B. *Women and Men Midwives: Medicine, Morality and Misogyny in Early America.* Westport, Conn., 1978.

——. *"Hydropathic Highway to Health": Women and Water-Cure in Antebellum America.* New York, Connecticut, 1986.

Douglass, William. *A Summary, historical and political, of the first planting, progressive improvements, and present state of British Settlements in North America.* 2 vols. London, 1760.

Dowling, Harry F. *Fighting Infection: Conquests of the Twentieth Century.* Cambridge, Mass., 1977.

Drotar, David L. *Microsurgery: Revolution in the Operating Room.* New York, 1981.

Duffy, John. *Epidemics in Colonial America.* Baton Rouge, Louisiana, 1953.

——. *Parson Clapp of the Strangers' Church of New Orleans.* Baton Rouge, La., 1957.

——. *The Rudolph Matas History of Medicine in Louisiana.* 2 vols. Baton Rouge, La., 1958–62.

——. *A History of Public Health in New York City, 1625–1866.* New York, 1968.

——. *A History of Public Health in New York City, 1866–1966.* New York, 1974.

——. *The Tulane University Medical Center: One Hundred and Fifty Years of Medical Education.* Baton Rouge, La., 1984.

——. *The Sanitarians: A History of American Public Health.* Urbana, 1990.

Duncan, Louis C. *Medical Men in the American Revolution, 1775–1783.* Carlisle Barracks, Pa., 1931.

Dutton, Diana B. *Worse than the Disease: Pitfalls of Medical Progress.* Cambridge, 1988.

Dwyer, Ellen. *Homes for the Mad: Life Inside Two Nineteenth-Century Asylums.* New Brunswick, N.J., 1987.

Epstein, Benjamin R., and Arnold Foster. *Some of My Best Friends.* New York, 1962.

Estes, J. Worth, and David M. Goodman. *The Changing Humors of Portsmouth: The Medical Biography of an American Town, 1639–1983.* Boston, 1986.

Etheridge, Elizabeth W. *The Butterfly Caste: A Social History of Pellagra in the South.* Westport, Conn., 1972.

Ettling, John. *The Germ of Laziness: Rockefeller Foundation and Public Health in the New South.* Cambridge, Mass., 1981.

Ewell, James. *The Medical Companion, or Family Physician.* Washington, D.C., 1827.

Fee, Elizabeth. *Women and Health: The Politics of Medicine.* Farmingdale, N.Y., 1983.

——. *Disease and Discovery: A History of the Johns Hopkins School of Hygiene and Public Health, 1916–1939.* Baltimore, 1987.

Fee, Elizabeth, and Daniel M. Fox, eds. *AIDS, the Burden of History.* Berkeley and Los Angeles, 1988.

Fishbein, Morris. *A History of the American Medical Association, 1847 to 1947*. Philadelphia, 1969.

Fitch, Jabez. *An Account of the Numbers that have died . . . within the Province of New Hampshire*. Boston, 1736.

Fitzpatrick, John C., ed. *The Writings of George Washington*. Washington, 1931.

Fleming, Donald. *William H. Welch and the Rise of Modern Medicine*. Boston, 1954.

Flexner, Abraham. *Medical Education in the United States and Canada: A Report to the Carnegie Foundation for the Advancement of Teaching*. New York, 1910.

Flexner, Simon, and James Thomas Flexner. *William Henry Welch and the Heroic Age of American Medicine*. New York, 1941.

Fortuine, Robert. *Chills and Fever: Health and Disease in the Early History of Alaska*. Fairbanks, Alaska, 1989.

Fosdick, Raymond B. *The Story of the Rockefeller Foundation*. New York, 1952.

Fox, Daniel M. *Health Policies, Health Politics: The British and American Experience, 1911–1965*. Princeton, 1986.

Fox, William L. *Dandy of Hopkins*. Baltimore, 1984.

Francis, J. W. *An Historical Sketch of the Origin, Progress, and Present State of the College of Physicians, of the University of the State of New-York*. New York, 1913.

Franke, Norman H. *Pharmaceutical Conditions and Drug Supply in the Confederacy*. Madison, Wis., 1955.

Franklin, Benjamin. *Some Account of the Pennsylvania Hospital*. Introduction by I. B. Cohen. Baltimore, 1954.

Furman, Bess. *A Profile of the United States Public Health Service, 1798–1948*. Washington, n.d.

Galishoff, Stuart. *Safeguarding the Public Health: Newark, 1895–1918*. Westport, Conn., 1975.

Gamble, Vanessa N. *The Black Community Hospital: Contemporary Dilemmas in Historical Perspective*. New York, 1989.

Garrison, Fielding H. *John Shaw Billings: A Memoir*. New York, 1915.

——. *An Introduction to the History of Medicine: With Medical Chronology, Suggestions for Study and Bibliographic Data*. 4th ed., rpt. Philadelphia, 1929.

——. *Contributions to the History of Medicine from the Bulletin of the New York Academy of Medicine, 1925–1935*. New York, 1966.

Gevitz, Norman. *The D.O.s: Osteopathic Medicine in America*. Baltimore, 1982.

——, ed. *Unorthodox Medicine in America*. Baltimore, 1988.

Gibson, John M. *Soldier in White: The Life of General George Miller Sternberg*. Durham, N.C., 1958.

Gifford, George, Jr., ed. *Physician Signers of the Declaration of Independence*. New York, 1976.

Gillett, Mary C. *The Army Medical Department, 1775–1818*. Washington, D.C., 1981.

——. *The Army Medical Department, 1818–1865*. Washington, D.C., 1987.

Gillson, Gordon E. *Louisiana State Board of Health: The Formative Years*. Baton Rouge, La., n.d.

———. *Louisiana State Board of Health: The Progressive Years*. Baton Rouge, La., 1976.

Goler, Robert I., and P. J. Imperato, eds. *Early American Medicine: A Symposium*. New York: Fraunces Tavern Museum, 1987.

Goodnow, Minnie. *Nursing History in Brief*. Philadelphia, 1939.

Gorovitz, Samuel. *Doctors' Dilemmas: Moral Conflict and Medical Care*. New York, 1982.

Green, Harvey. *Fit for America: Health, Fitness, Sport and American Society*. New York, 1986.

Green, Samuel A. *History of Medicine in Massachusetts*. Boston, 1881.

Grob, Gerald N. *The State and the Mentally Ill: A History of the Worcester State Hospital in Massachusetts, 1830–1920*. Chapel Hill, N.C., 1966.

———. *Mental Illness and American Society, 1875–1940*. Princeton, 1983.

———. *From Asylum to Community: Mental Health Policy in Modern America*. Princeton, 1991.

Gros, A. A., and N. V. A. Gerardin. *Rapport fait à la Société Médicale sur La Fièvre Jaune qui a regné d'une Manière Épidémique pendant l'Été de 1817*. New Orleans, 1818.

Gross, Samuel D. *A Discourse on the Life, Character, and Services of Daniel Drake, M.D. . . . January 27, 1853*. Louisville, Ky., 1853.

———. *Memorial Oration in Honor of Ephraim McDowell, "The Father of Ovariotomy."* Louisville, Ky., 1879.

Gunn, John C. *Gunn's Domestic Medicine, or Poor Man's Friend*. New York, 1853.

Haller, John S., Jr. *American Medicine in Transition, 1840–1910*. Urbana, 1981.

Haller, John S., Jr., and Robin M. Haller. *The Physician and Sexuality in Victorian American*. Urbana, 1974.

Hamer, Philip M. *The Centennial History of the Tennessee State Medical Association*. Nashville, Tenn., 1930.

Hamilton, Alice. *Exploring the Dangerous Trades: The Autobiography of Alice Hamilton*. New York, 1943.

Harden, Victoria A. *Inventing the NIH: Federal Biomedical Research Policy, 1887–1937*. Baltimore, 1986.

———. *Rocky Mountain Spotted Fever: History of a Twentieth-Century Disease*. Baltimore, 1990.

Hardie, James. *The Description of the City of New York*. New York, 1827.

Harris, Chapin A. *The Dental Art: A Practical Treatise on Dental Surgery*. Baltimore, 1839.

Harvey, A. McGehee. *Adventures in Medical Research: A Century of Discovery at Johns Hopkins*. Baltimore, 1974.

Hawke, David Freeman. *Benjamin Rush, Revolutionary Gadfly*. Indianapolis, 1971.

Hayward, Oliver S., and Elizabeth H. Thompson. *The Journal of William Tully*,

Medical Student at Dartmouth, 1808–1809. New York, 1977.

Heustis, Jabez W. *Physical Observations, and Medical Tracts and Researches, on the Topography and Diseases of Louisiana.* New York, 1817.

Hindle, Brooke. *The Pursuit of Science in Revolutionary America, 1735–1789.* Chapel Hill, N.C., 1956.

Historical Statistics of the United States: Colonial Times to 1957, A Statistical Abstract Supplement. Washington, D.C.: U.S. Government Printing Office, 1960.

Holley, Howard L. *A History of Medicine in Alabama.* University, Ala., 1982.

Hollingsworth, J. Roger. *A Political Economy of Medicine: Great Britain and the United States.* Baltimore, 1986.

Horine, Emmet Field. *Daniel Drake (1785–1852), Pioneer Physician of the Midwest.* Philadelphia, 1961.

Jacobson, Timothy C. *Making Medical Doctors: Science and Medicine in Vanderbilt since Flexner.* Tuscaloosa, Ala., 1987.

Jennett, Bryan. *High Technology Medicine: Benefits and Burdens.* Oxford, 1986.

Katz, Alfred H., and Jean S. Felton, eds. *Health and the Community: Readings in the Philosophy and Sciences of Public Health.* New York, 1965.

Kaufman, Martin. *Homeopathy in America: The Rise and Fall of a Medical Heresy.* Baltimore, 1971.

——. *American Medical Education: The Formative Years, 1765–1910.* Westport, Conn., 1976.

Kaufman, Martin, Stuart Galishoff, and Todd L. Savitt, eds. *Dictionary of American Medical Biography.* 2 vols. Westport, Conn., 1984.

Kelly, Howard A., and Walter L. Burrage. *American Medical Biographies.* Baltimore, 1920.

Kett, Joseph E. *The Formation of the American Medical Profession: The Role of Institutions, 1780–1960.* New Haven, Conn., 1968.

Keys, Thomas E. *History of Surgical Anesthesia.* New York, 1963.

King, Lester. *The Medical World of the Eighteenth Century.* Chicago, 1958.

Kohler, Robert E. *From Medical Chemistry to Biochemistry: The Making of a Biomedical Discipline.* Cambridge, 1982.

Konold, Donald E. *A History of American Medical Ethics, 1847–1912.* Madison, Wis., 1962.

Leavitt, Judith W. *Brought to Bed: Childbearing in America, 1750–1950.* New York, 1986.

Leavitt, Judith W., and Ronald L. Numbers, eds. *Sickness and Health in America: Readings in the History of Medicine and Public Health.* Madison, Wis., 1978.

Levine, Carol, and Robert M. Beatch, eds. *Cases in Bioethics.* Hastings-on-Hudson, N.Y., 1982.

Leyerle, Betty. *Moving and Shaking American Medicine: The Structure of a Socioeconomic Transformation.* Westport, Conn., 1984.

Long, Dorothy, ed. *Medicine in North Carolina: Essays in the History of Medical Science and Medical Service, 1524–1960.* 2 vols. Raleigh, N.C., 1972.

Lopate, Carol. *Women in Medicine.* Baltimore, 1968.

Ludmerer, Kenneth M. *Learning to Heal: The Development of American Medical Education.* New York, 1985.

McCrane, Reginald C. *The Cincinnati Doctors' Forum.* Cincinnati, 1957.

McCurdy, Edwin. *The History of South Carolina under the Proprietary Government, 1670–1719.* New York, 1897.

Marshall, Helen E. *Mary Adelaide Nutting, Pioneer of Modern Nursing.* Baltimore, 1972.

Massey, Edmund. *A Sermon against the Dangerous and Sinful Practice of Inoculation . . .* London, 1722.

Massie, J. Cam. *Treatise on the Eclectic Southern Practice of Medicine.* Philadelphia, 1854.

Mather, Cotton. *A Letter about a Good Management under the Distemper of Measles, etc.* Boston, 1739.

———. *The Angel of Bethesda.* Introduction by Gordon W. Jones. Barre, Mass., 1972.

Meckel, Richard A. *Save the Babies: American Public Health Reform and the Prevention of Infant Mortality, 1850–1929.* Baltimore, 1990.

Meigs, Charles D. *Females and Their Diseases.* Philadelphia, 1848.

———. *Obstetrics: The Science and the Art.* Philadelphia, 1849.

Miller, Genevieve. *Bibliography of the History of Medicine of the United States and Canada, 1939–1960.* Baltimore, 1964.

Milosh, Barbara. *"The Physician's Hand": Work Culture and Conflict in American Nursing.* Philadelphia, 1982.

Moldow, Gloria. *Women Doctors in Gilded-Age Washington: Race, Gender and Professionalization.* Urbana, 1987.

Moore, Harry A. *Public Health in the United States: An Outline with Historical Data.* New York, 1923.

Morais, Herbert M. *The History of the Negro in Medicine.* New York, 1967.

Morantz-Sanchez, Regina Markell. *Sympathy and Science: Women Physicians in American Medicine.* New York, 1985.

Morgan, John. *A Vindication of His Public Character in the Situation of Director-General.* Boston, 1777.

Murphy, Lamar R. *Enter the Physician: The Transformation of Domestic Medicine, 1760–1860.* Tuscaloosa, Ala., 1991.

Musto, David F. *The American Disease: Origins of Narcotic Control.* New Haven, 1973.

National Board of Medical Examiners, 75th Anniversary, Special Commemorative Annual Report. Philadelphia, 1990.

Nissenbaum, Stephen. *Sex, Diet and Debility in Jacksonian America: Sylvester Graham and Health Reform.* Westport, Conn., 1980.

Norwood, W. F. *Medical Education in the United States before the Civil War.* Philadelphia, 1944.

Numbers, Ronald. *Almost Persuaded: American Physicians and Compulsory Health Insurance, 1912–1920.* Baltimore, 1978.

——, ed. *The Education of American Physicians: Historical Essays.* Berkeley and Los Angeles, 1980.

——, ed. *Medicine in the New World: New Spain, New France and New England.* Knoxville, 1987.

Oldmixon, John. *The British Empire in America.* 2 vols. London, 1741.

Parascondola, John, ed. *The History of Antibiotics: A Symposium.* Madison, Wis., 1980.

Patterson, James T. *The Dread Disease: Cancer and Modern American Culture.* Cambridge, Mass., 1987.

Peckham, Howard H., ed. *The Toll of Independence: Engagements and Battle Casualties of the American Revolution.* Chicago, 1974.

Pepper, William. *Higher Medical Education, the True Interest of the Public and of the Profession: Two Addresses Delivered before the Medical Department of the University of Pennsylvania on Oct. 1, 1877 and Oct. 2, 1893.* Philadelphia, 1894.

——. *The Medical Side of Benjamin Franklin.* Philadelphia, 1910.

Pernick, Martin A. *A Calculus of Suffering: Pain, Professionalism, and Anesthesia in Nineteenth-Century America.* New York, 1985.

Powell, J. H. *Bring Out Your Dead.* Philadelphia, 1949.

Ravitch, Mark M. *A Century of Surgery: The History of the American Surgical Association.* 2 vols. Philadelphia, 1981.

Reiser, Stanley J. *Medicine and the Reign of Technology.* Cambridge, 1978.

Reverby, Susan B. *Ordered to Care: Dilemma of American Nursing, 1850–1945.* Cambridge, Mass., 1987.

Reverby, Susan B., and David Rosner, eds. *Health Care in America: Essays in Social History.* Philadelphia, 1979.

Risse, Guenter B., R. L. Numbers, and J. W. Leavitt, eds. *Medicine without Doctors.* New York, 1977.

Robbins, Christine Chapman. *David Hosack, Citizen of New York.* Philadelphia, 1964.

Robinson, Victor. *The Story of Medicine.* New York, 1943.

Rosen, George. *Fees and Fee Bills: Some Economic Aspects of Medical Practice in Nineteenth Century America.* Baltimore, 1946.

Rosenberg, Charles E. *The Cholera Years: The United States in 1832, 1849, and 1866.* Chicago, 1962.

——. *The Care of Strangers: The Rise of America's Hospital System.* New York, 1987.

Rosenfield, Peri. *Nursing Student Census, 1989.* New York, 1990.

Rosenkrantz, Barbara G. *Public Health and the State: Changing Views in Massachusetts, 1842–1936.* Cambridge, Mass., 1972.

Rosner, David. *A Once Charitable Enterprise: Hospitals and Health Care in Brooklyn and New York, 1885–1915.* Cambridge, 1982.

Rothstein, William G. *American Physicians in the Nineteenth Century: From Sects to Science.* Baltimore, 1972.

——. *American Medical Schools and the Practice of Medicine.* New York, 1987.

Savitt, Todd L. *Medicine and Slavery: The Diseases and Health Care of Blacks in Virginia.* Urbana, 1978.

Schlossman, Steven L., JoAnne Brown, and Michael Sedlak. *The Public School in American Dentistry.* Rand Publication Series. Santa Monica, Calif., 1986.

Seidel, Victor and Ruth, eds. *Reforming Medicine: Lessons of the Last Quarter Century.* New York, 1984.

Shafer, Henry Burnell. *The American Medical Profession, 1783 to 1850.* New York, 1936.

Shorter, Edwin. *The Health Century.* New York, 1987.

Shryock, Richard H. *American Medical Research, Past and Present.* New York, 1947.

——. *The History of Nursing: An Interpretation of the Social and Medical Facts Involved.* Philadelphia, 1959.

——. *Medical Licensing in America, 1650–1965.* Baltimore, 1967.

——. *Development of Modern Medicine.* New York, 1969.

Sicherman, Barbara. *Alice Hamilton: A Life in Letters.* Cambridge, Mass., 1984.

Simon, William. *History of the Baltimore College of Dental Surgery.* n.p., 1904.

Sims, J. Marion. *The Story of My Life.* New York, 1968.

Smith, George W. *Medicines for the Union Army: The United States Army Laboratories during the Civil War.* Madison, Wis., 1962.

Smith, William. *The History of the Province of New York.* London, 1776.

Spink, Wesley W. *Infectious Diseases. Prevention and Treatment in the Nineteenth and Twentieth Centuries.* Minneapolis, 1978.

Starr, Paul. *The Social Transformation of American Medicine: The Rise of a Sovereign Profession and the Making of a Vast Industry.* New York, 1982.

Stevens, Rosemary. *American Medicine and the Public Interest.* New Haven, 1971.

Stillé, Charles J. *History of the United States Sanitary Commission, Being the General Report of Its Works during the War of the Rebellion.* Philadelphia, 1866.

Stokes, Isaac N. *The Iconography of Manhattan Island.* 6 vols. New York, 1915–28.

Terris, Milton, ed. *Goldberger on Pellagra.* Baton Rouge, La., 1964.

Thacher, James. *A Military Journal during the American Revolutionary War, 1775–1783 . . .* Boston, 1823.

Thacher, Thomas. *A Brief Rule to Guide the Common People of New England how to order themselves and theirs in the Small Pocks, or Measles.* Boston, 1677.

Thomson, Samuel. *New Guide to Health, or Botanical Family Physician . . . to which is prefixed, A Narrative of the Life and Medical Discoveries of the Author.* 2d ed. Boston, 1825.

Thornton, Russell. *American Indian Holocaust and Survival: A Population History since 1492.* Norman, Okla., 1987.

Tilton, James. *Economical Observations on Military Hospitals and the Prevention of Diseases Incident to an Army.* Wilmington, Del., 1813.

Tomkins, Calvin. *Keepers of the Game.* Berkeley, 1978.

Toner, Joseph M. *Contributions in the Annals of Medical Progress and Medical Education. . . .* Washington, D.C., 1874.

———. *Medical Men of the Revolution with a Brief History of the Medical Department of the Continental Army. . . .* Philadelphia, 1876.

Torrey, E. Fuller. *Nowhere to Go: The Tragic Odyssey of the Homeless Mentally Ill.* New York, 1988.

Townsend, P. S. *An Account of the Yellow Fever as It Prevailed in the City of New York, in the Summer and Autumn of 1822.* New York, 1823.

Turner, James. *Animals, Pain, and Humanity in the Victorian Mind.* Baltimore, 1980.

Turner, Thomas B. *Heritage of Excellence: The Johns Hopkins Medical Institutions, 1914–1947.* Baltimore, 1974.

Ulrich, Laurel T. *A Midwife's Tale: The Life of Martha Ballard, Based on Her Diary, 1785–1812.* New York, 1990.

Velpeau, A.-A.-L.-M. *New Elements of Operative Surgery.* Edited by Valentine Mott. Translated by P. S. Townsend under the supervision of, and with notes and observations by, V. Mott. New York, 1847.

Viets, Henry R. *A Brief History of Medicine in Massachusetts.* Boston, 1930.

Vogel, Morris J. *The Invention of the Modern Hospital: Boston, 1870–1930.* Chicago, 1980.

Vogel, Morris J., and Charles E. Rosenberg, eds. *The Therapeutic Revolution: Essays in the Social History of Medicine.* Philadelphia, 1979.

Vogel, Virgil J. *American Indian Medicine.* Norman, Okla., 1977.

Walsh, James J. *History of the Medical Society of the State of New York.* Brooklyn, N.Y., 1907.

———. *A History of Medicine in New York: Three Centuries of Medical Progress.* 3 vols. New York, 1919.

Waring, Joseph I. *History of Medicine in South Carolina, 1670–1825.* Columbia, S.C., 1964.

———. *A History of Medicine in South Carolina, 1825–1900.* Columbia, S.C., 1967.

Warner, John Harley. *Medical Practice, Knowledge, and Identity in America, 1820–1885.* Cambridge, Mass., 1986.

Waterson, A. P., and Lise Wilkinson. *An Introduction to the History of Virology.* London, 1978.

Watson, Patricia Ann. *The Angelic Conjunction: The Preacher-Physicians of Colonial New England.* Knoxville, 1991.

Webster, Noah. *A Brief History of Epidemic and Pestilential Diseases . . . .* Hartford, Conn., 1799.

Welch, Henry, and Felix Marti-Ibanez. *The Antibiotic Saga.* New York, 1960.

Wesley, John. *Primitive Physick, or an easy and natural Method of Curing most Diseases.* 12th ed. Printed by Andrew Stewart, Philadelphia, 1764.

Whorton, James C. *Crusaders for Fitness: The History of American Health Reformers.* Princeton, 1982.

Williams, Ralph C. *The United States Public Health Service, 1798–1950.* Washington, 1951.

Wintrobe, Maxwell M. *Blood, Pure and Eloquent: A Story of Discovery, of People, and of Ideas.* New York, 1980.

Woodring, T. V. *Pioneer Medicine and Early Physicians in Nashville.* n.p., n.d.

Woodward, Joseph Janvier. *Outlines of the Chief Camp Diseases of the United States Armies.* Introduction by Saul Jarcho. New York, 1964.

Young, James Harvey. *The Toadstool Millionaires: A Social History of Patent Medicines in America before Federal Regulation.* Princeton, 1961.

——. *The Medical Messiahs: A Social History of Quackery in Twentieth-Century America.* Princeton, 1971; expanded paperback edition, Princeton, 1992.

——. *Pure Food: Securing the Pure Food and Drugs Act of 1906.* Princeton, 1989.

Index

Abel, John J., 232, 239
Acton, Lord, x
Adams, John, 51, 55
Adams, Samuel Hopkins, 317
African Americans, 304; in Civil War, 305–6; in medical schools, 306–7; as female medical students, 306; helped by foundations, 307; organize medical society, 307; in hospitals, 308–9; health conditions of, 335–36
Agramonte, Aristide, 174
AIDS, 345–47, 354–55
Alcohol, 181
American Association of University Professors, 325
American College of Surgeons, 258–59
American Institute of Homeopathy, 85
American Medical Association, 85–87, 125–26, 138, 150; on meteorological studies, 170; Council on Medical Education, 208–10; on contract medicine, 215–16; reform of, 218, 220, 222–25; code of ethics, 220, 224–25; supports public health measures, 225–27; on women, 290; on nursing, 297; on black medical schools, 306; on licensing, 315; fights quackery, 317; on health insurance, 318–19; ambivalence on public health, 337–38
American Medical College Association, 207–8
American Nurses Association, 299, 301
American Philosophical Society, 42
American Public Health Association, 330–31, 336
American Society of Dental Physicians, 113, 197
American Surgical Association, 199, 258; reorganized, 201
Amherst, Jeffrey, 3
Anarcha (slave), 102–3
Anesthesia, 110–19; in Civil War, 162; local, 195, 260
Aneurysms, 97–98
Animalculae theory, 21–22
Antibiotics, 240–42
Antiseptic procedures, 188–90
Apothecaries, 7–8
Appleton, Fannie, 116
Apprenticeship system, 38–39; training, 130–31, 148
Arnold, Richard, 138
Aseptic procedures, 189–90
Ashford, Bailey K., 176

Asylum for the Chronic Insane, 79
Atlanta Medical College, 208–9
Atwater, Wilbur O., 233
Augusta, Alexander T., 305
Avery, Oswald, 240, 248
Axelrod, Julius, 239, 243

Bailey, Charles, 264
Baker, Josephine, 295
Baldwin, Oliver B., 122
Ballard, Martha, 90
Baltimore College of Dental Surgery, 113, 195–97
Banting, Frederick, G., 233, 236
Barber surgeons, 7
Bard, John, 27, 32–34, 41, 100
Bard, Samuel, 27–28, 33–34, 37, 39, 131
Barker, Llewellys, F., 230
Bartlett, Josiah, 49
Barton, Edward H., 70, 75, 330
Bartram, John, 27
Baudelocque, Jean Louis, 104–5
Baumgartner, Leona, 295
Bayley, Richard, 132
Baynham, William, 100
Beach, Wooster, 83–84
Beaumont, William, 107–10
Bedloe's Island, 36
Bell, A. N., 216
Bell, John, 100–101
Bell, Whitfield, 46
Bellows, Henry W., 154
Benedict, Francis G., 233
Beriberi, 178–79
Berman, Alex, 87
Bernard, Claude, 230
Best, Charles H., 233, 236
Bevan, Arthur D., 261
Bigelow, Henry Jacob, 191–92

Bigelow, Jacob, 73
Billings, John Shaw: established Surgeon General's Library, 168–69; connection with Johns Hopkins, 205–6
Biochemistry, 233–48
Blackwell, Elizabeth, 286–87, 296
Blackwell, Emily, 287
Blake, Clarence J., 216
Blake, John, 127–28
Blalock, Alfred, 264, 295
Blanton, Wyndham B., 4, 217
Bleeding, 14–15, 70–77, 180
Bloodgood, Joseph C., 190
Blood transfusions, 199–201, 259–60
Bloomingdale Asylum, 78
Blue, Rupert, 177–78
Blue Cross–Blue Shield, 247
Bodley, Rachel, 291
Body-snatching, 132–33
Boerhaave, Hermann, 14
Bohun, Lawrence, 9
Bond, Thomas, 24, 29–30, 37
Boorstin, Daniel J., 11
Bordley, James, III, 237
Boston: smallpox epidemic, 20–21, fee bills, 141
Boston Female Medical College, 288
Boston University Medical Department, 288
Bouquet, Henry, 3
Bousfield, Midian Othello, 306, 308
Boyleston, Zabdiel, 20
Brandt, Allan M., 355
Broussais, François-Joseph-Victor, 72
Brown, Gustavus Richard, 74
Brown, John, abolitionist, 132–33
Brown, John, British physician, 14, 36, 64
Burnet, McFarlane, 266
Burrow, James G., 225, 318
Byrd, William, 45

Cancer, 16, 252–56, 345, 348

Cannon, Walter B., 198

Carrel, Alexis, 193, 237, 264–65; Dakin's solution, 201

Carroll, James, 174

Carter, Henry Rose, 174–75

Cartwright, Samuel H., 186, 278

Castle, William B., 236

Central Medical College, 287–88

Cesarean section, 102–7

Chadwick, James R., 290

Chaillé, Stanford E., 136

Chain, Ernest B., 240

Chalmers, Lionel, 41

Charity Hospital, 35–36, 133, 135; description of surgery, 98–99; antiseptic procedures, 189; cesarean section, 200; student residencies, 209–10

Charleston, S.C.: yellow fever, 27; fee bill, 41–43; banish physicians, 60–61

Charleston Medical School, 102, 287

Chicago Medical College, 204–5

Childs, H. H., 149

Chittenden, Russell, 233

Cholera, 75–77

Choppin, Samuel, 147

Chowning, William B., 175–76

Church, Benjamin, 49, 53–55

Cincinnati Eye Infirmary, 123

Civil War, Union and Confederate morbidity and mortality statistics, 151–52, 159–62

Clarke, William E., 113–14

Cleveland City Hospital, 308

Cleveland Medical College, 287

Clossy, Samuel, 132

Cobb, Montague, 309

Cochran, Jerome, 225

Cochran, John, 57, 59–60

Cohenheim, Julius, 206

Colden, Cadwallader: as botanist, 24–25; on yellow fever, 25; on sanitation, 25–26, 40, 46

Cole, Rufus, 230

College of Philadelphia, 28, 32–34

College of Physicians and Surgeons, 121, 131, 134, 137–38

Collip, James P., 232–33

Colton, Gardner, Q., 114–15

Confederate Medical Department, 158–66

Connecticut, medical societies, 43

Continental Medical Department, 49–50, 52–61

Contract system, 142–43, 215

Cooley, Denton, 265

Coolidge, William D., 198

Coons, Albert H., 252

Cooper, Ashley, 95, 98

Corning, James L., 195

Cox, Harold R., 250

Craik, James, 74

Cranston, John, 31–32

Crawford, Albert, 232

Crawford, Jane Todd, 100–101

Creole physicians, 71–73

Crick, Francis H. C., 249

Crile, George W., 193, 195, 201

Crosby, Albert W., 5

Cullen, William, 33, 64

Cumming, Kate, 164

Currie, James, 67

Curtis, Alva, 87

Cushing, Harvey W., 193, 195, 231, 261, 277

Cushing Institute, 172

Cystoscope, 199

Dakin, Henry D., 201

Dandy, Walter E., 193, 261

Dartmouth Medical College, 126, 131, 144

Davidge, John Beale, 134

Davis, Jefferson, 164

Davis, Marguerite, 234

Davis, Nathan Smith, 205

Davis, Paulina Wright, 289

Davy, Humphrey, 111

Dawson, W. C., 118

Debakey, Michael E., 253, 265

Delaporte, François, 175

Delery, Charles C., 147–48

Dentistry, 113–15, 195–98

Derham, James, 304

Diabetes, 233

Diagnosis Related Groups, 344

Dick, Elisha, 74

Dickson, Samuel H., 287

Diphtheria, 6, 22, 41, 335

Dispensaries, in New York City, 182

Dix, Dorothea Lynde, 78–79; Civil War role, 163, 297

Dixon, Edward, 204

Dock, Lavinia L., 298

Doctors' Riot, 131–32

Doering, E. J., 222

Doisey, Edward A., 235

Domagk, Gerhardt, 240

Domestic medical books, 92–94

Donaldson, H. H., 243

Donegan, Jane, 89

Douglass, William, 14–15, 39, 41, 44, 46; on inoculation, 21–22; on scarlet fever, 24

Dove, Robert, 304

Dow, Robert, 305

Dowling, Oscar, 336

Drake, Daniel, career, 121–24, 130, 141, 144

Dreckapotheke, 15–16

Drinker, Elizabeth Sandwich, 16–17

Dubos, Rene, 240

Duels, 146–48

Duncan, Louis C., 50

Dunglison, Robley, 109–10

Dupuytren, G., 95

Eastern Medical Board (Louisiana), 139

Eastern State Hospital, 77

Eclectic Medical Institute of Cincinnati, 84

Eclectics, 83–84, 87

Ehrlich, Paul, 240

Eisberg, Charles E., 263

Eliot, Charles W., 144–45, 205

"Elixir Sulfanilamide," 317

Elvehjem, Conrad A., 178, 234

Emerson, Haven, 244

Enders, John, 238, 252

Endocrinology, 231

Erlangen, Joseph, 243

Estes, J. Worth, 11, 15

Eustis, William, 55

Ewell, James, 93

Faraday, Michael, 111

Fauchard, Pierre, 145

Federation of State Medical Boards, 221

Fell, George H., 194–95

Fell-O'Dwyer apparatus, 195

Female Medical College of Pennsylvania, 288

Fenner, E. D., 138

Fermin, Giles, 9

Finlay, Carlos, 174–75

Finlay, Clement A., 153–55

Finley, Samuel, 63

Finney, J. M. T., 258

Fitch, Jabez, 22

Fitz, Reginald Heber, 194

Fleming, Alexander, 240
Flexner, Abraham, 136, 208–12, 276, 279, 293, 306
Flexner, Simon, 204, 251
Flint, Austin, 169–70; on changes in medicine, 179; on bleeding, 181
Flint Medical College, 306
Florey, Howard W., 240–41
Folk medicine, 16, 19, 91
Food and Drugs Act (1906), 317
Foster, Isaac, 57
Foster, John, 147
Fothergill, John, 24, 28–29, 63
Fox, Daniel M., 212
Franklin, Benjamin, 23–24, 28, 36, 91; assists young Americans, 63
Freedman's Bureau and Howard Medical School, 306
Freud, Sigmund, 244
Friendly Botanic Societies, 82, 87
French Clinical School, 71, 77
Fuller, Samuel, 9
Fulton, John E., 118
Funk, Casimer, 179, 234

Garden, Alexander, 26; expelled from Charleston, 61
Garfield, James A., 190–91
Garrett, Mary, 293
Garrison, Fielding H., on bleeding, 181
Gasser, Herbert, 243
Gavin, Frank, 311
Geiling, E. M. K., 239
Geneva Medical School, 287
Germ theory, 169–70
Gibbon, John H. Jr., 265
Gilman, Daniel Coit, 205–6
Goffman, Erving, 246
Goforth, William, 121–22, 130, 141
Goiter, 232

Goldberger, Joseph, 178–79, 234
Goldsmith, Oliver, 63
Goldstein, Cynthia, xi
Goodman, David M., 11
Goodpasture, Ernest W., 238
Goodyear, Charles, 197
Gorgas, William, 175
Goss, John, 67
Graham, Evarts H., 258–59
Graham, Sylvester, 88–89
Gram, Hans, 83
Greeley, Horace, 87
Gregory, Samuel, 288
Griscom, John H., 330
Gross, Samuel David, 124–25, 297; writings of, 192
Guillemin, Roger C. L., 243
Gunn, John C., 93–94
Guthrie, Charles C., 264–65
Guthrie, Samuel, 111–12
Gwinn, Mary, 293

Hahnemann, Samuel Christian, 82–85
Hall, Lyman, 49
Hall, Russell T., 89
Halleck, Henry W., 157
Halsted, William S., 190; on blood vessels, 193–95; at Johns Hopkins, 206, 277
Hamilton, Alexander (physician), 16
Hamilton, Alexander (statesman), 121
Hamilton, Alice, 295
Hamilton, Kitty and Penelope, 89
Hammond, William A.: reorganizes Union Medical Department, 155–56; court-martialed, 156–57, 165
Hampton, Isabel A. (Mrs. Hunter Robb), 298
Harding, Warren G., 178
Harkin, Dwight E., 264

Harris, Chapin A., 196–97
Harris, Elisha, 154, 330
Harris, Robert P., 106
Harrison, John, 135
Harrison, Ross G., 237
Hartline, H. K., 243
Harvard University Medical College, 13, 120, 125–26, 131, 136, 140, 144–45; examinations, 204–5; clinical clerkship, 209–10; admission of women, 288, 292; admission of Jews, 311
Harvey, A. McGehee, 237
Hayden, Horace H., 113, 196–97
Hayman, Henry, 116
Haynie, M. L., 73
Health insurance, 318–24, 341–44
Health Maintenance Organizations, 341–42
Heatley, Norman, 241
Helmholtz, Hermann, 185
Hematology, 236–37
Henderson, Lawrence J., 187
Hering, Constantine, 83
Herrick, Charles Judson, 243
Heustis, Jacob, 74
Hill-Burton Act, 309, 340
Hindle, Brooke, 62
Hippocrates, 278, 351
Hodge, H. L., 127
Holmes, Oliver Wendell, 73; on homeopathy, 84–85; on anesthesia, 116; biography, 125–26; on puerperal fever, 125–26
Holt, Emmett L., 259
Homeopathy, 83–87, 219–20
Hookworm, 176–77
Hooper Institute for Medical Research, 172
Hosack, David, 121, 130–31
Hospitals: colonial period, 34–38; changing status, 183–84; training nurses,

297–98. *See under name of hospital*
Hovey, George O., 292
Howard University Medical School, 306–7
Howell, W. H., 200, 259
Hudson, Robert P., 211
Huggins, Charles B., 253
Human Genome Project, 345
Hume, Joseph, 197
Humphreys, Alexander, 100
Hunt, Alexander, 135
Hunter, John, 28, 95; on dentistry, 195
Hunter, William (of London), 63, 90
Hunter, William (of Newport, R.I.), 32
Hurd, Henry M., 206
Hutchinson, James, 67
Hydropaths, 88–89
Hygienic Laboratory, 172–73

Immunochemistry, 252–56
Immunology, 265–66
Indians: health and medicine, 1–2; impact of smallpox on, 2–5. *See also* Native Americans
Inoculation, 20–22; hospitals, 38; in Revolutionary War, 51–52
Insane, 37, 77–79. *See also* Mental health
Insect vectors, 237–38
Irregular physicians, 350–51. *See* Eclecticism; Homeopathy; Hydropathy; Thomsonianism

Jackson, Charles A., 115, 118–19
Jackson, Chevalier, 262
Jackson, Clement, 11
Jackson, James, Jr., 73, 120
Jarvis, Edward, 330
Jefferson Medical College, 102, 123–25, 191
Jenner, Edward, 250
Jerne, Niels, 231
Jewell, Wilson, 330

Jews, in medicine, 310–14
"Jim Crow," 291
Johns Hopkins Medical School, 168, 171, 211, 345; founding of, 205–6
Johnson, Mary, 16
Johnson, Samuel, 63
Jones, John, 17, 33
Jones, Joseph, 151–52, 332
Julius Rosenwald Fund, 307

Kearsley, John, 27–28
Kearsley, John, Jr., 304
Keen, William W., 192
Kefauver, Estes, 317
Kefauver-Harris Drug Amendments, 317–18
Kells, Edmund C., 197–98
Kelly, Howard A., 206
Kelsey, Francis O., 317
Kendall, Edward C., 232
Kerfbyle, Johannes, 10
Kett, Joseph, 82
Kierstede, Roelof, 18
Kilborne, F. L., 171, 237
Kimball, O. P., 232
King, Elizabeth, 293
King's College Medical School (Columbia University), 27, 33–34, 37, 131; nursing course, 298–99
Kircher, Athanasius, 21–22
Knoxville Medical College, 306
Koch, Robert, 334
Koehler, Geörges J. F., 231
Krementz, Edward, 272
Kuhn, Adam, 33, 67
Kuhne, Willy, 206

Laetrile, 318
La Montagne, Johannes, 10
Lancisi, Giovanni Maria, 26
Landsteiner, Karl, 199–200, 256

Laser surgery, 270
"Laughing gas" parties, 113
Lavinder, C. H., 177
Lawson, Thomas, 110, 153–54
Lazear, Jesse, 174–75
Leach, R. B., 305
Lenhart, C. H., 232
Leonard Medical College, 306
Letterman, Jonathon, 156–58
Lettsom, John Coakley, 63
Lewis, Nolen D. C., 245
Lincoln, Abraham, 154
Lining, John, 27
Lister, Joseph, 188–89
Lithotomy, 17
Lloyd, James, 18
Loewi, Otto, 239
Logan, Samuel, 197
London Company, 3, 9–10
Long, Crawford W., 113–14, 118–19
Louisville Medical College, 306
Lovell, Joseph, 110
Lown, Bernard, 265
Lubove, Roy, 339
Lucas, Henry, 19
Ludmerer, Kenneth M., 211
Lunatic Asylum at Utica, 79
Luzenberg, Charles A., 98, 146–47
Lyme disease, 346
Lynk, Miles Vandahurst, 307

McArthur, L. L., 194
McBurney, Charles, 194
McCallum, William G., 232
McClellan, George B., 157
McCollum, Elmer V., 179, 234–35
McCormack, Joseph N., 224–25
McCormack Institute for Studying Infectious Diseases, 172
McDowell, Ephraim, 99–101
McFarlane, J. S., 146–47

McKean, Robert, 22–23
McKnight, Charles, 100
McLean, Jay, 200, 259
McLeod, J. R., 233
McNally, William, 253
Magendie, François, 230
Maggots, use in Civil War, 162–63
Maher, Walter B., 342
Malaria: in England and colonies, 4–5;
    Revolutionary War, 52; Civil War,
    161; in New York and New Jersey,
    333–34
Mall, Franklin P., 206
Malpractice, 222; increase in twentieth
    century, 324–26
Malt, Ronald A., 269
Marine, D., 232
Marshall, John, 97
Martin, Franklin H., 201
Maryland Medical College, 208–9
Maryland State Medical Society, 140
Massachusetts Committee on Public
    Safety, 53
Massachusetts Medical Society, 73, 120,
    140, 146; on women's issues, 289–90
Massachusetts Registration Act, 330
Massie, J. Cam, 94
Maston, Claudius H., 189
Masturbation, 186
Matas, Rudolph, 106, 174; on surgery,
    190; on vascular surgery, 192–93; on
    anesthesia, 195, 263
Mather, Cotton: on measles, 20; on
    inoculation, 22–23, 92
Mayo, Charles H., 191, 202
Mayo, William J., 191
Mayo, William W., 191
Mayo Clinic, 190, 201
Meade, Richard H., 264
Medawar, Peter B., 266

Medical and Chirurgical Faculty of
    Maryland, 186
Medical College of Georgetown, 306
Medical College of Louisiana, 128–29,
    135–36
Medical College of Ohio, 122–23, 125
Medical College of Philadelphia, 63, 131
Medical College of Virginia, 158
Medical Committee for Human Rights,
    309
Medical costs, 346–50
Medical degrees, colonial period, 30–34
Medical Department of the University of
    Louisiana, 135–36, 138
Medical education, 29. *See also medical
    school names*
Medical ethics, 279, 351–54
Medical fee bills, 17, 41–44, 106, 141–43,
    215
Medical history, 278–79
Medical licensure, 11, 38–40, 139–41,
    144, 218–21; weakness of, 314–16
Medical practice: colonial period, 16–17;
    early nineteenth century, 69–79; late
    nineteenth century, 179–81
Medical schools, 29–34; fees, 133–34,
    144; entrance requirements, 203–5,
    275; description of, 204–5; on public
    health, 278; on medical history, 278–
    79; on medical ethics, 279; on women,
    294–95. *See also* Women; *and under
    names of schools*
Medical Society of Boston, 41
Medical Society of Philadelphia, 42
Medical Society of the District of Colum-
    bia, 307
Medical Society of the State of New York,
    27
Medical specialties, rise of, 185, 215–16;
    in surgery, 261–62

Medical theories, 7, 13–14
Medicare and Medicaid, 340–43
Megapolensis, Samuel, 10
Meharry Medical College, 306–7
Meigs, Charles D., 117, 127
Mendel, Lafayette B., 235
Mental health, 244–46
Mercury, 70–77
Mering, Joseph von, 232
Merrick, Myra King, 288
Mesmer, Franz Anton, 23
Metcalf, John G., 117
Meyer, Adolph, 244
Miami University Medical College, 123
Microsurgery, 268–69
Middleton, Peter, 27, 32–34, 39, 44
Midwives, 10–11, 16, 40, 90–91, 117, 284–86
Miller, Willoughby Dayton, 197
Milosh, Barbara, 303
Milstein, César, 231
Minister-physicians, 8–9, 19–23, 43
Minkowski, Oscar, 232
Minot, George R., 236
Mitchell, John, 26–27, 65
Mitchell, John Kearsley, on germ theory, 169–70
Mitchell, S. Weir, 243
Mitchell, Samuel Latham, 131
Molecular biochemistry, 248–50
Moore, E. M., 199
Moore, George, 261
Moore, Harvey A., 244
Moore, Henry, 34
Moore, J. W., 244
Moore, Samuel Preston, 158–59, 165
Morantz-Sanchez, Regina M., 294
Morgagni, Giovanni, 28
Morgan, John, 28–29, 32–33, 39, 42, 48, 55–61, 63

Morton, William Thomas Green, 115–16, 118–19
Mott, Valentine, 73, 97–98
Moultrie, John, 41
Moultrie, William, 18
Muhlenburg, Henry Melchior, 19
Murphy, John B., 194, 201, 263
Murphy, Lamar R., 285
Murphy, William P., 236
Murray, John E., 266
Murray, Peter M., 308

National Association of Medical Colleges, 207
National Board of Health, 331
National Board of Medical Examiners, 208, 221, 315
National Health Service Corps, 343
National Health Survey, 339
National League of Nursing Education, 299
National Medical Association, 307–8
National Medical Convention (AMA), 137
National Sanitary Conventions, 330
Native Americans, 335. *See also* Indians
Neel, James V., 249
Neo-Thomsonianism, 87
Neurosciences, 243–44
New Amsterdam, 10, 34
Newark, N.J., 17
New Deal, 339
New England Female Medical College, 288
New England Medical College, 296
New Jersey Medical Society, 17, 40, 42–43, 59
New Orleans Polyclinic, 210
New Orleans School of Medicine, 138
Newport, R.I., 16

Newsom, Ella K., 164

Newton, Isaac, 13

New York City: seventeenth-century physicians, 10; medical licensure, 11, 40; yellow fever, 25; public health law, 26; cholera, 76; health boards, 121; fee bill, 141–42; bacteriological laboratory, 171–72; dispensaries, 62, 182; midwives, 286; health department, 330–31; health conditions, 330–31

New York Dispensary, 62

New York Hospital, 37–38

New York Infirmary for Women and Children, 287, 296

New York Medical Society, 141

New York Polyclinic, 210

New York State Medical Society, 137

New York Statistical Society, 330

Nightingale, Florence, 154, 163, 296

Nitze, Max, 199

Nixon, Richard M., 342

Nobel Prizes, 256

Noguchi, Hideo, 244

Nott, Josiah Clark, 73

Numbers, Ronald L., 319

Nurses: in Civil War, 163–64, 296–97; training of, 296–98; associations, 298–99; visiting nurses, 300–301; in military services, 301–2; professionalization of, 302–3; males as, 302

Nurse Society of Philadelphia, 296

Nutting, Mary Adelaide, 298

Obstetrics, 16, 18, 40, 90–91, 102–7; use of anesthesia, 116–18

Ochsner, Alton B., 253

O'Dwyer, Joseph, 194–95

Oldmixon, John, 44

Olitsky, Peter, 238

Olmsted, Frederick Law, 154

Ophthalmology, 261

Opie, Eugene L., 233

Opium, 180–81

Osborne, Thomas B., 235

Osler, William: on microscope, 170; bacteriological work, 169–70; on bleeding, 181; at Johns Hopkins, 206

Osteopathy, 220

Overton, James, 101

Paracelsus, 111

Paracentesis, 17

Parham, Frederick W., 189

Parish Medical School, 72

Parker, Willard, 73

Paschall, Elizabeth Coates, 17

Pauling, Linus, 236

Pearl, Raymond, 253

Peckham, Howard H., 51

Peebles, Thomas C., 252

Peer Review Organizations, 344

Pellagra, 234–35

Penicillin, 240–41

Pennsylvania Hospital, 24, 35–37, 77–78

Perkins, Elisha, 91–92

Pesthouses, 36

Pharmaceuticals, 15–16

Pharmacology, 239–40

Philadelphia: yellow fever epidemics, 27, 65; leading physicians, 28; Medical Society of, 42

Philadelphia Dispensary, 62

Phipps Institute, 172

Physical Society, 41

Physicians: categories of, 18–20; as ministers, 8–9, 19–23; as botanists, 24–27; public image of, 43, 47, 149–50; quarrels among, 149–50; studying abroad,

31–34, 168; status and income, 181–83, 185–86, 214–17, 314, 326–27; as moral arbiters, 185–86
Physick, Philip Syng, 97, 122
Physico-Medical Society of New Orleans, 129, 146–47
Physiology, 230–33
Pinel, Philippe, 77
Pittsburgh Sanitary Committee, 155
Pontiac, 3
Pope, Elijah, 113–14
Porcher, Francis P., 165
Portsmouth, N.H., 11, 44, 141
Post, John, 9
Post, Wright, 97–98
Potts, Jonathon, 57
Preston, Ann, 288
Prevost, François Marie, 105–7
Price, Roger, 6
Priestly, Joseph, 111
Pringle, John, 63
Proprietary medical schools, establishment of, 134–36
Prudden, T. Mitchell, 171
Psychiatry, 244–48
Public health: in eighteenth-century New York, 25–26; health boards, 149; bacteriological laboratories, 171; in medical schools, 278, 328; state and national boards, 330–31; health conditions, 330–32; use of railways, 336–37
Public health education, 336–37
Pupin, M. I., 198

Quackery, in colonies, 16, 44; in early nineteenth century, 91–92; in twentieth century, 315
Queen's College (Rutgers), 131
Queen Victoria, 117

Radiology, 198–99
Read, Widow, 91
Reagan administration, 247
Redman, John, 28, 63
Reed, Charles A. L., 218, 223
Reed, Walter, 174–75, 334
Reed Commission, 173–76, 237–38
Reverby, Susan, 299
Reynolds, Joshua, 63
Richmond, John Lambert, 107
Ricketts, Howard Taylor, 175–76, 250
Ricketts, 235
Rickman, William, 57–58
Riddell, John L., 128–29
Riggs, John M., 115
Rivers, Thomas M., 238
Robbins, Frederick C., 238
Robertson, Mason G., xi
Robertson Hospital, 164
Robinson, Morton, 222
Rockefeller Foundation, black medical education, 306–7
Rockefeller General Education Board, 307
Rockefeller Institute for Medical Research, 172; Sanitary Commission on hookworm, 176–77
Roentgen, Wilhelm Conrad, 198
Rogers, Coleman, 122
Rollins, William Herbert, 198
Romain, Charles V., 307
Romayne, Nicholas, 131
Roosevelt, Franklin D., 251
Rose, Apothecary, 8
Rosenberg, Charles, 184, 214
Ross, Ronald, 175
Rothstein, William G., 131, 283
Rouanet, Joseph, 147–48
Roudanez, L. C., 305
Rous, Peyton, 253

Royal College of Physicians, 7, 38
Royal Hospital (New Orleans), 35
Royal Society, 20
Rubber gloves, 190
Rush, Benjamin, 14, 16, 27–28, 33, 42, 49, 122, 130, 144, 146, 305; in Revolution, 57, 62–63; background and training, 62–63; political activities, 63–64; medical doctrine, 64–68, 71, 73–75; on insane, 77–78
Russell, James Earl, 298
Russell, Walter, 9

Sabin, Albert, 238, 251
St. Clair, Arthur, 49
St. Martin, Alexis, 108–9
Salk, Jonas, 251
Salmon, David E., 171, 250
Sanarelli, Giuseppe, 175
Scarlet fever, 6, 41
Schalley, Andrew V., 243
Schuppert, Moritz: on bleeding, 181; on antiseptic surgery, 189, 200
Semmelweis, Ignatz Philipp, 127
Senn, Nicholas, 192
Seton, Mother, 296
Sharon Medical Society, 43
Shattuck, Lemual, 330
Shelton, Jack, 342
Shew, Joseph, 89
Shippen, William, 29, 39
Shippen, William, Jr., 18, 29, 63, 90, 122; established medical school, 32–33; clash with John Morgan, 56–61
Shope, Richard E., 253
Shryock, Richard H., 39, 87, 89, 314
Simonds, J. C., 330
Simpson, James Young, 116
Sims, J. Marion, 99, 101–4, 144, 193–94
Sisterhood of St. Joseph, 296

Sisters of Charity, 296
Smadel, Joseph E., 252
Smallpox: in Central and South America, 2–4; against Indians, 3; in colonies, 5–6; in Revolutionary War, 51–52
Smith, Andrew H., 217
Smith, Elias, 81
Smith, J. Augustine, 149
Smith, James, 33
Smith, James McCune, 305
Smith, Nathan, 131
Smith, Stephen, 192
Smith, Theobald, 171, 237, 250
Smith, William, 16, 33
Snow, Edwin, 330
Société Médicale de la Nouvelle Orléans, 72
Society for the Promotion of Useful Knowledge, 27
Southern Medical Colleges Association, 208, 258
Spalding, Lyman, 131, 141
Specialists, impact on cost of medicine, 324–25
Specialty training, 275–78, in surgery, 201
Stanton, Edward M., 156–57
Starr, Paul, 228, 321, 349
Steenbock, Harry, 235
Stephens, Joanna, 270
Stern, M., 262
Sternberg, George M., 168; on bacteriology, 171; appoints yellow fever commission, 174–75, 238
Stevens, Alexander, 73
Stevens, Edward, 67
Stevens, Rosemary, 321
Stevenson, Sarah Hackett, 290
Stiles, Charles, 175–76
Stiles, Elizabeth Hubbard, 16

Stone, Warren, 76, 98–99, 135
Stout, Samuel H., 159
Stout, Samuel, 56
Stubbs, J. E., 222
Sulfa drugs, 240
Surgery, 17–18, 95–97, 200; abdominal,
    262–63; thoracic, 263–64; cardiovas-
    cular, 264–67
Surgical amphitheaters, 96
Sutherland, Earl W., 239
Sweet, Waterman, 91
Sydenham, Thomas, 14, 63
Szasz, Thomas, 246

Taussig, Helen B., 264, 295
Technology, diagnostic, 270–73
Tenant, John V. B., 33
Thacher, James, 48, 51, 55
Thacher, Thomas, 9, 92
Thalidomide, 317–18
Theiler, Max, 238, 251
Therapeutics, 70–77, 180–81
Thomas, E. Donnel, 266
Thomas, John, 49
Thomas, Lewis, 346–47
Thomas, M. Cary, 293
Thompson-McFadden Commission, 177
Thomson, Samuel, 81–82, 87
Thornton, Matthew, 49
Thorwald, Jurgen, 274
Tilton, James, 51
Todd, James, 327
Tompkins, Sally L., 164
Torrey, E. Fuller, 247
Trall, Russell T., 89
Transylvania Medical School, 122–23,
    131
Tuke, William, 77
Tulane University School of Medicine,
    135–36, 209–10. *See also* Medical Col-
lege of Louisiana; Medical Depart-
    ment of the University of Louisiana
Turner, Daniel, 32
Typhoid fever, in early Virginia, 4

Ulrich, Laurel T., 90–91
Ultrasound, 270
United States Marine Hospital Service,
    172–73. *See also* United States Public
    Health Service
United States Public Health Service:
    established 173–75; on Rocky Moun-
    tain spotted fever, 175–76; on hook-
    worm, 176–77; on pellagra, 177–79,
    338
United States Sanitary Commission,
    154–55
University of Baltimore, 113
University of Cincinnati Medical School,
    122–23, 125
University of Edinburgh, 31
University of Louisville Medical College,
    125
University of Maryland, 196–97; Medical
    College, 132, 134, 136
University of Michigan Medical College,
    203
University of Minnesota, Nursing
    School, 299
University of Pennsylvania Medical Col-
    lege, 122–24, 131, 136–38, 143–44;
    first university hospital, 206
University of West Tennessee Medical
    College, 306
Urology, 261–62
Ursuline Sisters of Rouen, 35

Van der Donck, Adriaen, 10
Vander Veer, Albert, 262
Variolation, 20–22

Vedder, Edward B., 178–79
Velpeau, A.-A.-L.-M., 95
Venable, James, 114
Venereal diseases, 338–39
Vermont State Medical Society, 137
Veterans Administration, 309
Virginia: early health conditions, 3–4, 16; first hospital, 34; medical licensure, 39–40
Virology, 250–52
Vitamins, 179, 234–35
Voegtlin, C., 232
Vogel, Virgil J., 2

Wagner-Murray-Dingell Bill, 321
Waksman, Selman A., 239, 241
Wald, George, 243
Walsh, James J., 41
Warner, John Harley, 145
Warren, John, 120
Warren, John Collins, 73, 115–16
Warren, Joseph, 49, 53, 120
Washington, George, 21, 63, 73–74
Waterhouse, Benjamin, 127–28, 146
Watson, James D., 249
Watts, John, 45
Webster, Noah, 6
Weekly Society of Gentlemen, 41
Weir, Robert F., 188–89
Welch, William H., 168, 206, 209–10, 239
Weller, Thomas H., 238
Wells, Horace, 114–15, 118–19
Wesley, John, 22, 92
Western [Medical] Board (Louisiana), 139
Whipple, George H., 236
White, William H., 244

Wiley, Harvey W., 317
Wilkerson, James, 49
Wilkinson, Will, 9
Williams, John R., 276
Williams, R. R., 179
Willoughby University Medical School, 149–50
Wilson, Louis B., 175–76
Winchester Medical College, 132–33
Wintrobe, M. M., 236
Wistar, Casper, 28, 122
Woman's Hospital of the State of New York, 104
Woman's Medical College of Baltimore, 293
Woman's Medical College of Pennsylvania, 288, 293
Women: as physicians, 16–17, 90–91, 290–94; fight for rights, 186–87; as medical students, 213, 285–90
Wood, Thomas, 32
Woodruff, Alice, 238
Woodward, Joseph J., 159
Woolcott, Oliver, 49
Worcester State Hospital, 78
Wotton, Henry, 9
Wyman, Walter, 173–75

Yale Medical College, 137
Yarrow, Rosalyn S., 243
Yellow fever: in colonies, 6, 25, 27; Reed Commission, 174–75; in 1905, 334
Young, Hugh, 262
Young, James Harvey, 92
Young, Thomas, 65

Zakrzewska, Marie, 287

JOHN DUFFY is Clinical Professor Emeritus (History of Medicine) at Tulane University School of Medicine and Professor Emeritus at the University of Maryland, where he was the Priscilla Alden Burke Professor of American History. A distinguished scholar of public health and medical history, Duffy is a past president of the American Association for the History of Medicine. He is the author of numerous articles and books, among them *The Rudolph Matas History of Medicine in Louisiana* (2 vols.), *A History of Public Health in New York City* (2 vols.), *Epidemics in Colonial America*, and *The Sanitarians: A History of American Public Health*.